The Great Psychotherapy Debate

Models, Methods, and Findings

The Great Psychotherapy Debate

Models, Methods, and Findings

Bruce E. Wampold
University of Wisconsin–Madison

2001

LAWRENCE ERLBAUM ASSOCIATES, PUBLISHERS
Mahwah, New Jersey   London

Lawrence Erlbaum Associates, Inc., Publishers
10 Industrial Avenue
Mahwah, NJ 07430

Cover design by Kathryn Houghtaling Lacey

Library of Congress Cataloging-in-Publication Data

Wampold, Bruce E., 1948–
The great psychotherapy debate : models, methods, and findings / Bruce E. Wampold.
p. cm.

Includes bibliographical references and index.
ISBN 0-8058-3201-7 (cloth : alk. paper)
ISBN 0-8058-3202-5 (pbk. : alk. paper)
1. Psychotherapy—Philosophy. 2. Psychotherapy—Evaluation.
I. Title.
RC437.5 .W35   2001
616.89'14'01—dc21   00-049020
                                                                      CIP

Books published by Lawrence Erlbaum Associates are printed on acid-free paper, and their bindings are chosen for strength and durability.

Printed in the United States of America
10 9 8 7 6 5

To those who have loved me, and to B.C.,
whose challenging support created
the opportunity for growth and exploration

Contents

Foreword

The "common factors" position on the effectiveness of psychotherapy—whose lineaments were sketched between fifty and thirty years ago by such scholars as Jerome Frank, Hans Strupp, Victor Raimy, and Lester Luborsky among others, and whose empirical foundations were laid scarcely more than 25 years ago—here attains its most forceful expression; and Bruce Wampold dons the mantel of foremost defender of a position with enormously important implications for mental health training, treatment, and public policy.

The common factors position (namely, that all of the many specific types of psychotherapeutic treatment achieve virtually equal—or insignificantly different—benefits because of a common core of curative processes) can move the focus of psychotherapy training and theory itself from therapist to client, from how the therapist "cures" to how the client "heals." The medical model of psychotherapy that Wampold so meticulously deconstructs in *The Great Psychotherapy Debate* has led us to accept a view of clients as inert and passive objects on whom we operate and whom we medicate. The implausibility that the great variety of specific ingredients in the multitude of psychotherapeutic approaches would yield indistinguishable outcomes is a strong clue that either it is instead a set of often unacknowledged common elements that is effective, or else it is a set of processes residing largely in the clients and merely mobilized by therapy that carries the power to improve clients' lives. This potential shift in perspective (from an emphasis on the differences among therapies to an awareness of the broad context in which therapeutic relationships are played out) can cause both therapists and theoreticians to reflect less on their interventions and more on clients' efforts at making themselves whole. The shift carries a threat of narcissistic injury.

The common factors versus specific ingredients debate is at the heart of policy questions about the scope of national health care, as well as private insurance. There are those health policy analysts who argue that any therapy that uses non-specific diagnoses and non-specific treatments is somehow bogus witchcraft lacking indications of when to begin and when to end, and its application should be excluded from third-party coverage. There are two sides to this question, obviously. This debate is not just about mental health treatment—although mental health has been a very central issue in it—but it is a debate that extends through all aspects of medical insurance. *The Great Psychotherapy Debate* may well come to serve as a model for the empirical research that will inform—or fundamentally challenge—the various sides in this important contest.

After nearly a century of marginally productive investigations based on a medical conception of psychotherapy, Professor Wampold is asking researchers to face the facts and move forward.

—Gene V Glass
Arizona State University

Preface

I am borne of two worlds. From about as long as I can remember, I loved mathematics, and the thrill of understanding deep structures and their beauty. Simple definitions leading to complex relationships; form and pattern expressed as chaos. The prime numbers, solid in definition, scattered seemingly at random. Rule governed, but complex and defying understanding. Mathematics, pure and pristine, yet finding application at every turn.

And the other world. The despair of losing unconditional and genuine love at the throw of a die. At five, I happily went into the woods to play, not knowing that I would never see my mother again. I struggled to understand that singularity, failing to understand that sheer rational logic would be insufficient.

For so many years, the wound to my soul that wouldn't heal, tugging at my consciousness, and created a world slightly out of focus. Along with the support of those who love and have loved me, psychotherapy provided the opportunity to explore, to see the wound from the inside out, to grieve, and to heal.

So, I approached this book from a personal perspective. Of course, I was drawn to a scientific understanding of psychotherapy, the same way I approached all academic endeavors. The natural inclination was to accept psychological treatments on the same basis as medical treatments—to embrace them as a clinical scientist. To a scientist, clinical trials, specific active ingredients, diagnoses, standardized treatments, and the aura of medicine, are all naturally attractive. Yet, the more I taught students about psychotherapy and the research that supports it, the more I realized that the medical model could not explain the preponderance of the research results. A scientist, above all else, listens carefully to the data, seeking a resonance of theory and results.

From my perspective, psychotherapy is a very personal and life changing experience, one that cannot be forced into a medical-like treatment without losing the essence of the endeavor. This perspective may be shaped by my experience. I would happily give up my perspective if the scientific evidence supported the current trend to conceptualize psychological treatments as analogues of medical treatments. On the contrary, however, the scientific evidence overwhelmingly supports a model of psychotherapy that gives primacy to the healing context, to the understanding of one's difficulties, to the faith in the therapy, and to the respect for the client's world view. The purpose of this book is to present the scientific evidence that supports a contextual, rather than a medical, model of psychotherapy.

The first chapter of this book presents two competing models of psychotherapy—the medical model and the contextual model. The medical model focuses on the specificity of treatments. In this model, theoretical explanations for disorders, problems, or complaints are formulated, treatments contain specific ingredients that are theoretically purported to be necessary for change, the therapist focuses on these specific ingredients, and researchers attribute the benefits of psychotherapy to those ingredients. The contextual model emphasizes the commonalities among therapies. All therapies involve the relationship of a client and therapist, each of whom believes in the efficacy of the treatment. The therapist provides the client with a rationale for the disorder and administers a procedure that is consistent with that rationale. The client discusses the most intimate details of his or her life, confident that the therapeutic relationship will continue. The particular specific ingredients contained in the treatment, according to the contextual model, are not responsible for therapeutic benefits. The debate between advocates of the two models has existed since the origins of psychotherapy, although phrased in many ways (e.g., as "common factors" versus "specific ingredients"). However expressed, this great debate separates practitioners and researchers into two camps, each confident that they know how and why psychotherapy works.

In chapter 2, various hypotheses that distinguish the two models are presented, along with a discussion of methods that can be used to test these hypotheses. The evidence related to the hypotheses is presented in chapters 3 through 8. Because understanding research methods is critical to interpreting findings from thousands of studies of psychotherapy, each chapter discusses research strategies and important details of design related to the hypotheses. Simply stated, the evidence overwhelmingly supports a contextual model of psychotherapy. Chapter 9 discusses the implications of accepting the contextual model and rejecting the medical model.

The defining feature of this book is that a scientific perspective is taken toward the great debate. I have strived to examine the results of thousands of studies and present them fairly and accurately. As I progressed with this project, the astonishing consistency of the results with the contextual model was surprising. It would be difficult to imagine how a scientist could examine these data and come to a different conclusion.

ACKNOWLEDGMENTS

I want to acknowledge those who have contributed to the thinking, writing, and understanding that have made this book possible. The ideas for this book emanated from my teaching a seminar on the research of individual interventions, and thus I thank the students who participated in the 951 seminars. Our clear and challenging discussions were invigorating; the students' diversity of perspectives widened the scope of my thinking. The Otsego group was also instrumental in the formulation of ideas and in encouraging me when I doubted that I could pull this project together. Don Atkinson has been a steadfast influence on my intellectual and personal development. R. Serlin's collaboration with regard to the effects of therapists, was critical in the development of chapter 8. M. J. Patton's suggestions helped clarify the opening arguments. L. McCubbin and S. Tierney provided critical suggestions regarding the presentation. D. Nelson provided valuable assistance in the preparation of the manuscript. Fenwick accorded lively company by my side on those long days at the computer, although he showed an indifferent attitude toward the content of the book.

1

Competing Meta-Models: The Medical Model Versus the Contextual Model

Understanding the nature of psychotherapy is a daunting task. There are over 250 distinct psychotherapeutic approaches, which are described, in one way or another, in over 10,000 books. Moreover, tens of thousands of books, book chapters, and journal articles have reported research conducted to understand psychotherapy and to test whether it works. It is no wonder, that faced with the literature on psychotherapy, confusion reigns, controversy flourishes, converging evidence is sparse, and recognition of psychotherapy as a science is tenuous.

Any scientific endeavor will seem chaotic if the explanatory models are insufficient to explain the accumulation of facts. If one were to ask prominent researchers to list important psychotherapeutic principles that have been scientifically established and generally accepted by most psychotherapy researchers, the list would indeed be short. On the other hand, an enumeration of the results of psychotherapy studies would be voluminous. How is it that so much research has yielded so little knowledge? The thesis of this book is that there is a remarkable convergence of research findings, provided the evidence is viewed at the proper level of abstraction.

Discovering the scientific basis of psychotherapy is vital to the efficient and humane design of mental health services. In the United States, psychotherapeutic services occupy a small niche in the enormous universe of health service delivery systems. The forces within this universe are compressing psychotherapy into a tiny compartment and changing the nature of the therapeutic endeavor. No longer can therapists conduct long-term therapy and expect to be reimbursed by health maintenance organizations (HMOs). In many venues, therapists can only be reimbursed for treating clients with particular mental disorders (i.e., clients who have been assigned particular diagnoses). A client in a troubled marriage who is experiencing the sequelae of this traumatic event (e.g., attenuated work performance, absenteeism, depression) must be assigned a reimbursable diagnosis, such as major depressive disorder, in order to justify treatment. Accordingly, a treatment plan must be adapted to the objective of alleviating the symptoms of depression with the insured patient rather than, say, resolving marital disagreements, changing lifelong patterns of relationships that are based on childhood attachments with parents, or improving the couples' communications.

The pressures of the health care delivery system have molded psychotherapy to resemble medical treatments. Psychotherapy, as often practiced, is laden with medical terminology—diagnosis, treatment plans, validated treatments, and medically necessary conditions, to name a few. The debate over prescription privileges for psychologists is about, from one perspective, how much psychologists want to conform to a medical model of practice. As "talk" treatments become truncated and prescriptive, doctoral level psychologists and other psychotherapy practitioners (e.g., social workers, marriage and family therapists) are economically coerced to practice a form of therapy different from what they were trained and different from how they would prefer to practice.

Sliding into the medical arena presumes that psychotherapy is best conceptualized as a medical treatment. In this book, the scientific evidence will be presented that shows that psychotherapy is incompatible with the medical model and that conceptualizing psychotherapy in this way distorts the nature of the endeavor. Cast in more urgent tones, the medicalization of psychotherapy might well destroy talk therapy as a beneficial treatment of psychological and social problems.

In this chapter, the medical model and its alternative, the contextual model, are presented. To begin, the definition of psychotherapy as well as terminology are presented. Second, the competing models are placed at their proper level of abstraction. Finally, the two models are explained and defined.

DEFINITIONS AND TERMINOLOGY

Definition of Psychotherapy

The definition of psychotherapy used herein is not controversial and is consistent with both the medical model and the contextual model, which are examined subsequently. The following definition is used in this book:

> Psychotherapy is a primarily interpersonal treatment that is based on psychological principles and involves a trained therapist and a client who has a mental disorder, problem, or complaint; it is intended by the therapist to be remedial for the client's disorder, problem, or complaint; and it is adapted or individualized for the particular client and his or her disorder, problem, or complaint.

Psychotherapy is defined as an interpersonal treatment to rule out psychological treatments that may not involve an interpersonal interaction between therapist and client, such as bibliotherapy or systematic desensitization based on tapes that the client uses in the absence of a therapist. The term *interpersonal* implies that the interaction transpires face-to-face and thus rules out telephone counseling or interactions via computer, although there is no implication that such modes of interacting are not beneficial. The adverb *primarily* is used to indicate that therapies employing adjunctive activities not involving a therapist, such as bibliotherapy, listening to relaxation tapes, or performing various homework assignments, are not excluded from this definition.

Presumably psychotherapy is a professional activity that involves a minimum level of skill, and consequently the definition requires that the therapist be professionally trained. Because the relationship between training and outcome in psychotherapy is controversial, the amount of training is not specified, but herein it is assumed that the training be typical for therapists practicing a given form of therapy.

Psychotherapy has traditionally been viewed as remedial, in that it is a treatment designed to remove or ameliorate some client distress, and consequently the definition requires that the client have a disorder, problem, or complaint. Moreover, the treatment needs to be adapted to help this particular client, although standardized treatments (i.e., those administered to a client with a disorder without regard for individual manifestations or client characteristics) are considered as they relate to the hypotheses of this book. The generic term *client* is used rather than the alternative term *patient* because the latter is too closely allied with a medical model.

Treatments that do not have a psychological basis are excluded. It may well be that nonpsychological treatments are palliative when both the client and the practitioner believe in their efficacy. Treatments based on the occult, indigenous peoples' cultural beliefs about mental health and behavior, New Age ideas (e.g., herbal remedies), and religion may be efficacious through the mechanisms hypothesized in the contextual model, but they are not psychotherapy and are not considered in this book. This is not to say that such activities are not of interest to social scientists in general and psychologists in particular; simply, psychotherapy, as considered herein, is limited to therapies based on psychological principles. It may turn out that psychotherapy is efficacious because Western cultures value the activity rather than because the specific ingredients of psychotherapy are efficacious, but that does not alter how psychotherapy should be defined.

Finally, it is required that the therapist intends the treatment to be effective. In the contextual model, therapist belief in treatment efficacy is necessary. In chapter 7, evidence that belief in treatment is related to outcome will be presented.

Terminology

The presentation that follows depends on a careful distinction between various components of psychotherapeutic treatments and their related concepts. Over the years, various systems for understanding these concepts have been proposed by Brody (1980), Critelli and Neuman (1984), Grünbaum (1981), A. K. Shapiro and Morris (1978), Shepherd (1993), and Wilkins (1984), among others. Although technical, the logic and terminology presented by Grünbaum (1981) is adapted to present the competing models because of its consistency and rigor.[1] Some time is spent explaining the notation and terms as well as substituting more commonly used terminology. Grünbaum's (1981) exposition is as follows:

> The therapeutic theory ψ that advocates the use of a particular treatment modality t to remedy [disorder] D demands the inclusion of certain *characteristic* constituents F in any treatment process that ψ authenticates as an application of t. Any such process, besides qualifying as an instance of t according to ψ, will typically have constituents C *other than* the characteristic ones F singled out by ψ. And when asserting that the factors F are remedial for D, ψ *may* also take cognizance of one or more of the non-characteristic constituents C, which I shall denominate as "incidental." (p. 159)

An example of a therapeutic theory (ψ) is psychodynamic theory; the particular treatment modality t would then be some form of psychodynamic therapy. The treatment (t) would be applied to remediate some disorder (D), such as depression. This treatment would contain some constituents (F) that are characteristic of the treatment that are consistent with the theory. At this point, it is helpful to make this concrete by considering Waltz, Addis, Koerner, and Jacobson's (1993) classification of therapeutic actions into four classes: (a) unique and essential, (b) essential but not unique, (c) acceptable but not necessary, and (d) proscribed. Waltz et al. provided exam-

---

[1]To some in the field, the terminology and the conceptual principles underlying their adoption are critically important: "I hope it is now apparent that there is no justification for the ineptitude of the customary terminology.... Workers in the field may be motivated to adopt the unambiguous vocabulary that I have proposed " (Grünbaum, 1981, p. 167). Although a case could be made for the various alternative models proposed, the important aspect is that a system be logical and consistent. It should be noted that the validity of the thesis of this book is not dependent on the adoption of a particular logical exposition.

ples, which are presented in Table 1.1, of these four therapeutic actions for psychodynamic and behavioral therapies. Grünbaum's (1981) characteristic constituents are similar to Waltz et al.'s unique and essential therapeutic actions.[2] Forming a contingency contract is a unique and essential action in behavioral therapy (see Table 1.1), and it is characteristic of the theory of operant conditioning. A term ubiquitously used to refer to theoretically derived actions is *specific ingredients*. Thus, characteristic constituents, unique and essential actions, and specific ingredients all refer to the same concept. For the most part, the term specific ingredients will be used in this book.

Grünbaum (1981) also referred to incidental aspects of each treatment that are not theoretically central. The common factor approach, which will be discussed later in this chapter, has identified those elements of therapy, such as the therapeutic relationship, that seem to be common to all (or most) treatments and therefore called them *common factors*. By definition, common factors must be incidental. However, there may be aspects of a treatment that are incidental (i.e., not characteristic of the theory) but not common to all (or most) therapies, although it is difficult to find examples of such aspects in the literature. Consequently, the term common factors will be used interchangeably with incidental aspects. In Waltz et al.'s (1993) classification, the "essential but not unique" and some of the " acceptable but not necessary" therapeutic actions (see Table 1.1) appear to be both theoretically incidental and common. For example, behavioral therapy and psychodynamic therapy, as well as most other therapies, involve establishing a therapeutic alliance, setting treatment goals, empathic listening on the part of the therapist, and planning for termination. Thus, incidental aspects and common factors are actions that are either essential but not unique or acceptable but not necessary. Because common factors is the term typically used in the literature, it is the prominent term used in this book, although *incidental aspects*, which connotes that these ingredients are not theoretically central, is used as well.

There is one aspect of the terminology that, unless clarified, may cause confusion. If treatment *t* is remedial for disorder *D* (in Grünbaum's terms), then, simply said, the treatment is beneficial. However, there is no implication that it is the characteristic constituents (i.e., specific ingredients) that are causal to the observed benefits. Thus, the language of psychotherapy must distinguish clearly cause and effect constructs (see Cook & Campbell, 1979). Specific ingredients and incidental aspects of psychotherapy are elements of a treatment that may or may not cause beneficial outcomes and

---

[2]"Characteristic constituents" and "unique and essential actions" are not identical because the word "essential" connotes that the ingredient is necessary for therapeutic benefits (i.e., is remedial). This is an empirical issue, and the question of whether a particular ingredient is a factor in creating beneficial outcomes is central to this book.

TABLE 1.1

Examples of Four Types of Therapeutic Actions

Psychodynamic Therapy	*Behavioral Therapy*
Unique and Essential (Specific Ingredients)	
1. Focus on unconscious determinants of behavior	1. Assigning homework
2. Focus on internalized object relations as historical causes of current problems	2. Practicing assertion in the session
3. Focus on defense mechanisms used to ward off pain of early trauma	3. Forming a contingency contract
4. Interpretation of resistance	
Essential But Not Unique	
1. Establish a therapeutic alliance	1. Establish a therapeutic alliance
2. Setting treatment goals	2. Setting treatment goals
3. Empathic listening	3. Empathic listening
4. Planning for termination	4. Planning for termination
5. Exploration of childhood	5. Providing treatment rationale
Acceptable But Not Necessary	
1. Paraphrasing	1. Paraphrasing
2. Self-disclosure	2. Self-disclosure
3. Interpreting dreams	3. Exploration of childhood
4. Providing treatment rationale	
Proscribed	
1. Prescribing psychotropic medications	1. Prescribing psychotropic medications
2. Assigning homework	2. Focus on unconscious determinants of behavior
3. Practicing assertion in the session	3. Focus on internalized object relations as historical causes of current problems
4. Forming contingency contracts	4. Focus on defense mechanisms used to ward off pain of early trauma
5. Prescribing the symptom	5. Interpretation of resistance

Note. From "Testing the Integrity of a Psychotherapy Protocol: Assessment of Adherence and Competence," by J. Waltz, M. E. Addis, K. Koerner, and N. S. Jacobson, 1993, *Journal of Consulting and Clinical Psychology, 61,* 620–630. Copyright © 1993 by the American Psychological Association. Reprinted with permission.

thus are putative causal constructs. A psychotherapy treatment contains both specific ingredients and incidental aspects, both, one, or none of which might be remedial. The term *specific effects* is used to refer to the benefits produced by the specific ingredients; *general effects* is used to refer to the benefits produced by the incidental aspects (i.e., the common factors). If both the specific ingredients and the incidental aspects are remedial, then there exist specific effects (i.e., the ones caused by the specific ingredients) and general effects (i.e., the ones caused by incidental aspects). If the treatment is not effective, then neither specific nor general effects exist, although specific ingredients and incidental aspects of psychotherapy are present. In sum, specific therapeutic ingredients cause specific effects, and incidental aspects cause general effects.

Having adopted certain terminology, it should be noted that the following terms used to describe specific ingredients and incidental factors as well as their effects are eschewed: active ingredients, essential ingredients, nonspecific ingredients, nonspecific effects, and placebo effects. Active ingredients and essential ingredients, terms often used to refer to specific ingredients, inappropriately imply that the specific ingredients are remedial (i.e., there exist specific effects); whether specific ingredients produce effects is an empirical question. Nonspecific ingredients and nonsepecific effects are avoided because they imply that the incidental factors act inferiorly vis-à-vis specific ingredients. Placebo effects, which are discussed in chapter 5, are often denigrated as effects produced by pathways that are irrelevant to the core elements of a treatment. For example, the therapeutic alliance, a common factor that has been shown to have potent beneficial effects (see chap. 6), is sometimes denigrated by referring to the effects it produces as nonspecific effects or placebo effects. The term general effects is used here because it is comparable linguistically and logically with its counterpart, specific effects.

Attention is now turned to placing the two models that are investigated in this book (viz., the medical model and the contextual model) at their proper level of abstraction.

LEVELS OF ABSTRACTION

As psychotherapy is an exceedingly complex phenomenon, levels of abstraction are indeterminable to some extent. Nevertheless, a short discussion of various levels is needed to understand the central thesis of this book. Four levels of abstraction are presented herein: therapeutic techniques, therapeutic strategies, theoretical approaches, and meta-theoretical models. These four levels are not unique, and it would be impossible to classify each and every research question and theoretical explication into one and only one of the levels. Some studies have examined questions that do not fit neatly into one of the levels, and some studies have examined questions that seem to span two or more levels. Nevertheless, it is necessary to understand how the thesis of this book, which contrasts the medical model with the contextual model, exists at a meta-theoretical level. At this level of abstraction, the vast array of research results produced by psychotherapy research creates a convergent and coherent conclusion. In this section, three levels of abstraction presented by Goldfried (1980) as well as a fourth, higher level, will be discussed. These levels of abstraction are summarized in Table 1.2

The highest level of abstraction discussed by Goldfried (1980) is the theoretical framework and the concomitant individual approaches to psychotherapy and their underlying, although sometimes implicit, philosophical view of human nature. In Grünbaum's terms, this is the level of the therapeutic theory ψ and the particular treatment modality t. Although Table 1.2 gives three examples of theoretical approaches to psychotherapy (cognitive–behavioral, interpersonal, psychodynamic), by one estimate there are over 250 approaches to psychotherapy if one considers the many variations proposed and advocated in the literature (Goldfried & Wolfe, 1996). At this level of abstraction, there is little agreement among researchers or practitioners. Advocates of a particular approach defend their theoretical positions and, to varying degrees, can cite research to support the efficacy of their endeavors. For example, recent reviews of research have found evidence to support behavioral treatments (e.g., Emmelkamp, 1994), cognitive treatments (e.g., Hollon & Beck, 1994), psychodynamic approaches (e.g., Henry, Strupp, Schacht, & Gaston, 1994) and experiential treatments (e.g., Greenberg, Elliott, & Lietaer, 1994). The plethora of research results emanating from clinical trials in which the efficacy of a particular treatment is established by comparisons with a no-treatment control or with another treatment is testimony to the importance of this level of abstraction. Unfortunately, the use of a particular approach seems to be divorced from this research:

> The popularity of a therapy school is often a function of variables having nothing to do with the efficacy of its associated procedures. Among other things, it depends on the charisma, energy level, and longevity of the leader; the number of students trained and where they have been placed; and the spirit of the times. (Goldfried, 1980, p. 996)

The lowest level of abstraction involves the techniques and actions used by the therapist in the process of administering a treatment. Well-articulated treatments prescribe the specific ingredients that should be used; consequently, techniques and approaches coincide, and therefore discussions of the efficacy of a particular treatment are related to the corresponding techniques. Psychodynamic psychotherapists make interpretations of the transference, whereas cognitive–behavioral therapists dispute maladaptive

TABLE 1.2

Levels of Abstraction of Psychotherapy and Related Research Questions

Level of Abstraction	Examples of Units of Investigation	Research Questions	Research Designs
Techniques (i.e., specific ingredients)	Interpretations Disputing maladaptive thoughts In vivo exposure	Is a given technique or set of techniques necessary for therapeutic efficacy? What are the characteristics of a skillfully administered technique?	Component designs Parametric designs Clinical trials with placebo controls Passive designs that examine the relationship between technique and outcome (within the corresponding treatment)
Strategies	Corrective experiences Feedback	Are strategies common to all psychotherapies? Are the strategies necessary and sufficient for change?	Passive designs that examine the relationship between technique and outcome (across various treatments)
Theoretical Approach	Cognitive–behavioral Interpersonal approaches Psychodynamic	Is a particular treatment effective? Is a particular treatment more effective than another treatment?	Clinical Trials with no treatment controls Comparative clinical trials (Tx A vs. Tx B)
Meta-Theory	Medical model Contextual model	Which meta-theory best accounts for the corpus of research results?	Research Synthesis

thoughts. Advocacy for the theoretical bases of cognitive–behavioral treatments is also advocacy for the actions prescribed by the treatment. As presented in Table 1.2, various research designs have been used to test whether techniques described at this level of abstraction are indeed responsible for positive therapeutic outcomes.

According to Goldfried (1980), a level of abstraction exists between individual approaches and techniques, which he labels clinical strategies. Clinical strategies "function as clinical heuristics that implicitly guide [therapist] efforts during the course of therapy" (Goldfried, 1980, p. 994). Goldfried's purpose of identifying this intermediate level of abstraction was to show that therapeutic phenomena at this level would exhibit commonalities across approaches and provide a consensus among the advocates of the various theoretical approaches. The two clinical strategies identified by Goldfried as generally common to all psychotherapeutic approaches are providing corrective experiences and offering direct feedback. The research questions at this level of abstraction are concerned with identifying the common strategies and identifying whether they are necessary and sufficient for therapeutic change. Although innovative and potentially explanatory, the strategy level of abstraction has not produced much research (Arkowitz, 1992), particularly in comparison with research devoted to establishing the efficacy of particular approaches.

The thesis of this book is situated at a level of abstraction beyond the theoretical perspectives that undergird the major approaches to psychotherapy. It is generally accepted that psychotherapy works (but just in case there is any doubt, this evidence is reviewed in chap. 3). However, the causal determinants of efficacy are not as well established. In more mundane terms, one might ask: What is it about psychotherapy that makes it so helpful? Explanations exist at each of the three lower levels of abstraction. During the course of presenting the research evidence, it will become clear that (a) logical impediments to understanding causal mechanisms exist at each of these levels of abstraction, and moreover (b) when viewed at these levels, the research evidence does not converge to answer the causality question. Consequently, a fourth level of abstraction is needed—theories about psychotherapeutic theories. In this book, two meta-theories are contrasted: the medical model and the contextual model.

The next sections of this chapter will define and explain the two meta-theories. At this juncture, it should be noted that these meta-theories have been explicated elsewhere. The contribution of this book is the presentation of the research evidence and the claim that this evidence conclusively supports the contextual model of psychotherapy.

MEDICAL MODEL

In this section, a brief history of the medical model is presented. This history serves to introduce the tenets of the medical model as well as to situate the medical model within the current psychotherapeutic context. Following the history, the tenets of the medical model are stipulated.

Brief History of the Medical Model of Psychotherapy

The origins of psychotherapy lie in the medical model. Sigmund Freud, in his practice as a physician, became involved with the treatment of hysterics. He believed that (a) hysteric symptoms are caused by the repression of some traumatic event (real or imagined) in the unconscious, (b) the nature of the symptom is related to the event, and (c) the symptom could be relieved by insight into the relationship between the event and the symptom. Moreover, from the beginning (as in his discussion of Anna O.), sexuality became central to the etiology of hysteria, with many symptoms associated with early sexual traumas. Freud experimented with various techniques to retrieve repressed memories, including hydrotherapy, hypnosis, and direct questioning, eventually promoting free association and dream analysis. From these early origins of psychoanalysis, the components of the medical model that are enumerated later were emerging: a disorder (hysteria), a scientifically based explanation of the disorder (repressed traumatic events), a mechanism of change (insight into unconscious), and specific therapeutic actions (free association).[3]

During his lifetime, Freud and his colleagues differed on various aspects related to theory and therapeutic action, creating irreconcilable rifts with such luminaries as Joseph Breuer, Alfred Adler, and Carl Jung, the latter two of whom were expelled from Freud's Vienna Psychoanalytic Society. As we shall see, the medical model is characterized by insistence on the correct explanation of a disorder and adoption of the concomitant therapeutic actions. Although Freud claimed that his theory was correct and supported by scientific evidence, the truth is that the empirical bases of Freudian psychoanalysis and competing systems (e.g., Adler's individual psychology or Jung's analytic psychology) were tenuous at best. Interestingly, as we shall see, interpersonal psychotherapy, which has become what is known as an empirically supported treatment, is derived from Sullivan's neo-Freudian interpersonal psychoanalysis.

Another historical thread of the medical model emanated from behaviorism. Although behavioral therapists often claim to reject the medical model, defined as a meta-theory, the medical model encompasses most, if not all, behavioral treatments. Behavioral psychology emerged as a parsimonious explanation of behavior based on objective observations. Ivan Petrovich Pavlov's work on classical conditioning detailed, without resorting to complicated mentalistic constructs, how animals acquired a conditioned response, how the conditioned response could be extinguished (i.e., extinction), and how experimental neurosis could be induced. John B. Watson and Rosalie Rayner's "Little Albert Study" established that a fear response could be conditioned by pairing an unconditioned stimulus of fear (viz., loud noise) with an unconditioned stimulus (viz., a rat) so that the unconditioned stimulus elicited the fear response (Watson & Rayner, 1920). Although Watson and Rayner did not attempt to alleviate Albert's fear, Mary Cover Jones (under the supervision of Watson) demonstrated that the classical conditioning paradigm could be used to desensitize a boy's fear of rabbits by gradually decreasing the proximity of the stimulus (i.e., the rabbit) to the boy.

---

[3]Over the years, Freud's conceptualizations evolved, encompassing drive theory (libidinal and aggressive motivations), sexual development, and the tripartite theory of personality (viz., id, ego, superego) and spawning additional techniques, such as interpretation of the transference.

A major impetus to behavioral therapy was provided by Joseph Wolpe's development of systematic desensitization. Wolpe, who like Freud was a medical doctor, became disenchanted with psychoanalysis as a method to treat his patients. On the basis of the work of Pavlov, Watson, Rayner, and Jones, Wolpe studied how eating, an incompatible response to fear, could be used to reduce phobic reactions of cats, which he had previously conditioned. After studying the work on progressive relaxation by physiologist Edmund Jacobson, Wolpe recognized that the incompatibility of relaxation and anxiety could be used to treat anxious patients. His technique, which was called *systematic desensitization*, involves the creation of a hierarchy consisting of progressively anxiety-provoking stimuli, which are then imagined by patients, under a relaxed state, from least to most feared.[4]

Although the explanation of anxiety offered by the psychoanalytic and classical conditioning paradigms differ dramatically, systematic desensitization has many structural similarities to psychoanalysis. It is used to treat a disorder (phobic anxiety), is based on an explanation for the disorder (classical conditioning), imbeds the mechanism of change within the explanation (desensitization), and stipulates the therapeutic action necessary to effect the change (systematic desensitization). So, although the psychoanalytic paradigm is saturated with mentalistic constructs whereas the behavioral paradigm generally eschews intervening mentalistic explanations, they are both systems that explain maladaptive behavior and offer therapeutic protocols for reducing distress and promoting more adaptive functioning. Proponents of one of the two systems would claim that their explanations and protocols are superior to the other. Indeed, Watson and Rayner (1920) were openly disdainful of any Freudian explanation for Albert's fears:

> The Freudians twenty years from now, unless their hypotheses change, when they come to analyze Albert's fear of a seal skin coat—assuming that he comes to analysis at that age—will probably tease from him the recital of a dream which upon their analysis will show that Albert at three years of age attempted to play with the pubic hair of the mother and was scolded violently for it. (p. 14)

Given this brief introduction, the components of the medical model are now presented.

---

[4]There is evidence that the effects of systematic desensitization are not due to the purported classical conditioning explanations offered (e.g., Kirsch, 1985). The general finding that the purported explanations for various generally accepted efficacious treatments have not been verified empirically is discussed in chapter 5.

Components of the Medical Model

As conceptualized for the purpose of this book, the medical model has five components.

Client Disorder, Problem, or Complaint.   The first component of the medical model of psychotherapy is a client who is conceptualized to have a disorder, problem, or complaint. In medicine, the patient presents with a set of signs and symptoms that are indicative of a medical disorder. The analogous system in psychotherapy is the taxonomy of disorders developed in the *Diagnostic and Statistical Manual of Mental Disorders* (e.g., *DSM–IV*, American Psychiatric Association, 1994). Those who adhere to this taxonomy use signs and symptoms to provide a diagnosis for the patient in much the same way as physicians do.

As framed in this book, the medical model of psychotherapy does not require that a diagnosis be assigned to the client. It is sufficient that there is a system that identifies any aspect of the client that is amenable to change and that can be described in a way understandable to those who subscribe to a given therapeutic approach. For example, a behavioral psychotherapist could identify a social skills deficit as the presenting problem. To the behavioral psychotherapist, a social skill deficit is clearly not a mental disorder, yet it is a problem and as such qualifies as a component of the medical model of psychotherapy.

Psychological Explanation for Disorder, Problem, or Complaint. The second component of the medical model is that a psychological explanation for the client's disorder, problem, or complaint is proposed. The various psychotherapeutic approaches offer widely different theoretical explanations for a particular disorder. In medicine, there is greater convergence on the causes of a particular disorder. For example, few medical experts would disagree on the medical explanations of tuberculosis, diabetes, Down's syndrome, or angina. Of course there are medical disorders for which alternative explanations exist, but medical researchers recognize these differences and seek to collect evidence that will rule in or out various explanations.

For most psychological disorders, many alternative explanations exist. For example, depression may be due to irrational and maladaptive thoughts (cognitive therapies), lack of reinforcers for pleasurable activities (behavioral therapies), or problems related to social relations (interpersonal therapies). The important aspect of the medical model of psychotherapy is that some psychological explanation exists for the disorder, problem, or complaint.

Mechanism of Change.   The medical model of psychotherapy stipulates that each psychotherapeutic approach posit a mechanism of change. Generally speaking, psychoanalytic therapists make the unconscious conscious, cognitive therapists alter maladaptive thoughts, interpersonal therapists improve social relations, and family therapists disrupt destructive family dynamics. It is probably safe to say that the exposition of every psychotherapeutic approach contains a statement of the mechanism of change.

Specific Therapeutic Ingredients. To varying degrees, psychotherapeutic approaches prescribe specific therapeutic actions. The trend over the past few decades has been to explicate these actions in manuals, carefully laying out the specific ingredients that are to be used in treating a client.

Specificity. To this point, the medical model stipulates that the client presents with a disorder, problem, or complaint; the therapist ascribes to a particular theoretical orientation, which provides an explanation for the disorder, problem, or complaint and a rationale for change; and the therapist provides treatment that contains specific therapeutic ingredients that are characteristic of the theoretical orientation as well as the explanation of the disorder, problem, or complaint. Specificity, the critical aspect of the medical model, implies that the specific therapeutic ingredients are remedial for the disorder, problem, or complaint. That is, in a medical model, the specific ingredients are assumed to be responsible (i.e., necessary) for client change or progress toward therapeutic goals. Specificity implies that specific effects will be overwhelmingly larger than the general effects.

Medical Model of Psychotherapy Versus Medical Model in Medicine

It is important to discriminate between the medical model of psychotherapy and the medical model in medicine. Essentially, the medical model of psychotherapy is an analogue to the medical model in medicine, rather than a literal adoption.

The medical model in medicine contains the same components as the medical model of psychotherapy except that the theories, explanations, and characteristic techniques are physiochemically based. Specificity, in medicine, is established by demonstrating the efficacy of a technique as well as the physiochemical basis of the technique:

> The professional question for organized medicine was not whether [alternative] treatments were efficacious, but whether they involved physiochemical causes. For example, mesmerism was discredited not on the basis of efficacy issues but

because its adherents failed to demonstrate physical mechanisms involving magnetic fluids. (Wilkins, 1984, p. 571)

It is important to note that in medicine it is recognized that extraphysiochemical effects are present. That is, the model takes into account that treatments contain ingredients that are not characteristic of the explanatory theory and that these incidental factors may, in and of themselves, be partially remedial for a given disorder. For example, the medical patient's belief that a drug is beneficial will increase its potency. In medicine, these effects are called placebo effects and are presumed to be caused by nonphysiochemical (i.e., psychological) processes. Although these extraphysiochemical effects are recognized in medicine, they are simply uninteresting (Wilkins, 1984). The left panel of Figure 1.1 illustrates the specific physiochemical effects as well as the placebo effects in medicine. In medicine, placebos are used to control for the nonphysiochemical effects. As is discussed briefly in this section and then developed in chapter 5, psychotherapy analogues to medical placebos are not possible, and the attempt to rule out effects due to incidental factors are rendered problematic.

The medical model of psychotherapy differs from the medical model in medicine primarily because in psychotherapy the effects due to specific therapeutic ingredients and the effects due to incidental factors are both psychological, creating conceptual as well as empirical ambiguities. However, in medicine it is possible to deliver a purely physiochemical treatment. For example, a patient may inadvertently take a substance that purportedly is remedial for their disorder, or a surgery may be performed on a comatose patient. In psychotherapy, the specific ingredients cannot be de-

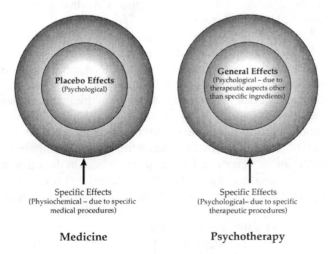

FIG. 1.1.   Medical models in medicine and in psychotherapy.

livered without the incidental ingredients. A therapeutic relationship is always present in psychotherapy and affects the manner in which the specific ingredients are delivered. In psychodynamic therapy, an interpretation will be more powerful when made by a therapist with a strong alliance with the client. The fact that the effects due to specific ingredients and common factors are psychological makes both of these effects interesting and relevant to psychotherapists. Accordingly, psychotherapy research has been devoted to both of these effects.

In the medical model in medicine, the focus is clearly on physiochemical effects, and psychological effects are considered as nuisance. Although in the medical model of psychotherapy there are two types of psychological effects, adherents of the medical model, including advocates of particular theoretical approaches, give primacy to specific ingredients and their effects. That is, medical model adherents recognize that general effects exist, but find them relatively uninteresting and believe that the preponderance of the therapeutic effect is due to specific ingredients. For example, a cognitive–behavioral advocate is interested in how cognitive schemas are altered and how this alteration is beneficial and is relatively uninterested with incidental aspects, such as the therapeutic relationship, and their effects.

To summarize, the medical model of psychotherapy presented herein takes the same form as the medical model in medicine but differs in that (a) disorders, problems, or complaints are held to have psychological rather than physiochemical etiology; (b) explanations for disorders, problems, or complaints and rationale for change are psychologically rather than physiochemically based; and (c) specific ingredients are psychotherapeutic rather than medical. Because the medical model of psychotherapy requires neither physiochemical nor mentalistic constructs, strict behavioral interventions would fit within this model.

There are areas for which the demarcation of the medical model of psychotherapy and the medical model in medicine becomes ambiguous. Some disorders that were thought to be psychological have been shown to have a clear and unambiguous physiochemical etiology. For example, general paresis was considered a psychologically based disorder until it was understood to be caused by the spirochete responsible for syphilis. Other disorders are clearly organic, but psychological treatments are nevertheless effective; behavioral interventions to manage the problems associated with autism or attention deficit disorder are of this type. On the other hand, attempts have been made to locate the physiochemical processes involved with the placebo effect in medicine, an attempt that is directed toward transforming a nuisance psychological process into a specific physiochemical and medical one. As a final instance of the crossover between psychotherapy and physiochemical models, it has been shown that psychotherapy affects brain chemistry (e.g., Baxter et al., 1992). These crossovers create some ambiguity regarding the distinctiveness of the two medical models and raise the specter of a false mind–body dualism; nevertheless, these theoretical ambiguities are not central to the thesis of this book.

Current Status of the Medical Model of Psychotherapy

The brief history presented earlier demonstrated that the roots of psychotherapy are planted firmly in the medical model. It is apparent that the psychotherapy research community has continued to adhere to the medical model. Two recent developments in psychotherapy research, psychotherapy treatment manuals and empirically supported treatments, have constrained psychotherapy research to the medical model, effectively stifling alternative meta-theories.

Psychotherapy Treatment Manuals.   A treatment manual contains "a definitive description of the principles and techniques of [the] psychotherapy, … [and] a clear statement of the operations the therapist is supposed to perform (presenting each technique as concretely as possible, as well as providing examples of each)" (Kiesler, 1994, p. 145). The purpose of the treatment manual is to create standardization of treatments, thereby reducing variability in the independent variable in clinical trials, and to ensure that therapists correctly deliver the specific ingredients that are characteristic of the theoretical approach. With regard to the latter point, manuals enable "researchers to demonstrate the theoretically required procedural differences between alternative treatments in comparative outcome studies" (Wilson, 1996, p. 295). Credit for the first treatment manual is usually attributed to Beck, Rush, Shaw, and Emery (1979), who delineated cognitive–behavioral treatment for depression. The proliferation of treatment manuals since Beck et al.'s manual in 1979 has been described as a "small revolution" (Luborsky & DeRubeis, 1984). Treatment manuals have become required for the funding and publication of outcome research in psychotherapy: "The treatment manual requirement, imposed as a routine design demand, chiseled permanently into the edifice of psychotherapy efficacy research the basic canon of standardization" (Kiesler, 1994, p. 145).

It is straightforward to understand how the treatment manual is imbedded in the medical model. The typical components of the manual—which include defining the target disorder, problem, or complaint; providing a theoretical basis for the disorder, problem, or complaint, as well as the change mechanism; specifying the therapeutic actions that are consistent with the theory; and the belief that the specific ingredients lead to efficacy—are identical to the components of the medical model. In chapter 7, the research evidence is presented relative to the question of whether using manuals results in better therapy outcomes.

Empirically Supported Treatments. The second development in psychotherapy research is the identification of empirically supported treatments (ESTs). The emphasis in the 1990s on managed care in medicine and related health areas, including mental health, created the need to standardize treatments and provide evidence of efficacy. As diagnostic related groups (DRGs), which allowed fixed payment per diagnosis, became accepted in the medical community, psychiatry responded with psychopharmacological treatments (i.e., drugs) for many mental disorders; the medical model in medicine was making significant inroads in the treatment of mental disorders. A task force of Division 12 (Clinical Psychology) of the American Psychological Association (APA) reacted in a predictable way: "If clinical psychology is to survive in this heyday of biological psychiatry, APA must act to emphasize the strength of what we have to offer—a variety of psychotherapies of proven efficacy" (Task Force on Promotion and Dissemination of Psychological Procedures, 1995, p. 3). Accordingly, to identify treatments that would meet the criteria of being empirically validated (the term originally used), the task force developed criteria that if satisfied by a treatment, would result in the treatment being included on a list published by the Task Force. Although the criteria have evolved, they originated from the criteria used by the Food and Drug Administration (FDA) to approve drugs. The criteria stipulated that a treatment would be designated as empirically validated for a particular disorder provided that at least two studies showed superiority to groups that attempted to control for general effects and were administered to a well-defined population of clients (including importantly the clients' disorder, problem, or complaint) using a treatment manual.

The first attempt to identify treatments that satisfied the criteria netted 18 well-established treatments (Task Force on Promotion and Dissemination of Psychological Procedures, 1995). Revisions to the list were made subsequently (Chambless et al., 1996; 1998) and included such treatments as cognitive behavior therapy for panic disorder, exposure treatment for agoraphobia, behavior therapy for depression, cognitive therapy for depression, interpersonal therapy for depression, multicomponent cognitive–behavioral therapy for pain associated with rheumatic disease, and behavioral marital therapy for marital discord. Recently, a special issue of the *Journal of Consulting and Clinical Psychology* was devoted to a discussion of ESTs and the identification of empirically supported treatments for adult mental disorders, child and adolescent disorders, health related disorders (viz., smoking, chronic pain, cancer, and bulimia nervosa), and marital distress (Baucom, Shoham, Mueser, Daiuto, & Stickle, 1998; Beutler, 1998; Borkovec &

Castonguay, 1998; Calhoun, Moras, Pilkonis, & Rehm, 1998; Chambless & Hollon, 1998; Compas, Haaga, Keefe, Leitenberg, & Williams, 1998; Davison, 1998; DeRubeis & Crits-Christoph, 1998; Garfield, 1998; Kazdin & Weisz, 1998; Kendall, 1998; Persons, Burns, & Perloff, 1998).

It is abundantly clear that the EST movement is deeply imbedded in a medical model of psychotherapy. First, the criteria are clear that to be designated as well-established empirically validated treatments, the treatments should be directed toward a disorder, problem, or complaint: "We do not ask whether a treatment is efficacious; rather, we ask whether it is efficacious for a specific problem" (Chambless & Hollon, 1998, p. 9). Although use of the *DSM* as the nosology for assigning disorders is not mandated, Chambless and Hollon indicated the *DSM* has "a number of benefits" for determining ESTs; those who have reviewed research in order to identify ESTs typically use the *DSM* (e.g., DeRubeis & Crits-Christoph, 1998).

The requirement that only treatments administered with a manual are certifiable as an EST further demonstrates a connection between ESTs and the medical model because, as discussed earlier, manuals are intimately tied to the medical model. The lists of empirically supported treatments are predominated by behavioral and cognitive–behavioral treatments, which may reflect the fact that such treatments are easier to put in the form of a manual than are experiential or psychodynamic treatments.

A third perspicuous aspect of the EST movement is the criteria, which were patterned after the FDA drug approval criteria that require that evidence is needed relative to specificity as well as efficacy. According to the EST criteria, specificity is established by demonstrating superiority to pill or psychological placebo or by showing equivalence to an already established treatment.[5] Clearly, specificity, a critical component in the medical model of psychotherapy undergirds the EST movement.[6] Indeed, the motivation to adopt a medical model in order to bolster the status of psychotherapy was evident from the beginning:

> We [The Task Force] believe establishing efficacy in contrast to a waiting list control group is not sufficient. Relying on such evidence would leave psychologists at a serious disadvantage vis à vis psychiatrists who can point to numerous double-blind placebo trials to support the validity of their interventions. (Task Force on Promotion and Dissemination of Psychological Procedures, 1995, p. 5)

---

[5]It has been pointed out that the designs stipulated in the criteria are insufficient to establish specific effects because the control groups do not control for general effects (Wampold, 1997), a point that is discussed further in chapter 5.

[6]Interestingly, some of those involved with the EST movement have recommended dropping the specificity requirement: "Simply put, if a treatment works, for whatever reason, ... then the treatment is likely to be of value clinically, and a good case can be made for its use" (Chambless & Hollon, 1998, p. 8). Nevertheless, treatments that could demonstrate specificity as well as efficacy would be "highly prized," indicating the continued belief that specificity remains central as is discussed later in this chapter.

CONTEXTUAL MODEL

Although the medical model is pervasive in the academic community and, as has been shown, is now required de facto for examining outcomes in psychotherapy, a small but persistent group of researchers has resisted adopting the model. Practitioners have increasingly felt enormous pressure to conform to the medical model as reimbursements require diagnoses, treatment plans, and all of the other trappings of the medical model. Nevertheless, practitioners have not, for the most part, constrained their treatments to the dictates of manuals, and they are reluctant to shape their treatments to a unitary theoretical approach.

In this section, an alternative to the medical model, which will be labeled the contextual model of psychotherapy, is presented. First, a brief history of alternatives to single theoretical approaches is presented.

Brief History of Alternatives to Allegiance to Single Theoretical Approaches

According to Arkowitz (1992), dissatisfaction with individual theoretical approaches spawned three movements: (a) theoretical integration, (b) technical eclecticism, and (c) common factors. The contextual model is a derivative of the common factors view.

Theoretical Integration. Theoretical integration is the fusion of two or more theories into a single conceptualization. Although earlier attempts were made to explain psychoanalysis with learning theory, Dollard and Miller's (1950) seminal book *Personality and Psychotherapy: An Analysis in Terms of Learning, Thinking, and Culture* was the first true integration of two theories that provided an explanation of behavior (in this case neuroses; Arkowitz, 1992). Because behavior therapy was not well developed at this time, Dollard and Miller's work was considered theoretical and provided little direction for an integrated treatment. Following the introduction of behavioral techniques (e.g., systematic desensitization), behavior therapists were generally more interested in remarking on the differences rather than the similarities of the two theories. Nevertheless, during the 1960s and 1970s, psychodynamic therapists shed the orthodoxy of psychoanalysis and became more structured, more attentive to coping strategies in the here-and-now, and more inclined to assign responsibility to the client (Arkowitz, 1992). At the same time, behavior therapists were allowing mediating constructs such as cognitions into their models and began to recognize the importance of factors incidental to behavioral theories, such as the therapeutic relationship.

The softening of the orthodoxy of both psychodynamic and behavioral approaches set the stage for Wachtel's (1977) integration of psychoanalysis and behavior therapy, *Psychoanalysis and Behavior Therapy: Toward an Integration*. Wachtel, in this and other writings, demonstrated how psychodynamic and behavior explanations could stand together to explain behavior and psychological disorder and how interventions from the two theories could facilitate therapeutic change, both behavioral and intrapsychic. The essence of the integration was nicely summarized by Arkowitz (1992):

> From the psychodynamic perspective, he [Wachtel] emphasized unconscious processes and conflict and the importance of meanings and fantasies that influenced our interactions with the world. From the behavioral side, the elements included the use of active-intervention techniques, a concern with the environmental context of behavior, a focus on the patient's goals in therapy, and a respect for empirical evidence.... Active behavioral interventions may also serve as a source of new insights (Wachtel, 1975), and insights can promote changes in behavior (Wachtel, 1982). (Arkowitz, 1992, pp. 268–269)

Since Wachtel's seminal work, psychotherapy integration has grown in popularity, with new integrations and refinements of others. The central issue for psychotherapy integration is to avoid having the integrated theory become a unitary theory of its own and to generate hypotheses that are distinct from the theories on which the integration is based (Arkowitz, 1992). The latter point is particularly relevant here because the purpose of this book is to review the empirical evidence to test whether it supports the medical model or an alternative. It is vital for empirical testing that the two meta-theories generate different predictions, and for that reason, theoretical integration does not provide a viable alternative to the medical model.

Technical Eclecticism.   The guiding light of technical eclecticism is Paul's question: "What treatment, by whom, is most effective for this individual with that specific problem, under which set of circumstances, and how does it come about?" (Paul, 1969). Technical eclecticism is dedicated to finding the answer to Paul's questions for as many cells as possible in the matrix created by crossing client, therapist, and problem dimensions. The search is empirically driven, and theory becomes relatively unimportant. The two most conspicuous systems for technical eclecticism are Arnold Lazarus' *Multimodal Therapy* (see, e.g., Lazarus, 1981) and Larry Beutler's *Systematic Eclectic Psychotherapy* (see, e.g., Beutler & Clarkin, 1990). Essentially, technical eclecticism is focused on the lowest level of abstraction—techniques (see Table 1.2). As such, it involves one aspect of the medical model, specific treatments for specific disorders, but shies away from the explanatory aspects of the medical model. Consequently, it would be impossible to derive hypotheses that would differentiate technical eclecticism from a medical model basis for the efficacy of psychotherapy. Nevertheless, some of the empirical evidence generated by technical eclecticism applied at the strategy level of abstraction (see, e.g., Beutler & Baker, 1998) is cited in chapter 5 as evidence for the contextual model.

Attention is now turned to the common factor approach, which forms the basis of the contextual model.

Common Factors

By the 1930s, psychoanalytic therapies had proliferated, with various theoretical variations advocated by such luminaries as Karen Horney, Alfred Adler, Carl Jung, and Harry Stack Sullivan (Cushman, 1992). The advocate of each therapeutic approach was encouraged by treatment successes, which quite naturally were interpreted as evidence to support the theory and the characteristic therapeutic actions. In 1936, Rosenzweig realized that each of the advocates were singing the same refrain and used an *Alice in Wonderland* metaphor to refer the equivalence in outcomes: "At last the Dodo said, 'Everybody has won, and all must have prizes.'" The general equivalence of outcomes in psychotherapy has now been firmly labeled as the Dodo Bird effect (which is the focus of chap. 4).

To Rosenzweig, the conclusion to be drawn from the general equivalence of psychotherapy outcomes was clear:

> The proud proponent, having achieved success in the cases he mentions, implies, even when he does not say it, that his ideology is thus proved true, all others false.... [However] it is soon realized that besides the intentionally utilized methods and their consciously held theoretical foundations, there are inevitably certain *unrecognized factors* in any therapeutic situation—factors that may be even more important that those being purposely employed. (Rosenzweig, 1936, p. 412)

In terms of the terminology used in this chapter, Rosenzweig was arguing against specificity and for the aspects of the therapy that are not central to the theoretical approach.

Since Rosenzweig proposed that common elements of therapy were responsible for the benefits of psychotherapy, attempts have been made to identify and codify the aspects of therapy common to all psychotherapies. Goldfried (1980), as mentioned previously, discussed the strategy level of abstraction in order to propose that when considered at this level, psychotherapies had particular strategies in common (see Table 1.2). Castonguay (1993) noted that focusing on therapist actions, such as therapeutic strategies, ignored other common aspects of psychotherapy. He distinguished three meanings that can be applied to understanding common factors in psychotherapy. The first meaning, which is similar to Goldfried's strategy level of abstraction, refers to global aspects of therapy that are not specific to any one approach (i.e., are common across approaches), such as insight, corrective experiences, opportunity to express emotions, and acquisition of a sense of mastery. The second meaning pertains to aspects of treatment that are auxiliary to treatment and refer primarily to the interpersonal and social factors. This second meaning encompasses the therapeutic context and the therapeutic relationship (e.g., the working alliance). The third meaning of the term involves those aspects of the treatment that influence outcomes but are not therapeutic activities or related to the interpersonal–social context. This latter meaning includes client expectancies and involvement in the therapeutic process.

In an attempt to bring coherence to the many theoretical discussions of common factors, Grencavage and Norcross (1990) reviewed publications that discussed commonalities among therapies and segregated commonalities into five areas: client characteristics, therapist qualities, change processes, treatment structures, and relationship elements. Table 1.3 presents the three most frequent elements in each category. These elements span the three meanings given by Castonguay (1993) as discussed earlier.

The common factor model proposes that there exists a set of factors that are common to all (or most) therapies, however identified and codified, and that these common factors are responsible for psychotherapeutic benefits rather than the ingredients specific to the particular theories. In terms of Figure 1.1, the common factor model claims that the area of the outer, specific effect ring would be small in comparison with that of the area for general effects. Statistically, one could say that a large proportion of the variance would be due to common factors, and a small proportion of the variance would be due to specific ingredients—in chapter 9, the variance due to these sources is estimated.

The common factor model is a diffuse model in that it stipulates that (a) there are a set of common factors and (b) these factors are therapeutic. There are more comprehensive models that contain common factors components, and although these models are often lumped into the common factor camp (e.g., Arkowitz, 1992), they are, from the standpoint of this book, distinct, as will be discussed later in this chapter. The alternative to the medical model, which is called the contextual model of psychotherapy, is presented next.

Definition of Contextual Model

The model presented in this section is called a contextual model because it emphasizes the contextual factors of the psychotherapy endeavor. Various

TABLE 1.3

Common Factors Gleaned From the Literature
by Grencavage and Norcross (1990)

Category	Commonalities
Client characteristics	Positive expectation–hope or faith; Distressed or incongruent client; Patient actively seeks help
Therapist qualities	General positive descriptors; Cultivates hope–enhances expectations; Warmth–positive regard
Change processes	Opportunity for catharsis–ventilation; Acquisition and practice of new behaviors; Provision of rationale
Treatment structures	Use of techniques–rituals; Focus on "inner world"–exploration of emotional issues; Adherence to theory
Relationship elements	Development of alliance–relationship (general); Engagement; Transference

Note. Only the three most frequent commonalities found by Grencavage and Norcross (1990) are presented here. From "Where Are the Commonalities Among the Therapeutic Common Factors?" by L. M. Grencavage and J. Norcross, 1990, *Professional Psychology: Research and Practice, 21,* pp. 374–376. Copyright © 1994 by the American Psychological Association. Adapted with permission.

contextual models of psychotherapy have been proposed (e.g., Brody, 1980; Frank & Frank, 1991). As was true for the medical model, there are philosophy-of-science distinctions that can be made amongst the variations; these distinctions are important to theoreticians and philosophers of science, but are relatively unimportant from the standpoint of this book. For the purpose of the present argument, the working model adopted is the one proposed by Jerome Frank in the various editions of his seminal book, *Persuasion and Healing* (Frank & Frank, 1991). Because space permits only a brief synopsis of the model, the reader is encouraged to read the original.

Frank's Model.   According to Frank and Frank (1991), "the aim of psychotherapy is to help people feel and function better by encouraging appropriate modifications in their assumptive worlds, thereby transforming the meanings of experiences to more favorable ones" (p. 30). Persons who present for psychotherapy are demoralized and have a variety of problems, typically depression and anxiety. That is, people seek psychotherapy for the demoralization that results from their symptoms rather than for symptom relief. Frank has proposed that "psychotherapy achieves its effects largely by directly treating demoralization and only indirectly treating overt symptoms of covert psychopathology" (Parloff, 1986, p. 522).

Frank and Frank (1991) described the components shared by all approaches to psychotherapy. The first component is that psychotherapy involves an emotionally charged, confiding relationship with a helping person (i.e., the therapist). The second component is that the context of the relationship is a healing setting, in which the client presents to a professional who the client believes can provide help and who is entrusted to work in his or her behalf. The third component is that there exists a rationale, conceptual scheme, or myth that provides a plausible explanation for the patient's symptoms and prescribes a ritual or procedure for resolving them. According to Frank and Frank, the particular rationale needs to be accepted by the client and by the therapist, but need not be "true." The rationale can be a myth in the sense that the basis of the therapy need not be "scientifically" proven. However, it is critical that the rationale for the treatment be consistent with the worldview, assumptive base, and attitudes and values of the client or, alternatively, that the therapist assists the client to become in accord with the rationale. Simply stated, the client must believe in the treatment or be lead to believe in it. The final component is a ritual or procedure that requires the active participation of both client and therapist and is based on the rationale (i.e., the ritual or procedure is believed to be a viable means of helping the client).

Frank and Frank (1991) discussed six elements that are common to the rituals and procedures used by all psychotherapists. First, the therapist combats the client's sense of alienation by developing a relationship that is maintained after the client divulges feelings of demoralization. Second, the therapist maintains the patient's expectation of being helped by linking hope for improvement to the process of therapy. Third, the therapist provides new learning experiences. Fourth, the clients' emotions are aroused as a result of the therapy. Fifth, the therapist enhances the client's sense of mastery or self-efficacy. Sixth, the therapist provides opportunities for practice.

It is important to emphasize the status of techniques in the contextual model. Specific ingredients are necessary to any bona fide psychotherapy whether conceptualized as a medical model treatment or a contextual model treatment. In the contextual model, specific ingredients are necessary to construct a coherent treatment that therapists have faith in and that provides a convincing rationale to clients. This point is cogently articulated by Frank in the preface to the most recent version of his model (Frank & Frank, 1991):

> My position is not that technique is irrelevant to outcome. Rather, I maintain that, as developed in the text, the success of all techniques depends on the patient's sense of alliance with an actual or symbolic healer. This position implies that ideally therapists should select for each patient the therapy that accords, or can be brought to accord, with the patient's personal characteristics and view of the problem. Also implied is that therapists should seek to learn as many approaches as they find congenial and convincing. Creating a good therapeutic match may

involve both educating the patient about the therapist's conceptual scheme and, if necessary, modifying the scheme to take into account the concepts the patient brings to therapy. (p. xv)

Interestingly, Frank's recognition that in the contextual model, a viable treatment must have a consistent, rational explanatory system was first articulated in 1936 by Rosenzweig:

> It may be said that given a therapist who has an effective personality and who consistently adheres in his treatment to a system of concepts which he has mastered and which is in one significant way or another adapted to the problem of the sick personality, then it is of comparatively little consequence what particular method that therapist uses.... Whether the therapist talks in terms of psychoanalysis or Christian Science is from this point of view relatively unimportant as compared with the *formal consistency* with which the doctrine employed is adhered to, for by virtue of this consistency the patient receives a schema for achieving some sort and degree of personality organization. (Rosenzweig, 1936, pp. 413–415)

Comments on the Contextual Model.   The first important point to make is the distinction between the common factor model and the contextual model. Common factor models contain a set of common factors, each of which makes an independent contribution to outcome. Although Frank and Frank (1991) discussed components common to all therapies, the healing context and the meaning attributed to it by the participants (therapist and client) are critical contextual phenomena. According to Frank and Frank, provision of new learning experiences, as an example, will not be therapeutic unless the client perceives the therapy to be taking place in a healing context in which he or she as well as the therapist believe in the rationale for the therapy; the therapist delivers therapeutic actions consistent with the rationale; the client is aroused and expects to improve; and a therapeutic relationship has been developed. In a contextual conceptualization of common factors, specific therapeutic actions, which may be common across therapies, cannot be isolated and studied independently. As we shall see (primarily in chap. 5), many researchers who ascribe to the medical model design control groups to rule out common factors, naive to the contextual factors critical to a contextual model.

It is vital to understand the status of the contextual model vis-à-vis other psychotherapeutic theories. Previously, Grünbaum 's (1981) system was adapted to explain the medical model. Interestingly, Grünbaum considers Frank's model as another theory with characteristic ingredients:

> Frank credits a treatment–ingredient *common* to the rival psychotherapies with such therapeutic efficacy as they do possess.... He is tacitly classifying as "incidental," rather than as "characteristic," all those treatment factors that he deems to be therapeutic. In adopting this latter classification, he is speaking the

classifactory language employed by the theories underlying the various thera-pies, while denying their claim that the treatment ingredients they label "charac-teristic" are actually effective. (Grünbaum, 1981, p. 161—162)

According to this interpretation, the contextual model is a theory on the same level of abstraction as behavioral, psychodynamic, and interpersonal theories, obviating its status as a meta-theory. There are a number of (inter-related) arguments that mitigate against classifying the contextual model as a psychotherapeutic theory rather than a meta-theory. First, the characteris-tic ingredients of a psychotherapeutic theory are unique to that theory or are shared by a few closely related theories, whereas the common ingredients discussed by Frank and other common factor conceptualizations are shared by all theoretical approaches. In this sense, all treatments are characteristic of the contextual model. Second, the contextual factors and common ingre-dients of the contextual model, which are considered incidental by psychotherapeutic theories, cannot be removed from the treatments pre-scribed by the various theories. Third, the contextual model dictates that a treatment be administered but that the particular components of that treat-ment are unimportant relative to the belief of the therapist and the client that the treatment is rational and efficacious. The contextual model states that the treatment procedures used are beneficial to the client because of the meaning attributed to those procedures rather than because of their specific psychological effects.

If one considers the contextual model to be at the same level of abstrac-tion as other psychotherapeutic theories, then one could design studies comparing a particular approach—for instance, cognitive–behav-ioral—with a contextual model approach. This is not possible, however, be-cause one cannot construct a manualized contextual model treatment. In another sense, all treatments are examples of contextual model treatments in that they all contain the features of the contextual model. So, when one compares cognitive–behavioral treatment for depression with an interper-sonal treatment for depression, one is also comparing a cognitive–behav-ioral model with a contextual model. If the two treatments are equally effective, is it because of their respective specific ingredients or because both are instances of contextual model treatments? This is the central ques-tion answered by this book.

A final point that causes confusion in the design of comparison groups in psychotherapy outcome research is the status of Rogerian therapy. This ap-proach to therapy, which is now called person-centered therapy, fits the de-scription of a theoretical approach subsumed under the medical model in many ways. It contains a clear theory of the person and therapeutic change as well as techniques for facilitating such change (e.g., Rogers, 1951). Al-though the techniques are generally not directed toward a specific disorder, as is typical of the medical model, the person-centered therapist conceptualizes the nature of client problems within the humanistic explanatory system. Moreover, client-centered approaches have been adapted and tested with various populations, illustrated by Rogers's work with individuals with schizophrenia (Rogers, Gendlin, Kiesler, & Truax, 1967). Many equate client-centered therapy with common factors because of the emphasis on relationship and therapeutic process, but client-centered and other experiential therapists provide a level of treatment more sophisticated and complex than simple empathic responding. As will be shown in chapter 5, attempts to control for common factors by using Rogerian or nondirective therapy are flawed.

Status of Contextual Model

As mentioned previously, the medical model definitely holds the superordinate position in academia, particularly in the research environment. However, there are conspicuous examples of contextual model and common factor approaches that are supported by research evidence, such as Sol Garfield's *Psychotherapy: An Eclectic–Integrative Approach* (1995). Clearly, however, adherents of a contextual model or common factor approach are considered "soft" or unscientific by medical model adherents. Consider Donald Klein's criticism of psychotherapy as a treatment for depression:

> It is remarkably hard to find differences between the outcomes of credible psychotherapies or any evidence that a proposed specific beneficial mechanism of action has anything to do with therapeutic outcome.... These findings ... are inexplicable on the basis of the therapeutic action theories propounded by the creators of IPT [interpersonal therapy] and CBT [cognitive–behavioral therapy]. However they are entirely compatible with the hypothesis (championed by Jerome Frank; see Frank & Frank, 1991) that psychotherapies are not doing anything specific: rather, they are nonspecifically beneficial to the final common pathway of demoralization, *to the degree that they are effective at all* [italics added].... The bottom line is that if the Food and Drug Administration (FDA) was responsible for the evaluation of psychotherapy, then no current psychotherapy would be approvable, whereas particular medications are clearly approvable. (Klein, 1996, pp. 82–84)

Klein clearly denigrates any psychotherapeutic effects that are not specific. Moreover, any benefits of psychotherapy that may be attributable to a "demoralization pathway " is so suspect that it casts doubts about the efficacy of psychotherapy generally, in spite of the overwhelming evidence of the benefits of the psychotherapeutic enterprise. Chambless and Hollon (1998), who recognized the importance of demonstrating efficacy regardless of the causal mechanisms, nevertheless believe that " treatments found to be superior to conditions that control for such nonspecific processes or to another bona fide treatment are *even more highly prized and said to be effi-cacious and specific* [italics added]" (p. 8). Clearly, they value effects at-tributable to specific ingredients, demonstrating the tendency to value the presumably scientific medical model of psychotherapy over a contextual model. Parloff (1986), as well, noted the disrespect given to general effects:

> Some mechanisms of change are, *ipso facto*, less acceptable than others. If the seemingly positive effects of psychotherapy are attributable primarily to such mechanism as "suggestion," "placebo," "attention," or "common sense" advice, then the credibility of psychotherapy as a profession is automatically impugned. (pp. 523–524)

Clinical "scientists" are so enamored with the medical model of psycho-therapy that they begrudgingly acknowledge that benefit could accrue through mechanisms other than those characteristic of theoretical ap-proaches, and they denigrate such mechanisms much in the way that medi-cal researchers recognize but are uninterested in nonspecific effects.

It might be informative to know whether practitioners subscribe to a medical model or a contextual model of psychotherapy. Numerous sur-veys have been conducted to determine the theoretical orientation of prac-titioners (see Garfield & Bergin, 1994, for a summary; see also Jensen & Bergin, 1990; Norcross, Prochaska, & Farber, 1993). On all such surveys, whether the respondents are psychologists, social workers, or psychia-trists, practitioners indicate that, relative to any single theoretical ap-proach, they ascribe to an eclectic orientation. However, it is difficult to know whether these responses indicate an allegiance to a theoretical inte-gration of two theories and the concomitant characteristic ingredients or to a rejection of the orthodoxy of theoretical approaches and the medical model. Jensen and Bergin (1990) asked respondents who indicated that they practiced eclecticism to indicate the combinations of theoretical ap-proaches used in their practice; most therapists indicated that they used dynamic, cognitive, and behavioral approaches. In these surveys, the de-gree to which those who endorse a single theoretic approach adhere to the manualized version of these treatments is unknown, although most sus-pect that adherence to a manual is doubtful. However, therapists believe that the expertness of their therapeutic technique as opposed to more rela-tionship-oriented constructs lead to successful outcomes (Eugster & Wampold, 1996; Feifel & Eells, 1963). Interpretation of these results is difficult because both the medical model and the contextual model recog-nize that therapists will have a theoretical rationale for client distress and will implement interventions that are consistent with that explanation. However, it is clear that practitioners do not share the orthodoxy of theo-retical approach with advocates or developers of these approaches.

CONCLUSIONS

In this chapter, two competing meta-models were presented. The medical model proposes that the ingredients characteristic of a theoretical approach are the important sources of psychotherapeutic effects. Developments in psychotherapy research (viz., manualization of treatments and empirically supported treatments) have assumed the medical model is true and have progressed accordingly. The contextual model, which emphasizes a holistic common factors approach, provides an alternative meta-theory for psychotherapy.

The purpose of this book is to examine the research evidence to determine whether it is consistent with one of the two meta-theoretic models. In the next chapter, a series of hypotheses that discriminates between the two models will be discussed. The following chapters examine each of the hypotheses.

2

Differential Hypotheses
and Evidentiary Rules

The medical model and the contextual model provide two very different conceptualizations of psychotherapy. The medical model of psychotherapy patterns itself after the medical model in medicine, has the trappings of a scientific endeavor, and is the darling of those who see themselves as rigorous, serious clinical researchers. To question the validity of the medical model is to entertain the thought that psychotherapy is a "touchy-feely" movement supported by well-intentioned but soft-headed practitioners who want to ignore scientific evidence and be guided by their clinical judgement and intuition. But what if the scientific evidence casts doubt on the very edifice that has "science" written on its front door?

For years, there has been a nagging suspicion that the medical model may not be able to account for many research results that have appeared in the literature. For example, the ubiquitous and robust finding that all psychotherapies intended to be therapeutic are equally efficacious (see chap. 4) is incompatible with the specificity component of the medical model because it suggests that all specific ingredients are equally potent and all theoretical orientations equally valid. Nevertheless, adherents to the medical model, in various ways, dismiss these results. Some would say that the results are ipso facto incorrect:

If the indiscriminate distribution of prizes carried true conviction ... we end up with the same advice of everyone—"Regardless of the nature of your problem seek any form of psychotherapy." This is absurd. We doubt even the strongest advocates of the Dodo Bird argument dispense this advice. (Rachman & Wilson, 1980, p. 167)

31

Others would claim that if researchers continue searching, meaningful differences among treatments will appear:

> So long as better mental health status is important, no amount of prior failures to rise above the results of some baseline should obstruct further efforts, and the omnibus significance test used by Wampold et al. [that resulted in no differences among treatments] represents just such an obstruction. (Howard, Krause, Saunders, & Kopta, 1997, p. 223)

Still others claim that the severity of the treated disorder affects the results:

> With mild conditions, the nonspecific effects of treatments (therapeutic alliance, positive expectations about change, etc.) are likely to be powerful enough in themselves to affect both primary and secondary outcomes, leaving little room for the specific factors to play much of a role. (Crits-Christoph, 1997, pp. 217)

The argument has also been made that the attention of research has not been sufficiently specific:

> Research has not yet identified each therapy 's narrow range of maximal effectiveness. The apparent homogeneity of effects merely reflects averaging each therapy 's results across heterogeneous clients, therapists, and settings. (Stiles, Shapiro, & Elliott, 1986, p. 168)

A variation of the claim that homogeneity of efficacy is due to insufficient examination of interaction between treatments and client characteristics is the contention that the *DSM* system identifies syndromes rather than single disease entities with known etiology:

> If one assumed that depressive symptoms were one possible endpoint from a number of etiological pathways and that any group of persons with depression contained a number from each pathway, then comparative outcome studies are forever doomed to get equivalent results because those who might have had a biological cause might respond to medication but not those were interpersonally unskilled, and so on. So far there is little evidence that there are common etiological pathways that describe a uniform course or response to treatment for any reasonable proportion of the *DSM–IV* categories. (Follette & Houts, 1996, p. 1128)

As well, there are those who argue that issues related to the measures used to assess outcome mitigate against finding differences among treatments:

> The apparent equivalence of outcomes could reflect a failure of comparative outcome studies to measure the particular changes that differentiate treatments.... These authors [behaviorists] have alleged that such imprecise measurement is bound to obscure differences among the effects of different therapies. (Stiles et al., 1986, p. 170)

Not uncommon, one treatment may be superior to another on the target measures that were not a focus of treatment. (Crits-Christoph, 1997, p. 216)

Another argument suggests that treatments are insufficiently standardized
to generate differences:

[Another] challenge to the findings of outcome equivalence argues that differences in technique's effectiveness may have been obscured by shortcomings in
the operationalization of treatment variables for research. Therapists in comparative studies may have had different, unclear, or mistaken ideas of what each
treatment consisted of and so may have failed to deliver the distinct treatment
methods consistently. Clearly, one cannot attribute the presence or absence of
differences in effectiveness to the treatments themselves without evidence that
they were delivered as intended and they included the crucial components responsible for therapeutic benefit. (Stiles et al., 1986, p. 169)

Each of these perspectives offers alternative explanations for the uniform efficacy result. Although each of these explanations is plausible, there
is no evidence that they are correct. In fact, quite the opposite is true—there
is evidence that these alternative explanations are false (see chap. 4).

Over the years, research results that are not consistent with the medical
model conceptualization of psychotherapy have appeared. However, these
results have been discounted for various reasons, much as the uniform efficacy result has been dismissed. Whenever a meta-theory is unquestioned,
discordant results can be accommodated by various ad hoc explanations.
The geocentric model of the solar system worked perfectly well for centu-
ries, relying on excessively complex formulations, until Galileo proposed
the heliocentric model, which explained the movement of the planets parsi-
moniously. The contention of this book is that the research evidence is consistent with a contextual model of psychotherapy rather than a medical
model and that if science is grounded in theories that accord parsimoni-
ously with research evidence, the medical model will be rejected.

The contextual model and other common factor approaches are dismissed
as being "soft" or unscientific. There have been various attempts to justify
common factor or contextual models on the basis of scientific evidence.
Frank and Frank (1991) cited much research to support their contextual
model. Hubble, Duncan, and Miller (1999) recently edited a popular book
The Heart & Soul of Therapy: What Works in Therapy that attempted to empirically support a number of common factors in therapy. However, each of
the attempts, however convincing they are, supports contextual models by selectively citing studies, by relying on evidence from analogues (e.g., derived
from other cultures or from medical studies), or by using alternative research
paradigms (e.g., qualitative research). The case for the contextual model presented in this book relies primarily on the corpus of psychotherapy evidence,
most of it generated from studies guided by the medical model (e.g., clinical

trails), obviating any contention that the evidence is "soft" or biased. Simply put, this systematic review of the evidence will show that the medical model cannot support the weight of its own evidence.

The first section of this chapter outlines hypotheses in six areas that bear on the validity of the medical model and the contextual model of psychotherapy. The second section discusses the evidentiary rules for testing these hypotheses.

DIFFERENTIAL HYPOTHESES

The hypotheses relative to the medical and contextual models of psychotherapy in six areas are discussed briefly. In each of the chapters that presents the evidence, the hypotheses are explored in greater detail. The hypotheses as well as the chapters in which they are investigated are presented in Table 2.1.

Absolute Efficacy

Absolute efficacy refers to the effects of a treatment in comparison to no treatment. Determination of absolute efficacy answers the question, "Does Treatment A produce better outcomes than no treatment?" Absolute efficacy is typically deduced from a treatment–control group clinical trial, which contrasts a treatment condition with a no-treatment control group (e.g., a waiting-list control group). The limitations of the results from these designs with regard to differentiating the medical model and the contextual model are readily apparent: If Treatment A is deemed to be efficacious (i.e., found to be superior to a no-treatment control group), were the positive outcomes due to the specific ingredients or the incidental aspects of the therapy? That is, are the effects specific or general?

Clearly, both the medical model and the contextual model predict that psychotherapy will be efficacious, albeit through different mechanisms. In this sense, the establishment of absolute efficacy does not favor one meta-theory over the other. For several reasons the evidence relative to absolute efficacy is presented (see chap. 3). First, if psychotherapy does not produce positive outcomes, there is little reason to debate the validity of various models. Second, the seeds of various other hypotheses lie in the fertile ground of clinical trials— for example, the early meta-analyses devoted to absolute efficacy raised questions about therapeutic aspects such as relative efficacy, allegiance, therapist effects, and so forth. Third, the establishment of absolute efficacy provides the opportunity to demonstrate the usefulness of research synthesis for answering complex questions related to psychotherapy outcomes.

In chapter 3, it will be shown that psychotherapy is remarkably efficacious for a variety of disorders, problems, or complaints, and for a variety of

TABLE 2.1

Differential Hypotheses for Medical Model and Contextual Model

Hypothesis Name	Medical Model Prediction	Contextual Model Prediction	Chapter
Absolute efficacy	Psychotherapy efficacious	Psychotherapy efficacious	3
Relative efficacy	Variation in efficacy • Dodo bird conjecture false	Uniform efficacy • Dodo bird conjecture true	4
Specific effects	Evidence of specific effects • dismantling studies show effects • demonstration of mediating processes or temporal relationships • Theoretical interactions with Tx present • Tx > Placebo > No Tx	No evidence of specific effects • dismantling studies show no effects • no evidence of mediating processes or temporal relationships • Non-theoretical interactions with Tx present • Tx > Placebo > No Tx	5
General effects	Evidence of general effects • general effects < specific effects	Evidence of general effects • general effects > specific effects	6
Allegiance and adherence	Adherence critical Allegiance unimportant	Adherence unimportant (but coherence important) Allegiance critical	7
Therapist effects	Therapist effects relatively small • Tx effects > therapist effects	Therapist effects relatively large • Tx effects < therapist effects	8

persons. The history of establishing outcomes is traced from Eysenck's (1952) claim that the rate of success of psychotherapy does not exceed the rate of spontaneous remission, to M. L. Smith and Glass's (1977) landmark meta-analysis of outcomes in psychotherapy, to the present status of outcomes in psychotherapy.

Relative Efficacy

Relative efficacy refers to the effects produced by the comparison of two treatments and answers the questions, "Does Treatment A produce better outcomes than Treatment B?" Relative efficacy is deduced from comparative outcome studies in which one treatment is contrasted with another. The medical model predicts that there will be variation in efficacy among psychotherapeutic treatments because the specific ingredients characteristic of the various theoretical approaches differ and therefore are not equally beneficial. Cognitive–behavioral advocates hypothesize that depression is a result of maladaptive cognitions, which, if disputed by the therapist, will be palliative. Less valid explanations of the etiology should lead to less efficacious treatments. The medical model stipulates that specific ingredients are indeed responsible for the positive effects of psychotherapy and presumably some of these ingredients are more efficacious than others (and some even will be harmful). Consequently, there will be variation in the efficacy of various treatments.

On the other hand, the contextual model predicts that treatments intended to be therapeutic, regardless of the specific ingredients included in the treatment, will be efficacious. Another way to conceptualize uniform efficacy is to say that all psychotherapies are instances of the contextual model, and therefore all treatments should produce equivalent outcomes. That is, all bona fide treatments possess the proper context and common factors necessary to produce beneficial outcomes. Thus, under the contextual model, treatments are uniformly efficacious.[1] With regard to relative efficacy, the two models make divergent predictions—variation in efficacy (medical model) versus uniform efficacy (contextual model).

When Rosenzweig hypothesized in 1936 that the positive outcomes of psychotherapy were due to various commonalities, he subtitled his article with a quote from *Alice in Wonderland* to indicate the equivalence of outcomes: "At last the Dodo said, 'Everybody has won and all must have prizes.'" In 1975, Luborsky, Singer, and Luborsky (1975) reviewed comparative studies and again alluded to the Dodo bird in the subtitle: "Is it true that 'Everyone has won and all must have prizes'?" Since 1975, the general equivalence of outcomes in psychotherapy has been called the *Dodo bird effect*. Consequently, the hypothesis that psychotherapies are uniformly effective is referred to as the *Dodo bird conjecture*. The medical model predicts that the Dodo bird conjecture is false, whereas the contextual model predicts that it is true.

In chapter 4, the accumulating evidence relative to the Dodo bird conjecture is presented. Luborsky et al.'s (1975) original review sets the stage for a series of meta-analyses that addressed this issue. With few exceptions, the results are consistent with the hypothesis that psychotherapies are uniformly efficacious, supporting the contextual model meta-theory. The various meta-analyses of comparative studies are used to estimate the variance in outcomes due to specific ingredients, although that estimate is revised in

---

[1]Although the contextual model predicts that outcomes will be homogeneous across treatments, the model predicts that there will be variation due to other sources, such as therapists, allegiance, and quality of the therapeutic alliance.

chapter 8, when it is shown that treatment effects are statistically contaminated by therapist effects.

Specific Effects

The medical model stipulates that the beneficial effects of psychotherapy are due, to a large extent, to the specific ingredients. If this is so, demonstrable evidence of the psychological processes related to the specific ingredients should be detectable. Although specificity is difficult to establish, there are a number of research strategies that can be used to isolate the effects of specific ingredients.

One strategy to identify specific effects is the dismantling design in which a treatment is compared with a condition that receives the treatment minus one or a few purportedly critical ingredients. If the treatment package is found to be superior to the treatment without the ingredients, then the ingredient or ingredients are responsible, in part, for the positive outcome produced by the treatment package. The medical model predicts that when the specific ingredients of a treatment are removed, the treatment will be significantly less effective, whereas the contextual model, which does not give primacy to the particular ingredients, predicts that removing one or a few ingredients will not attenuate efficacy. The contextual model also predicts that adding a theoretically crucial ingredient, which is tested with an additive design, will not augment the benefits of treatment. In chapter 5 the evidence produced by component designs (i.e., dismantling and additive designs) is reviewed. Across all of the component designs used in psychotherapy research, adding or subtracting a specific ingredient has been found to have no effect on outcome.

Another strategy to establish specificity is to show that a psychological change process is occurring as predicted. More technically, specificity requires that the hypothesized change mechanism mediates the treatment effects. For example, cognitive–behavioral treatment for depression is expected to alter cognitions that will then reduce depressive symptomatology. Such a result is further strengthened if other treatments (say, interpersonal treatment for depression) do not show the same mediating relationship (Wampold, 1997). Another way to demonstrate change process is to examine the temporal relationship between administration of a specific ingredient and outcome. If specific ingredients are remedial, as predicted by the medical model, then change will not occur prior to the administration of the ingredient, but will occur reliably thereafter. In chapter 5, it will be shown that attempts to establish specificity by examining mediating or temporal relations have generally failed. In addition, such attempts sometimes yield evidence for mediation and temporal relationships that support certain common factors.

One of the medical model explanations for uniform efficacy results is that differences among therapies are obscured by various patient characteristics. For example, as argued in the introduction of this chapter by Follette and Houts (1996), depression is a syndrome for which etiology varies across the population of depressed persons, and treatments must be specific to particular clients' depression—cognitive–behavioral treatment for clients whose depression is cognitively based, psychopharmacology for those whose depression is biologically based, interpersonal therapy for those whose depression is socially based, and so on. This is a reasonable hypothesis that, if confirmed, would account for the Dodo bird effect and support the medical model. Various terms have been associated with designs that test for such differential effects: matching studies, aptitude (i.e., person characteristics) × treatment interactions, and moderating variables. Essentially, in these designs, the medical model predicts interactions between treatment and client characteristics that are explicitly predicted by psychotherapeutic theory. Little evidence has been found for the existence of such interactions, however.

Some interactions between client characteristics and treatments, if empirically verified, support the contextual model. One of the key elements of the contextual model is that the treatment should be in accord with the beliefs of the client. For example, some clients will naturally feel more inclined to accept a behavioral rationale for their disorder, problem, or complaint; feel more comfortable with behavioral therapy; and form an alliance with a behavioral therapist. Other clients, however, will be more inclined to accept an intrapsychic explanation, feel more comfortable with a dynamic therapy, and form an alliance with a dynamically oriented psychotherapist. The contextual model therefore predicts interactions between treatments and various client characteristics related to acceptance of or belief in various treatments. Some evidence exists for such interactions, although it is not particularly convincing.

In chapter 5, research designs used to detect interactions between treatments and person characteristics will be discussed. It will be shown that there are methodological as well as conceptual issues that make it difficult to detect interactions. Nevertheless, the theoretical based interactions predicted by the medical model are virtually nonexistent, whereas some interactions based on a contextual model conceptualization have been detected.

A final design used to control for general effects in psychotherapy research is to use various control groups that supposedly are composed of all of the common factors and none of the specific factors. The logic of designs using these control groups (originally called placebo controls, but also referred to as alternative treatments or nondirective counseling) is clearly based in the medical model. Indeed, adherents of the medical model claim that the superiority of a treatment to a placebo type control is evidence of the specificity of the treatment. Because medical model adherents recognize that specificity does not rule out the presence of general effects, they predict that treatments with efficacious specific ingredients will be superior to placebo treatments, which in turn will be superior to no treatment.

In chapter 5, the logical problems inherent in placebo treatments in psychotherapy are discussed. It will be shown that placebo treatments in psychotherapy are not analogues of placebo treatments in medicine and are not able to control for the general effects produced by incidental aspects of psychotherapies. Essentially, the problem is that placebo treatments in psychotherapy are not identical to active treatments with the specific ingredients "invisibly" removed. Consequently, double-blinding is impossible. Moreover, in psychotherapy the specific ingredients and the incidental factors are of the same type (i.e., psychological) and thus are inseparable.

The contextual model requires that treatments contain rationales and techniques that both the client and the therapist believe are therapeutic. It is not possible to design a placebo treatment that can be delivered blind to the therapist and therefore is deficient solely on that account. Placebos are deficient vis-à-vis the contextual model on a number of other accounts as well, as discussed in chapter 5. Nevertheless, from the contextual model perspective, placebo conditions contain some of the common factors. Consequently, the contextual model makes exactly the same prediction as the medical model, namely that treatments intended to be therapeutic will be superior to placebo treatments, which in turn will be superior to no treatment.

General Effects

General effects are produced by the aspects of therapy that are incidental to the respective theories. The contextual model predicts that the effects of therapy consist primarily of general effects. The contextual model stipulates that features of the psychotherapy context are vital to the success of the endeavor and therefore it is not possible to isolate a set of common factors and test whether each one is related to psychotherapeutic outcome. Nevertheless, there is persuasive evidence that some common factors are related demonstrably, reliably, and consequentially to outcomes. In chapter 6, evidence is presented to show that the relationship between the client and therapist is related to outcomes across various types of psychotherapies and that this relationship is therapeutic (i.e., the relationship causes the outcomes rather than improvement in therapy causing a better relationship).

As mentioned previously, the medical model posits that there will be general effects. The issue is the relative size of general and specific effects. Adherents of the medical model claim that the general effects are relatively small in comparison with the specific effects. As noted earlier, the empirical evidence shows that the specific effects are small, if they exist at all (see chap. 4). In ~~~~~~~~~~~~~~ using the most liberal estimate of specific ~~~~~~~~~~~~~~~~~~~ estimate of general effects, general effe~~~~~~~~~~~~~~~~~~ as much of the variance in outcomes as d~~~~~~~~~~~~~~

Allegiance and Adherence

Adherence is defined as the "extent to which a therapist used interventions and approaches prescribed by the treatment manual, and avoided the use of interventions and procedures proscribed by the manual" (Waltz, Addis, Koerner, & Jacobson, 1993, p. 620). Essentially adherence ratings are measures of the degree to which therapists provide the specific ingredients of a treatment. Clearly, according to the medical model, adherence should be related to outcome because provision of the specific ingredients is hypothesized to be critical to the success of therapy. The contextual model prediction relative to adherence is more complicated. The contextual model requires the delivery of ingredients consistent with a rationale, which appears to require adherence. Yet the contextual model is less dogmatic about the ingredients and allows eclecticism, as long as there is a rationale that underlies the treatment and that rationale is cogent, coherent, and psychologically based. Sol Garfield (1992), a prominent proponent of a common factor approach, discussing the results of a survey of eclectic therapists, described well adherence in a contextual model context:

> These eclectic clinicians tended to emphasize that they used the theory or methods they thought were best for the client. In essence, procedures were selected for a given patient in terms of that client's problems instead of trying to make the client adhere to a particular form of therapy. An eclectic therapy thus allows the therapist potentially to use a wide range of techniques, a view similar to my own in most respects.... This approach is clearly opposite to the emphasis on using psychotherapy manuals to train psychotherapists to adhere strictly to a specific form of therapy in order to ensure the integrity of the type of psychotherapy being evaluated. (p. 172)

Thus, according to the contextual model, adherence to a manualized treatment is not required and is not thought to be related to outcome. Therefore, adherence to a manual is important in the medical model but relatively unimportant in the contextual model. In chapter 7, it is shown that adherence has not generally been found to be related to outcome.

Allegiance is the degree to which the therapist delivering the treatment believes that the therapy is efficacious. In practice settings, when therapists are free to choose among various therapies for a particular client, presumably they use the one that they feel is most efficacious given their training, expertise, and inclination. The situation is not the same in many clinical trials. In studies that compare two psychotherapies, therapists often deliver treatments in each of the conditions, in what is referred to as a *crossed design* (see chap. 8 for a detailed discussion of therapist effects in crossed and nested designs). These therapists typically are associated, in one way or another, with the laboratory invo   loping one of the treatments, and they consequently have an all   During the clinical trial, these therapists are train   erapies even though they do not have alle

Belief in the efficacy of tr   he client, is a central element of the cor   he contextual model makes a clear predic   rapist is positively related to outcome—   e therapy, the better the outcome. On the   laces emphasis on the specific ingredients, which, if deriv   in the treatment protocol, should produce positive outcomes regardless of the allegiance of the therapist.

Typically, the degree of allegiance of therapists is not measured directly. However, through various indirect means, such as the allegiance of the researcher and the therapist's place of training or practice, allegiance of the therapist can be inferred. In chapter 7, it will be shown that allegiance appears to have an enormously large impact on outcome, which supports the contextual model. As well, allegiance effects are shown to be sufficiently large and therefore, if not taken into account, will affect the conclusions that are made about various treatments.

Therapist Effects

Therapist effects refer to the degree to which therapists vary in the outcomes they produce, apart from the effects due to treatments. The medical model predicts that the variance due to treatments will be greater than the variance due to therapists, particularly if therapists adhere to treatment manuals. In the medical model, the emphasis is on the particular treatment and delivery of the specific ingredients, and therefore it is desired that therapists are homogeneous.

The contextual model, on the other hand, predicts that the variability due to treatments will be small compared with the variability due to therapists within treatment. It is believed that there is natural variability in the competence of therapists generally and that this general competence is critical to the outcome of therapy. The personal characteristics of the therapist and the relationship between the therapist and the client are central to the client's attempt to make sense of his or her issue and to feel empowered to change.

The difference in the models can be summed up in the following way. The medical model results in the advice, "Seek the best treatment for your condition"; for example, "For depression, cognitive–behavioral treatment is indicated; the particular therapist is relatively unimportant." On the other hand, the contextual model suggests that you "Seek a good therapist who uses an approach that makes sense to you"; for example, "See Dr. X because he or she successfully treats people who are similar to you and because you believe in his or her approach to psychotherapy."

Generally, therapist effects have been ignored in clinical trials. This may be due to the fact that clinical trials are typically conducted by medical model adherents, who are much less interested in therapist effects than in treatment effects. The relative size of therapist effects is critical to testing the validity of the medical model vis-à-vis the contextual model. In chapter 8, attempts to estimate therapist effects will be discussed and it will be shown that these effects are larger than treatment effects.

Unfortunately, ignoring therapist effects in clinical trials leads to overestimations of treatment effects. In chapter 8, the ways in which therapists, as a research factor, are handled in clinical trials, will be discussed. The consequence of ignoring therapist effects in the various experimental designs is that treatment effects are overestimated, and statistical tests of differences among treatments are too liberal. Thus, the effects due to treatments presented in chapter 4 are actually overestimations, and adjusted estimates will be derived.

EVIDENTIARY RULES

Chapters 3 through 8 present the evidence relative to the hypotheses discussed earlier and presented in Table 2.1. The remainder of this chapter discusses the rules used to accept and present this evidence. There are several reasons why care is needed in this endeavor.

Simply put, there are too many research studies to present and discuss each one. Even if this were possible, however, the corpus of studies would have a divergence of conclusions: Some studies support Premise X, whereas others do not. Should Premise X be accepted, rejected, or held in abeyance? The worst state is when advocates of Premise X cite the studies that are supportive of it and the opponents of Premise X cite the studies that refute it, causing an irreconcilable debate, each side defending the studies cited and criticizing the quality of the studies used by the other side:

> If a result of a study is contrary to prior beliefs, the strongest holders of those prior beliefs will tend to martial various criticisms of the study's methodology, come up with alternative interpretations of the results, and spark a possibly long-lasting debate. (Abelson, 1995, p. 11)

On the basis of statistical theory and hypothesis-testing conventions, the scientific community is willing to accept a 5% chance of falsely rejecting the null hypothesis. Therefore, even if a certain null hypothesis is true, 5% of studies will yield results that demonstrate otherwise. Consequently, even an impartial reviewer will face difficulty if unanimity of results is required to reach a conclusion. Moreover, making sense from a corpus of studies is complicated by such issues as power (and thus sample size), reliability and validity of measures, fidelity of treatments, selection and assignment of participants, attrition, and statistical analyses. To identify and investigate robust conclusions from a corpus of studies, researchers have developed various methods to quantitatively synthesize results. These methods, which have often been called *meta-analyses* (the term that is used throughout this book), allow a reviewer to test hypotheses on the basis of the aggregated evidence from all germane primary studies, avoiding the selective citation and subjective criticism problems that exist otherwise. The perspicuous advantages of meta-analysis, as well as the rudiments of the method, are discussed in the next section. Because of these advantages, the findings produced by meta-analyses are considered the most persuasive evidence that can be used to discriminate between the medical model and the contextual model.

As useful as meta-analyses prove to be, there is additional evidence that is also informative because either meta-analyses do not exist in an area or the evidence would profitably supplement the meta-analyses. In order of persuasiveness, the following sources of evidence are used in this book:

1. meta-analyses that bear directly on the hypothesis,
2. comprehensive studies bearing directly on the hypotheses,
3. well-conducted studies bearing directly on the hypothesis, and
4. well-conducted studies or meta-analyses bearing indirectly on the hypothesis.

The second tier of evidence includes large, well-funded, institutionally supported, multi-site comprehensive studies such as the National Institute of Mental Health Treatment of Depression Collaborative Research Program (Elkin et al., 1989), Project MATCH (Project Match Research Group, 1997), or Sloane, Staples, Cristol, Yorkston, and Whipple's (1975) early, but exemplary, comparative outcome study. These projects, as a result of the financial and institutional support, have design elements that control for various threats to validity, have large sample sizes, involve experts in the field as principle investigators and as consultants, use review boards, and are well scrutinized by the scientific community. However, even these features have not inoculated the studies' conclusions against criticism, as was evident from the reactions to the National Institute of Mental Health Treatment of Depression Collaborative Research Program (e.g, Elkin, Gibbons, Shea, & Shaw, 1996; Jacobson & Hollon, 1996a, 1996b; Klein, 1996). Nevertheless, the conclusions that can be drawn from these studies set them above studies with fewer participants and less adequate designs. Moreover, it appears that the results of these exemplary studies are consistent with meta-analyses.

There are some studies that address critical questions for which there are neither meta-analyses (nor sufficient numbers of studies on which a meta-analysis could be conducted) nor comprehensive studies. These studies, when well conducted, offer important supporting evidence. A single study cannot provide conclusive evidence because there is always the chance that the null hypothesis was falsely rejected (Type I error) or was falsely retained (Type II error); moreover, every study will have some threats to validity.

The lowest tier of evidence used herein includes well-designed studies or meta-analyses that are indirectly related to the hypotheses that discriminate between the medical and the contextual model. Because these studies cannot stand alone and because they do not address directly the hypothesis, evidence derived from these studies is necessarily tenuous. However, these studies can provide support for a particular position.

At all tiers, care will be taken to avoid selecting studies (either primary or meta-analytic) that fail to support the thesis of this book. That is, contradictory evidence is cited when it exists.

In presenting the evidence at the various tiers, cognitive–behavioral treatment of depression figures prominently for several reasons. First, the manual for cognitive–behavioral treatment of depression (Beck et al., 1979) was one of the first manuals and has resulted in standardization of this treatment. Moreover, this treatment is well accepted as being efficacious, appearing on the original list of empirically validated treatments (Task Force on Promotion and Dissemination of Psychological Procedures, 1995) and all subsequent such lists. Finally, it is safe to say that cognitive–behavioral treatment of depression is the most widely used research treatment. Consequently, many well-conducted studies of cognitive–behavioral treatment of depression directed at efficacy and specificity as well as meta-analyses have appeared in the literature. If the medical model of psychotherapy fails for this treatment, it is unlikely to be maintained for less standardized and efficacious treatments.

The following sources of evidence are not considered scientific and are avoided:

1. poorly designed studies,

2. opinions (including those of researchers, clinicians, or clients), and

3. logical arguments that are not empirically supported.

Research design and statistical methods are essential tools for making scientific inferences in the social sciences. Without appropriate knowledge of the methods used to study psychotherapy, many results must be taken on faith rather than on understanding. One of the predicates of this volume is that conclusions must be evaluated in the context of the methods (research design as well as statistics) used; appropriate design and statistical treatment of data tend to reveal truth, whereas inappropriate methods tend to obscure it. The evaluation of the validity of research in psychotherapy involves expert opinion guided by the principles of design and statistics. Throughout this volume, the evidence cited is explained in detail so that the validity of the conclusions can be deduced. However, an understanding of social science research design and statistics is needed to evaluate the presentation of evidence in this book so that the conclusions made need not be taken on faith alone. Because meta-analysis results are given evidentiary primacy and because this method is often not found in the core curriculum of training programs related to psychotherapy, a brief introduction to this topic follows.

Meta-Analysis

In this section, the rudiments of meta-analysis are explained. The reader familiar with the method as well as its advantages and caveats can move directly to chapter 3 without loss of continuity. Statistical treatments of meta-analytic methods exist and should be consulted for a comprehensive understanding of the topic (e.g., Cooper & Hedges, 1994; Hedges & Olkin, 1985; Hunter & Schmidt, 1990; Rosenthal & Rubin, 1984). Meta-analysis is a generic term used to describe a collection of methods. Because of its adoption by many meta-analysts, the methods (and much of the notation) developed by Hedges and Olkin (1985) are discussed.

Overview and Example.   Meta-analysis is a quantitative method to aggregate similar studies in order to te   st proposes a hypothesis about some rel   ., psychotherapy is more effective than   s that bear on that hypothesis, aggreg   a meta-analytic algorithm, and tests the   e described by progressing through an ex   e- fulness of meta-analysis for testing hy

Suppose that researchers are interes   a newly developed psychotherapy is effic   l- dress this question might well involve comparing the treatment with a no-treatment control group. In such an experiment, participants who met the study criteria (including some criteria that are related to the disorder, problem, or complaint for which the treatment was targeted) would be randomly assigned to two conditions, one of which receives the treatment

(treatment group) and one of which does not (e.g., a waiting-list control group). At the end of treatment, the appropriate areas of mental health or psychological functioning are assessed. The null hypothesis in such a case would be

$$\mathbf{H_0}\text{: } \boldsymbol{\mu}_T = \boldsymbol{\mu}_C .$$

That is, the population mean of those treated is equal to the population mean of those untreated (here the subscript C is used to refer to the control group, the participants of which are assumed to be selected from the population of people who do not receive the treatment). Assuming that lower scores indicate better mental health or psychological functioning (as would be the case for a scale that measures depression), the alternative hypothesis is that the treatment is superior to no treatment:

$$\mathbf{H_0}\text{: } \boldsymbol{\mu}_T < \boldsymbol{\mu}_C .$$

Now suppose that the first study conducted to test the efficacy produced a statistically significant test statistic (most likely a t statistic for independent groups) at an alpha level of .05. That is, the decision would be made to reject the null hypothesis and declare that the treatment was efficacious.[2] Two problems exist in declaring absolutely that the treatment is superior to no treatment. First, the decision to reject the null hypothesis carries with it a probability of making an incorrect decision (i.e., a Type I error), which in this experiment was set to .05. That is, there is the possibility (i.e., 5% chance), due to sampling error, that the null hypothesis is true and that the treatment is not efficacious. The second problem is that there inevitably will be flaws in the study, which could be used to invalidate the study.

Clearly, it would be helpful to replicate the study. Suppose that a second study was conducted to test the same hypothesis, using the same treatment and experimental design. Further, suppose that, in this study, the null hypothesis was not rejected, as the t statistic was insufficiently large. Now there is a quandary relative to declaring that the treatment is efficacious: For, if only a box score is kept, the game is tied one to one. There will be an inclination to look for differences between the two studies that can explain the discrepancy. For example, the samples may have been systematically different in terms of geographic region, age, or the proportion of male and female participants. Suppose that one of the apparent differences in the two studies is that the first study used many more participants, 300 in the first study compared with 20 in the second, as shown in Table 2.2. Advocates of

---

[2]Here the term *efficacious* is used to denote that the treatment produced an effect vis-à-vis the control group. In chapter 3, this term, as well as the term *effective*, is defined rigorously.

the treatment might claim that the study with 300 participants is "superior" to a study with only 20 participants, and thus, from these two studies, one should "believe" in the first study and conclude that the treatment is efficacious. A cogent counterargument might be made, however, that the study with 300 participants has the power to detect very small effects that, although reliable, have very little clinical significance.

It might be tempting to seek resolution relative to the efficacy of this treatment by examining additional studies that compared the treatment with a control group. Suppose that the extent of such studies is shown in Table 2.2. Of the eight studies, suppose that three were conducted by researchers who had allegiance to the treatment (e.g., were developers of the treatment, advocates of its use, or both). Now the picture is even more confusing, as only three of the eight studies yielded statistically significant t values, and two of those three were conducted by researchers with allegiance. However, it should be realized that the power of the t test to detect reasonably large effects is not great for samples of fewer than 50, so it is not surprising, even if there was an effect, that it should go undetected in some of the studies in Table 2.2. Even if one uses the liberal criterion that only one third of studies need to detect an effect in order to declare that an effect exists, 10 studies, each with 40 participants, will fail to meet that criterion over half the time if a true effect of medium size exists! (Hedges & Olkin, 1985, p. 50). All told, counting the number of studies that produce statistical significance is a particularly poor way to determine whether an effect exists in the population.

Effect Size.   Meta-analysis is based on the size of the effect produced by each study. A common index of effect size is the standardized difference between means, defined as

$$g = (M_T - M_C)/s \ , \tag{2.1}$$

where g is the effect size, M_T is the sample mean of the treatment group, M_C is the sample mean of the control group, and s is the standard deviation derived from pooling the standard deviations of the treatment and control group.[3] For the eight studies in Table 2.2, the value of g varied from .053 to .862. Later in this chapter, various ways to interpret the size of effects will

---

[3] Credit for developing a measure of effect size that is not dependent on the metric used in particular studies is attributed to Glass (1976), although Glass used the standard deviation of the control group rather than the pooled standard deviation, a point that is discussed further in chapter 3. The pooled estimate gives a better estimate when the variances in the two groups are homogeneous. Note that in the studies used in this example, the metric of the outcome measures were the same, but the beauty of the effect size measure is that studies using different metrics can be synthesized.

TABLE 2.2

Individual Studies Testing Whether a Treatment is Efficacious

No.	Allegiance	Treatment Group M	SD	Control Group M	SD	Sample Size	t	g	d	$\hat{\sigma}^2(d)$
1	No	14.1	6.3	15.6	5.9	300	2.13*	.246	.245	.013
2	Yes	11.1	6.2	15.6	6.4	20	1.60	.714	.684	.212
3	No	12.2	5.9	14.0	5.8	100	1.54	.308	.305	.040
4	No	12.6	6.2	15.1	7.0	70	1.58	.378	.374	.058
5	Yes	10.0	6.0	14.9	6.3	120	4.36*	.797	.791	.036
6	No	14.1	5.7	15.3	6.1	40	0.64	.203	.199	.100
7	Yes	10.0	5.9	15.0	5.7	120	4.72*	.862	.856	.036
8	No	14.6	5.5	14.9	5.9	50	0.19	.053	.052	.080

Note. For these studies, it is assumed that the sample size of the treatment group is equal to the sample size of the control group. The meta-analytic aggregate statistics are as follows: $d_+ = .421$; $\hat{\sigma}^2(d_+) = .005$; $\hat{\sigma}^2(d_+) = .071$; 95% CI for $\delta = (.282, .560)$.
*$p < .05$.

be discussed; at this point it will suffice to note that .053 is negligible, and .862 is rather large. It is important to note that effect size and statistical significance yield different conclusions. In Study 1, the effect size was quite small ($g = .246$), yet the difference between the groups was statistically significant because the sample size and hence the power to detect an effect were large. On the other hand, Study 2, which was thought to demonstrate that the treatment was not efficacious, produced a rather large effect size ($g = .714$); in this case, power to detect a true effect, should it exist, was low, as there were only 20 participants in the experiment.

The effect size index g is a sample statistic. However, the interest is in the true (i.e., population) effect size δ, which is defined as

$$\delta_i = (\mu_{T_i} - \mu_{C_i})/\sigma_i \qquad (2.2)$$

where, for study i, μ_{T_i} and μ_{C_i} are the population means for treatment group and the control group, respectively, and σ_i is the population standard deviation (assuming homogeneity of variance). Assume for the moment that the effect sizes across k studies are constant and denoted by δ (i.e., $\delta = \delta_1 = \delta_2 = \ldots = \delta_k$). The goal is to estimate population effect size δ from individual studies and from the corpus of studies.

The sample effect size g is a biased estimator of δ. A good approximation of the unbiased estimator, which will be denoted by d, is given by

$$d \cong (1 - \frac{3}{4N - 9})g , \tag{2.3}$$

where N is the total number of participants in the study (Hedges & Olkin, 1985, p. 81). As can be seen by examining Equation 2.3 or its application in Table 2.2, the bias in g is relatively small, especially for studies with at least moderate sample sizes. Many meta-analyses cited as evidence in this book fail to correct for this bias, but because the bias is small, the conclusions are not greatly affected.

The estimated variance of d is given by

$$\hat{\sigma}^2(d) = (n_T + n_C)/n_T n_C + d^2/2(n_{T + n_C}) , \tag{2.4}$$

where n_T and n_C are the sample sizes of the treatment and control group, respectively (Hedges & Olkin, 1985). Note that the variance is dependent on the sample size. The larger the sample size, the smaller the variance of the estimate of the effect size—which makes sense, as larger studies produce more precise estimates. These estimates for each study are found in the right-most column of Table 2.2.

Aggregated Effect Size as Estimate of Population Effect Size.   Although each study provides an independent estimate of the population effect size δ, a more efficient estimator can be obtained by aggregating over the eight studies. Hedges and Olkin (1985, pp. 110–111) derived an estimator of δ that is weighted by the inverse of the variances of the d_is, therefore giving more weight to studies with smaller variances. This strategy gives more weight to studies with larger sample sizes. The estimator of δ suggested by Hedges and Olkin (1985, p. 111) is given by the following:

$$d_+ = \sum_{i=1}^{k} \frac{d_i}{\hat{\sigma}^2(d_i)} / \sum_{i=1}^{k} \frac{1}{\hat{\sigma}^2(d_i)} \tag{2.5}$$

Applying this formula to the eight studies in Table 2.2 yields $d_+ = .421$. The estimate of the population effect size for this treatment, based on aggregating the effect sizes from the eight studies, is .421.

There are several questions that must be answered about this estimate. The primary question is whether this value is sufficiently large to reject the hypothesis that the population effect size is zero. More technically, the null hypothesis is

$$H_0: \delta = 0$$

This test is approached via confidence intervals. The variance of the estimate is given by the following formula (Hedges & Olkin, 1985, p. 113):

$$\hat{\sigma}^2(d_+) = \left(\sum_{i=1}^{k} \frac{1}{\hat{\sigma}^2(d_i)}\right)^{-1} \tag{2.6}$$

In the present example, $\hat{\sigma}^2(d_+) = .005$. Using the normal approximation, the 95% confidence interval has the following bounds:

$$\delta_L = d_+ - 1.96\, \hat{\sigma}(d_+) \quad \text{and} \quad \delta_U = d_+ + 1.96\, \hat{\sigma}(d_+) \tag{2.7}$$

For the continuing example,

$$\delta_L = .421 - 1.96\sqrt{.005} = .282, \quad \text{and}$$

$$\delta_U = .421 + 1.96\sqrt{.005} = .560$$

Because the 95% confidence interval does not contain zero, the null hypothesis that $\delta = 0$ is rejected at the $\alpha = .05$ level.

The conundrum relative to whether the eight studies supported the efficacy of the treatment that existed when the studies were heuristically examined is now easily settled. The null hypothesis that the population effect size is zero is rejected, and it is concluded that the treatment is efficacious. Meta-analysis has permitted the aggregation of effect sizes over several studies in order to estimate the population effect size. Notice that the variance of d_+ is quite small, and smaller than the variance of the estimate for any single study. The power of meta-analysis is that estimates at the meta-analytic level are formed essentially from combining the samples of the individual studies, yielding precise estimates.

Two critical points about the aggregation strategy used in this hypothetical meta-analysis need to be made. First, as mentioned earlier, the aggregated estimate of the population effect size was calculated by using the inverse of the variance of the individual estimates. It is statistically inefficient simply to take the arithmetic average (i.e., the mean) of the individual ds and then test the null hypothesis by using the standard deviation of the ds.

A second point it that the aggregation method (i.e., Equation 2.5) assumes that the d_is are independent. In the example, each d_i was derived from separate and presumably independent studies. Typically, however, studies in psychotherapy use multiple outcome measures, and the outcome measures within studies are not independent. Unfortunately, early meta-analysts calculated an effect size for each outcome measure within each study and meta-analyzed them as though they were independent, thereby distorting various test statistics.

Interpretation of Effect Sizes.   There are several ways to interpret an effect size. In the present example, the aggregate effect size was .421. That is, the difference between the mean of the treatment group and the mean of the control group was equal to almost one half of one standard deviation. Another way to interpret the effect size is to convert it to the proportion of variability accounted for by the treatment, a familiar statistic in the regression context. Using the relationship that

$$r^2 \cong d^2/(d^2 + 4) \ , \qquad (2.8)$$

where r is a correlation coefficient, the treatment in the present example accounts for $(.421)^2/[(.421)^2 + 4] = .042$ of the variability in outcomes (i.e., about 4%).

A third way to interpret the size of an effect is to compare them with the benchmarks set by Cohen (1988) for the social sciences. On the basis of a review of social science research, Cohen stipulated the following standards:

large effect: $d = .80$
medium effect: $d = .50$
small effect: $d = .20$

Although these designations (viz., large, medium, and small effect) are arbitrary and blind to the particular thesis being investigated, they provide a linguistic descriptor for effects. In the present example, the treatment effect size would be classified as slightly smaller than a medium effect.

A fourth way to interpret effect sizes is to examine the overlap of the control and treatment distributions. As noted by Glass (1976), the effect size is the mean of the treatment group in the control group distribution, as shown in Figure 2.1. That is, the cumulative normal distribution of the effect size represents the proportion of the control group population who are worse off than the average person in the treatment population. In the present example, the value of the standard normal cumulative distribution for $z = .421$ is .66. That is, the average person in the treatment group is better off than 66% of those who are untreated.

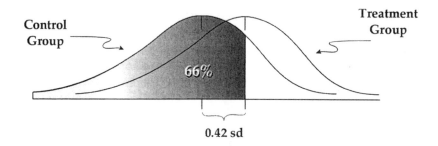

FIG. 2.1.   Overlapping treatment and control group distributions.

A final way to interpret an effect size is to calculate the success rates for people who are treated and those who are untreated. Rosenthal and Rubin (1982) suggested a "binomial effect size display," calculated as shown in Table 2.3. Such a display assumes that the overall success rate is .50 and suffers from a number of statistical problems, but nevertheless it is an interesting way to demonstrate the potency of a treatment. In the present case, the treatment would increase the success rate from 40% for those untreated to 60% for those receiving the treatment.

Table 2.4 summarizes the various ways to interpret effect sizes through the range typical of psychotherapy studies. For the most part, the effect size discussed in this book is Hedges and Olkin's (1985) d, and the reader should consult Table 2.4 for interpretive information. For example, if a d of 0.5 were obtained for a treatment–no treatment comparison, then a medium effect would have been obtained, the average treated person would have better outcomes than 70% of untreated persons, 6% of the variance in outcome would be attributed to treatment, and 62% of treated persons would have successful outcomes.

TABLE 2.3

Binomial effect size display (adapted from Rosenthal & Rubin, 1982):
Proportion of Successes and Failures as a Function of r

	Outcome	
Group	*Failure*	*Success*
Control	.50 + r/2	.50 – r/2
Treatment	.50 – r/2	.50 + r/2

TABLE 2.4

Effect Sizes With Various Interpretations

d	Cohen's Designation[a]	Proportion of Untreated Controls Less Than Mean of Treated Persons[b]	Proportion of Variability in Outcomes Due to Treatment[c]	Correlation Coefficient[d]	Success Rate of Untreated Persons[e]	Success Rate of Treated Persons[f]
.0		0.500	0.000	.000	0.500	0.500
.1		0.540	0.002	.050	0.475	0.525
.2	Small	0.579	0.010	.100	0.450	.550
.3		0.618	0.022	.148	0.426	0.574
.4		0.655	0.038	.196	0.402	0.598
.5	Medium	0.691	0.059	.243	0.379	0.621
.6		0.726	0.083	.287	0.356	0.644
.7		0.758	0.109	.330	0.335	0.665
.8	Large	0.788	0.138	.371	0.314	0.686
.9		0.816	0.168	.410	0.295	0.705
1.0		0.841	0.200	.447	0.276	0.724

[a]See Cohen (1988).

[b]See Glass (1976).

[c]$r^2 = d^2/(d^2 + 4)$; see Rosenthal (1994, p. 239), for example.

[d]$r = \sqrt{r^2}$. In this instance, r is a point-biserial correlation coefficient.

[e]Assuming overall success rate of .50, success rate of untreated persons = $0.50 - r/2$; see Rosenthal & Rubin (1982).

[f]Assuming overall success rate of .50, success rate of treated persons = $0.50 + r/2$; see Rosenthal & Rubin (1982).

Homogeneity.   One of the criticisms of meta-analysis is that aggregation occurs over studies that may be dissimilar in many different ways. Consequently, it is argued that the studies are not answering the same research question, in that they are not estimating a common population parameter. However, the issue of whether the studies are indeed similar can be answered empirically. If the set of k studies are drawn from the same population, then each study will be estimating the same population effect size δ; the effect size estimates d_i from the k studies will vary predictably because of sampling error. If there exists a common population effect size for the k studies, then the effect sizes are said to be homogenous. Homogeneity can be expressed as a null hypothesis:

$$\mathbf{H_0}: \delta_1 = \delta_2 = \ldots = \delta_k$$

The alternative hypothesis is that the studies are heterogenous (at least one δ_i differs from another).

Hedges and Olkin (1985, p. 123) provided a large sample test of homogeneity. The statistic

$$Q = \sum_{i=1}^{k} \frac{(d_i - d_+)^2}{\hat{\sigma}^2(d_i)} , \qquad (2.9)$$

which, when compared with a chi-square distribution with $k - 1$ degrees of freedom, is sufficiently large, the null hypothesis of homogeneity is rejected. Failure to reject the homogeneity hypothesis provides evidence against the claim that the meta-analysis is invalid because it combines "apples and oranges." If the homogeneity hypothesis is rejected, it makes little sense to test the hypothesis $H_0: \delta = 0$, because it would appear that there is no common δ.

For the example of the eight studies presented in Table 2.2, $Q = 14.22$, which is sufficiently large to reject the null hypothesis of a common population effect size underlying the eight studies; (the critical value at $\alpha = .05$ for $\chi^2(7)$ is 14.07. Therefore, although the aggregate effect size for the eight studies was sufficiently large to reject the null hypothesis that the population effect is zero, it is difficult to interpret in light of the heterogeneity of effect sizes. Given heterogeneity, the task is to identify categories of studies that produce different effects. That is, are there apples and oranges such that the apple studies produce larger (or smaller) effects than the oranges?

Categorical Models.   Often there are groups of studies in a meta-analysis that are thought to differ in some important way. The meta-analyst might predict that the effects for the groups differ in some predictable way. For instance, the researcher might hypothesize that (a) studies with reactive outcome measures would produce larger effects than nonreactive outcome measures, (b) better designed studies would produce larger effects than poorer designed studies, or (c) studies using experienced therapists would produce larger effects than studies using inexperienced therapists. Hedges and Olkin (1985, p. 154) derived a between-groups test based on a goodness-of-fit statistics:

$$Q_B = \sum_{i=1}^{p} \frac{(d_{i+} - d_{++})^2}{\hat{\sigma}^2(d_{i+})} \qquad (2.10)$$

where p is the number of groups, d_{i+} is the aggregate effect size estimate for group i (calculated according to Equation 2.5 for the studies in group i), $\hat{\sigma}^2(d_{i+})$ is the estimate of the variance of d_{i+} (using Equation 2.6), and d_{++} is the aggregate effect size estimate for all of the studies. The statistic Q_B is compared with a chi-square distribution with $p - 1$ degrees of freedom. If Q_B is sufficiently large, then the null hypothesis of equality of effect size among groups is rejected. This test is an omnibus test in the same way that the F test in analysis of variance (ANOVA) is used to test for differences in means among groups.

In the continuing example, suppose that it is hypothesized that the allegiance of the researcher to the treatment results in large effects. The null hypothesis is that the population effect size for studies with researcher allegiance is equal to the population effect size for studies without researcher allegiance. The following group statistics can be calculated:

Researcher Allegiance (Group 1) $d_{1+} = .813$ $\hat{\sigma}^2(d_{1+}) = .017$
No Researcher Allegiance (Group 2) $d_{2+} = .251$ $\hat{\sigma}^2(d_{1+}) = .007$

Using Equation 2.9, $Q_B = 13.17$, which, when compared with a chi-square distribution with 1 degree of freedom, is sufficiently large to reject the null hypothesis that the population effect sizes for the two types of studies are equal. Clearly, those studies for which there was allegiance to the treatment produced larger effects than the studies conducted by researchers with no allegiance.

It should be noted that meta-analysts frequently compare groups of studies by running traditional parametric tests. In this example, a t test between the allegiance and no-allegiance studies could have been conducted using the sample effect sizes as measures. However, there is no statistical justification for this test, and moreover, being able to estimate the variance of each sample effect size, the goodness-of-fit test is more powerful.

Testing Strategies and Other Strategies.   Hedges and Olkin (1985) suggested the following strategy. First, ignore categories within studies, and test for homogeneity. If the null hypothesis of homogeneity cannot be rejected or if the Q statistic is small, do not test for between-categories differences; simply estimate the population effect size by d_+, and form the confidence interval for δ (which provides a test against zero). If the homogeneity hypothesis is rejected, then partition the studies into categories in some meaningful way, preferably with a priori hypotheses. Perform tests of between-groups differences with Q_B, and test for within-category homogeneity. If within-category homogeneity exists, then d_{i+} is the estimate of the category effect size and Q_B tests between category differences. If a category is not homogeneous, then it could be partitioned further, although such partitions should be theoretically driven to the extent possible.

A number of other meta-analytic procedures exist, including aggregating correlation coefficients, testing comparisons, examining the relationship between effect sizes and continuous variables (i.e., regression models), adjusting for unreliability of measures, and testing random and fixed effects. Some of these methods have been used to aggregate psychotherapy studies and are described when these meta-analyses are presented.

Meta-Analytic Usefulness.   Through the hypothetical example of eight studies, the power and flexibility of meta-analysis has been demonstrated. Attempting to make sense from a large number of studies is difficult if not impossible and leaves open the possibility that studies can be selectively reviewed to support a particular point. Mann (1994) described a number of instances, which are presented in Table 2.5, for which conclusions made by expert reviewers were later shown conclusively by meta-analysis to be wrong. The first of these instances, psychotherapy efficacy, is the subject of chapter 3. For a more complete history of meta-analysis and its usefulness in psychology, education, medicine, and policy, see Hunt (1997).

CONCLUSIONS

In this chapter, the research to be reviewed relative to the medical model and the contextual model was outlined. Meta-analysis has been shown to be a powerful method to objectively synthesize this research, and the basics of this method were reviewed. Meta-analytic evidence as well as evidence from other exemplary studies is used in this book to test hypotheses in the following areas:

- Absolute efficacy
- Relative efficacy
- Specific effects
- General effects
- Allegiance and adherence
- Therapist effects

TABLE 2.5

Meta-Analysis Confounds the Experts

Subject	Conclusion of Expert Reviewer	Meta-Analysis
Psychotherapy	Worthless (Eysenck, 1965).	Positive results, but little differences between varying approaches (M. L. Smith and Glass, 1977).
Delinquency prevention	Programs have no consistent positive effects (National Academy of Sciences Panel on Rehabilitative Techniques, 1981).	Many programs have modest good effects; skill-oriented, nonpsychologically oriented ones may have more modest effects. Punitive schemes are counterproductive (Lipsey, in press).
School funding	Surprisingly little direct impact on educational outcome (Hanushek, 1989).	Important to educational outcome (Hedges et al. 1994).
Job Training	Effectiveness subject to bitter dispute.	Women show modest positive effects from programs that help and find work, men from basic education; current systems do not match people and programs well (Cordray and Fischer, 1994).
Reducing anxiety in surgical patients	Inconclusive, but thought to have little potential for reducing length of stay and costs (Schwartz and Mendelson, 1991).	Inexpensive 30–90 minute preparation sessions can reduce length of stay with sharp impact on costs (Devine, 1994).

Note. Reprinted with permission from "Can Meta-Analysis Make Policy?" by C. C. Mann, 1994, *Science, 266*, p. 960. Copyright © 1994 by American Association for the Advancement of Science.

3

Absolute Efficacy: The Benefits of Psychotherapy Established by Meta-Analysis

Because it is now generally accepted that psychotherapy is efficacious, many have forgotten the "tendentious and adversarial" (M. L. Smith, Glass, & Miller, 1980, p. 7) debate about the benefits of psychotherapy that cast a pallor over the psychotherapy community from the early 1950s to the middle 1980s. On the one side were those who contended that the rate of success of psychotherapy was less than or equal to the rate of "spontaneous remission." The most notable advocates of this position were Hans J. Eysenck (1952; 1954; 1961; 1966) and S. Rachman (1971; 1977), both of whom were advocates of behavior therapy (as distinct from psychotherapy) as a paragon of scientific activity. On the other side were defenders of traditional psychotherapy, such as Saul Rosenzweig (1954), Allen Bergin (1971; Bergin & Lambert, 1978), and Lester Luborsky (1954; Luborsky, Singer, & Luborsky, 1975), who contended that Eysenck's and Rachman's claims for the ineffectiveness of psychotherapy were flawed and that the evidence supported the benefits of psychotherapy. In 1977, the first meta-analysis of psychotherapy outcomes, conducted by Mary Lee Smith and Gene V Glass (Smith & Glass, 1977), was published and changed the nature of the debate dramatically. Smith and Glass found that psychotherapy was remarkably beneficial and that the contentions of the various detractors were empirically unsupportable. In spite of criticisms of this particular meta-analysis, its sequel (viz., M. L. Smith et al., 1980), and

58

meta-analysis as a method (e.g., Eysenck, 1978, 1984; Wilson & Rachman, 1983), the efficacy of psychotherapy has now been firmly established and is no longer a subject of debate. Interestingly, the estimate of the effect size produced in the early meta-analyses has turned out to be remarkably robust.

The first section of this chapter discusses briefly the research designs that are used to establish efficacy. The focus is on the inadequacy of these designs to separate specific effects from general effects. The second section summarizes the period preceding meta-analysis in which the debate about the benefits of psychotherapy were particularly intemperate. Besides providing a historical background, the problems inherent with heuristic reviews of the literature are illustrated vividly. The third section of the chapter presents the meta-analyses that have been directed toward establishing efficacy.

RESEARCH DESIGNS FOR ESTABLISHING EFFICACY

Absolute efficacy refers to the effects of treatment vis-à-vis no treatment and accordingly is best addressed by a research design where treated participants are contrasted with untreated participants. In the prototypical design to test for efficacy, participants meeting the study criteria (e.g., meeting the diagnostic criteria for depression) are randomly selected from a population and then randomly assigned to one of two groups, a treatment group and a no-treatment control group. The no-treatment group is often a waiting-list control group, as the participants are promised the treatment at the conclusion of the study (assuming that the treatment proves to be efficacious). The scores of participants who have been treated are assumed to be representative of the hypothetical population of persons who meet the study criteria (e.g., are depressed) and who receive treatment. The scores of the control group participants are assumed to be representative of the hypothetical population who meet the study criteria and who do not receive the treatment. As discussed in chapter 2, the null hypothesis in such a case would be as follows:

$$\mathbf{H_0}: \mathbf{\mu}_T = \mathbf{\mu}_C \quad ,$$

where μ_T is the mean of the population of treated persons and μ_C is the mean of the population of untreated persons. (C is used to refer to the control group, the participants in which are assumed to be selected from the population of people who do not receive the treatment.) If the null hypothesis is rejected, it is concluded that the treatment is efficacious.

This design fits the description of a randomized posttest-only control group design (for a discussion of such designs in the psychotherapy area, see Heppner, Kivlighan, & Wampold, 1999; Kazdin, 1998). In those cases in which it is advantageous to administer a pretest, the design becomes a randomized pretest–posttest control group design. Because either design (posttest-only or pretest–posttest) examines the efficacy of the treatment as a package, such designs are often referred to as *treatment package* designs (Kazdin, 1994). As well, such designs would be instances of a *clinical trial*.

The essence of the logic of a treatment package design is that the only differences between the two groups (and by inference, the two populations) is that one has received the treatment and the other has not; consequently, any obtained difference is evidence that the treatment is efficacious. It should be noted that a de facto requirement for funding and publication of treatment package studies is that the treatment be guided by a manual and that adherence to the manual be monitored.

Any experiment has threats to validity and the treatment package design is no exception (see Cook & Campbell, 1979; Heppner et al., 1999; Kazdin, 1998). One of the criticisms of treatment package designs is that the waiting-list control group provides an inadequate control because the expectation of receiving therapy in the future invalidates the assumption that this group is representative of untreated individuals. More specifically, it has been claimed that untreated individuals are likely "to seek help from friends, family members, teachers, priests, or quacks …. They discuss their problems with all sorts of people who although mostly untrained, nevertheless provide a certain amount of support" (Eysenck, 1984, p. 50); those in a waiting-list control group however, would forego such informal help. Eysenck (1984) claimed that consequently the effects of treatments are overestimated because improvements of the waiting-list control group are suppressed vis-à-vis untreated individuals, who have no promise of future treatment. Such a claim rests on the assumptions that (a) seeking support informally is decreased as a result of being on a waiting-list control group, and (b) such informal treatment is efficacious; neither of these assumptions has been verified.[1] In spite of the logical possibility of this threat to the validity of treatment package designs, this design has been labeled as the "'gold standard' for measuring whether a treatment works" (Seligman, 1995, p. 22).

It is now time to explain the distinction between two terms, *efficacy* and *effectiveness*, which are used in reference to the benefits of psychotherapy. Efficacy refers to the benefits of psychotherapy that are derived from comparisons of the treatment and a no-treatment control in the context of a well-controlled clinical trial. That is, if a treatment is found to be superior to a waiting-list control group in a treatment package design, then the treat-

---

[1] If such informal help is a significant factor in the improvement of persons with a disorder, problem, or complaint, it would provide evidence for a contextual model of psychotherapy as opposed to a medical model, a seemingly contradictory position for Eysenck, who attacked psychotherapy as being unsubstantiated scientifically.

ment is said to be efficacious. Effectiveness, on the other hand, refers to the benefits of psychotherapy that occur in the practice context—that is, how effective are the treatments administered to clients who present to therapists in the community? Many have contented that a clinical trial creates an artificial context that is not representative of how treatments are administered in the practice context, and consequently the establishment of the efficacy of psychotherapy does not ipso facto imply that the treatments are beneficial to clients (i.e., are effective). The delivery of treatments in clinical trials and in practice vary along several dimensions, including (a) the degree to which the treatment is guided by a manual; (b) the homogeneity of the clients, particularly around the typical lack of comorbidity in trials; (c) the training and supervision of the therapist; and (d) the monitoring of outcomes. In chapter 7, the data on effectiveness is reviewed as it relates to adherence to manuals.

The important issue is to realize that the evidence obtained from treatment package designs that compare a treatment with a no-treatment condition cannot discriminate between the medical model and the contextual model of psychotherapy. If a particular treatment is found to be efficacious with such designs, it is not possible to know whether the effects were due to the specific ingredients or the incidental factors of the treatment. In other words, is the efficacy composed of specific effects or general effects (or both)? Certainly, advocates of a treatment will claim that the benefits are due to the specific ingredients.

The context is now set for reviewing the evidence about the absolute efficacy of psychotherapeutic treatments. The history is presented in two parts, the period prior to meta-analytic analysis of treatment package design and the period thereafter.

HEURISTIC REVIEWS RELATIVE TO ABSOLUTE EFFICACY: INFERENTIAL CHAOS

The early history of psychotherapy was distinguished by proponents' belief that the treatments of various psychodynamic and eclectic therapies were beneficial. Because claims were "scientifically" justified by case studies and uncontrolled experiments, proponents were free to justify their existence polemically:

> Rivalry among theoretical orientations has a long and undistinguished history in psychotherapy, dating back to Freud. In the infancy of the field, therapy systems, like battling siblings, competed for attention and affection in a "dogma eat dogma" environment.... Mutual antipathy and exchange of puerile insults between adherents of rival orientations were much the order of the day. (Norcross & Newman, 1992, p. 3)

Clearly, research was needed to examine the efficacy of psychotherapy so that claims could be made based on empirical evidence rather than the quality of one's rhetoric. In 1952, Eysenck sought to provide the evidence.

Eysenck (1952): The First Attempt to Review Literature to Examine Efficacy

In 1952, Eysenck sought to "examine the evidence relating to the actual effects of psychotherapy, in an attempt to seek clarification on a point of fact" (p. 319) by reviewing 24 studies of psychodynamic and eclectic psychotherapy. Unfortunately, these studies did not use a control group. Realizing that "in order to evaluate the effectiveness of any form of therapy, data from a control group of nontreated patients would be required" (p. 319), he used the spontaneous remission rate derived from two other sources, one of severe neurotics in state mental hospitals who received "in the main custodial care, and very little if any psychotherapy" (p. 319), and one based on psychoneurotic disability claimants treated by general practitioners. That is, the recovery rates derived from 24 studies were compared with the recovery rates derived from two separate sources. Eysenck made the following conclusion:

> Patients treated by means of psychoanalysis improve to the extent of 44 percent; patients treated eclectically improve to the extent of 64 percent; patients treated only custodially or by general practitioners improve to the extent of 72 percent. There thus appears to be an inverse correlation between recovery and psychotherapy; the more psychotherapy, the smaller the recovery rate.... [The data] fail to prove that psychotherapy, Freudian or otherwise, facilitates the recovery of neurotic patients. (Eysenck, 1952, p. 322)

Eysenck's findings were damning. This comprehensive and purportedly objective review of the literature had shown that psychotherapy was not effective and might even be harmful! The conclusions, which were widely cited and reported in the press, were challenged by proponents of psychotherapy (e.g., Bergin, 1971; Bergin & Lambert, 1978; Luborsky, 1954; Rosenzweig, 1954). Although there were many problems with Eysenck's method, the most conspicuous and dangerous one was that participants were not randomly assigned to the treatment and control groups (i.e., to the 24 treatment groups and the 2 control groups), creating unknown differences between the treatment and the controls other than the presence or absence of treatment. Luborsky (1954) commented on this threat to validity:

> I do not believe Eysenck has an adequate control group nor that comparisons of groups can be made within the experimental group.... To conclude as he does, Eysenck must assume patients do something they do not do: randomly self-select themselves to psychiatrists, general practitioners, and state hospitals. (p. 129).

Clearly, trying to compare clients from one study with clients from another study creates confounds of unknown magnitude. As discussed later, the determination of relative efficacy (see chap. 4) suffers from similar attempts to make cross-study comparisons.

Eysenck's (1952) attempt to objectively examine the efficacy of psychotherapy by reviewing the literature opened the door to several additional attempts to review the literature in order to prove one's point, as discussed in the next section.

Eysenck's Sequels and Other Attempts to Prove a Point

Eysenck, emboldened by his "success" in proving the failure of psychotherapy, published two additional reviews that attempted to demonstrate the inadequacy of psychodynamic and eclectic psychotherapy and to establish the efficacy of behavior therapy (Eysenck, 1961; Eysenck, 1966). Rachman (1971) followed suit. Not to be deterred, the proponents of psychotherapy published their own reviews (Bergin, 1971; Luborsky et al., 1975; Meltzoff & Kornreich, 1970). Needless to say, the two sides came to very different conclusions: Eysenck and Rachman concluded that psychodynamic and eclectic psychotherapy were not efficacious, whereas Bergin, Metzoff and Kornreich, and Luborsky concluded otherwise.

How is it that these two sets of reviewers, having available essentially the same set of studies to review, can come to such different conclusions? The answer to this question reveals the inadequacies of heuristic reviews, which rely on subjective criteria for inclusion and non-meta-analytic methods for aggregation. The problems incurred by the two sides of this debate were discussed by M. L. Smith et al. (1980) and partially revealed in a table they developed that summarized the controlled studies that were included in the reviews mentioned in this section (and which is shown in Table 3.1 herein).

Several points related to the studies listed in Table 3.1 need to be made. First, the table only summarizes the controlled studies (i.e., psychotherapy vs. control) that were reviewed. Comparisons with nonequivalent control groups persisted, with Eysenck (1961) sticking to a spontaneous remission rate of about two thirds, whereas Bergin (1971) determined the rate to be about one third, a figure that makes the benefits of psychotherapy more apparent. However, in either case, the comparisons are flawed because treatment and control participants were not comparable. The remaining comments are restricted to the reviews of controlled studies.

The second point is that determining the effects of psychotherapy by counting the number of studies that are statistically significant is problematic, as was illustrated in chapter 2. Bergin (1971), for example, found that 37% of the controlled studies showed a positive result and concluded that "it now seems apparent that psychotherapy, as practiced over the past 40

TABLE 3.1

Summary of Controlled Studies in Major Pre-Meta-Analytic Reviews

| Reviewer | Date | Number of Studies (% of Total) | | | | |
		Positive	Null[a]	"Mixed" or "In doubt"	Impeached	Total
Eysenck	1961	0	3 (75%)	0	1[b]	4
Eysenck	1966	0	7 (87%)	0	1[b]	8
Bergin	1971	22	15 (25%)	23[c]	0	60
Rachman	1971	1	5[d] (22%)	0	17[e]	23
Meltzoff & Kronreich	1970	81	20 (20%)	0	0	101
Luborsky, Singer, & Luborsky	1975	7	2 (22%)	0	0[f]	9[g]

Note.   Smith, Mary Lee, Gene V Glass, and Thomas I. Miller. *The Benefits of Psychotherapy.* Table 2.1 © 1980. The Johns Hopkins University Press. Adapted with permission.

[a]Includes studies in which treated groups did not significantly differ from controls, in which controls were superior, in which treated groups did not exceed baseline.

[b]Disallowed because of methodology (positive results).

[c]Fifteen studies were "in doubt," and 8 were not included in table for unknown reasons (mixed results).

[d]Treatments for children, psychotics, and behavioral treatments are excluded from this table.

[e]Seventeen studies were impeached (15 positive and 2 null results).

[f]Number impeached is unknown because of method of reporting and excluding studies on the basis of low design quality.

[g]Behavioral treatments and treatments on psychotics are excluded from summary table.

years, has had an average effect that is modestly positive" (p. 263). What is a modest effect? Heuristic reviews lead to ambiguity, and thus reviewers have great latitude in assigning verbal descriptions to the results.

The third and most important point is that the reviewers used different sets of studies on which to make their conclusions. For the most part, the reviewers did not indicate how studies were culled from the literature. Moreover, reviewers applied rules, often in inconsistent ways, to remove studies from their database due to flaws in design. In 1970, Meltzoff and Kornreich reviewed 101 studies, classifying studies as having either "adequate" or "questionable" designs (both designs are included in Table 3.1). No studies were "impeached"—that is, excluded—because of flaws in design. On the other hand, Rachman (1971), publishing at nearly the same time, reviewed only 23 studies, 17 of which were impeached. Interestingly, of the 17 studies impeached, 15 showed positive results! The judgments made by Rachman seem to be biased or, at least, arbitrary.[2] For example, studies were impeached because of inconsistent effects of dependent measures (three measures showed positive outcomes whereas one did not[3]), failure of positive results at termination to be maintained at follow-up, use of unpublished tests, and graphical presentation of the results.

The reviews of the controlled studies presented in Table 3.1 present a tremendous dilemma for the scientific understanding of psychotherapy. Having available the same corpus of research studies, prominent researchers reached dramatically different conclusions. Moreover, the conclusions were consistent with the reviewers' preconceived positions—evidence at the service of a point of view rather than at the service of science. The reviews discussed lacked (a) systematic selection of studies from the literature, (b) objective and empirically based criteria for inclusion, and (c) statistically justified means to aggregate the results of the studies. Thus, the reviews could be called heuristic. The pre-meta-analytic reviews of the efficacy of psychotherapy demonstrate the inconsistencies that characterize heuristic reviews.

In 1977, meta-analysis came to the rescue of psychotherapy, as is shown in the next section.

META-ANALYSES OF TREATMENT PACKAGE DESIGNS: ORDER FROM CHAOS

In the period following the heuristic reviews of psychotherapy research, Eysenck's indictment of psychotherapy cast a pallor over the field:

> Most academics [had] read little more than Eysenck's (1952, 1966) tendentious diatribes in which he claimed to prove that 75% of neurotics got better regardless of whether or not they were in therapy—a conclusion based on the interpretation of six controlled studies. The perception that research shows the inefficacy of psychotherapy has become part of the conventional wisdom even within the profession. (M. L. Smith & Glass, 1977, p. 752)

In 1977, M. L. Smith and Glass attempted to settle the efficacy issue using meta-analysis.

---

[2]Moreover, the criteria used by Rachman to impeach studies were different for psychotherapy and for behavior therapy, creating a further bias (see M. L. Smith, Glass, & Miller, 1980, chap. 2).

[3]Meta-analytic strategies for multiple dependent measures are discussed later in this chapter and in chapter 4.

M. L. Smith and Glass (1977) and M. L. Smith et al. (1980)

The goal of Smith and Glass's (1977) meta-analysis was to aggregate the results of all studies that compared psychotherapy and counseling with a control group or with a different therapy group in order to quantitatively estimate the size of the psychotherapy effect. They used various well-described search strategies to locate 375 published and unpublished studies (i.e., dissertations or presentations). No studies were excluded because of design flaws, but design characteristics, as well as many other features of the studies, were coded so that the relation between these features and effect size could be investigated.

For each dependent variable in each study, a sample effect size was calculated, using the following formula:

$$ES = (M_T - M_C)/s_C$$

where ES is the sample effect size, M_T is the mean of the dependent variable for the treatment group, M_C is the mean of the dependent variable for the control group, and s_C is the standard deviation of the control group. This statistic is similar to g defined in chapter 2, except that the denominator of the statistic used by M. L. Smith and Glass (1977) was the standard deviation of the control group rather than the pooled standard deviation (see Glass, 1976; cf Hedges & Olkin, 1985). Under the assumption of homogeneity of variance, the statistic used by Smith and Glass is less efficient than those currently used. As the statistical theory for meta-analysis of effect size measures was in its infancy, aggregation methods used by Smith and Glass consisted simply of taking the arithmetic average of the ES measures to obtain an aggregate effect size.

The findings were clear-cut. The 375 studies produced 833 effect size measures (more than 2 per study), and yielded an average effect size of .68. Interpretation of this effect can be made by consulting Table 2.4. This effect would (a) be classified as between a medium and large effect in the social sciences, (b) mean that the average client receiving therapy would be better off than 75% of untreated clients, (c) indicate that treatment accounts for about 10% of the variance in outcomes, and (d) translate into a success rate of 34% for the control group compared with success rate of 66% for the treatment group. Smith and Glass made a simple but astoundingly important conclusion: "The results of research demonstrate the beneficial effects of counseling and psychotherapy" (p. 760). If this result were to stand up to various challenges, then it would show rather convincingly that the critics of psychotherapy were wrong.

In 1980, M. L. Smith et al. published a sequel to M. L. Smith and Glass (1977), with an expanded set of studies and a more sophisticated analysis.

An extensive search was made in order to find all published and unpublished controlled studies of counseling psychotherapy through 1977. In all, 475 studies were found, which produced 1766 effect sizes, calculated in the same manner as by Smith and Glass. The arithmetic average of the effect sizes was .85, larger than that found previously. An effect size of .85 is a large effect in the social sciences, and means that the average client receiving therapy would be better off than 80% of untreated clients, that the treatment accounts for over 15% of the variance in outcomes, and that the success rate would change from 30% for the control group to 70% for the treatment group (see Table 2.4).

It should be noted that there were many other findings in M. L. Smith and Glass's (1977) and M. L. Smith et al.'s (1980) meta-analyses, but discussion of those conclusions is presented as they relate to the various hypotheses tested in this volume.

Challenges to the Early Meta-Analyses

Not surprisingly, those who had sought to demonstrate that psychotherapy was not beneficial (e.g., Eysenck and Rachman) criticized the results of these meta-analyses (and subsequent meta-analyses) as well as meta-analysis in general (Eysenck, 1978, 1984; Rachman & Wilson, 1980; Wilson, 1982; Wilson & Rachman, 1983). These criticisms are briefly reviewed herein.

One criticism is that meta-analysis aggregates studies that vary in quality, giving weight to poorly conceived studies and misleading results. Of course, as demonstrated in the heuristic reviews, the alternative is to have reviewers exclude studies that, in their judgment, are flawed; but this process leads to a systematic impeachment of studies that do not support preconceived positions. The strategy used by M. L. Smith and Glass (1977; M. L. Smith et al., 1980) was to include all controlled studies regardless of quality, objectively rate the quality of the studies (i.e., with specific criteria and multiple raters), and see whether quality was related to outcome. Not all the results are discussed herein, but, for example, consider internal validity of the study. The effect sizes for studies with low, medium, and high internal validity were .78, .78, and .88, respectively. Although the difference between the best designed studies (viz., high internal validity) and the poorer designed studies (viz., low and medium internal validity) was small (viz., .10), the conclusion was that the better designed studies produced larger effects and, consequently, excluding poorer studies would have increased the aggregate effect size, exactly opposite to what was contented by the critics! Essentially, the meta-analyst treats quality of the research design as an empirical question that can be answered with the analysis. Of course, if all studies are poor, the results of a meta-analysis may be bogus, but then again so would the results of any other attempt to make sense of the studies.

Another criticism of meta-analysis is that it is atheoretical, creating simply a fact or facts that accumulate without form or structure. The truth is that meta-analysis can be used in a theoretically driven way to discover truth as well as can a primary study. Certainly, primary studies and meta-analyses can be used atheoretically—for example, to determine whether Treatment A is efficacious. On the other hand, meta-analyses can be addressed to establish the veracity of two competing theories, such as the way that analyses are used in this volume.

A third criticism is that meta-analyses aggregate "apples and oranges," a point addressed in chapter 2. For example, the meta-analyses discussed herein lump together a wide variety of approaches to psychotherapy, and therefore the conclusion is a gross one. Unfortunately, when these early meta-analyses were conducted, tests of homogeneity of effect sizes had not been developed and therefore were not used to see whether "one size fits all." However, M. L. Smith and Glass (1977; M. L. Smith, Glass, & Miller, 1980) did segregate studies by treatment to determine whether effect sizes differed by treatment; the results of this analysis are discussed in the context of relative efficacy (chap. 4). Although various apples-and-oranges arguments have been leveled against various meta-analyses, the veracity of the criticism could be empirically tested by conducting a between-groups test of the apples and the oranges. That is, are the effects produced by apples different from the effects produced by oranges?

A final criticism leveled at meta-analysis is around the criteria used for various ratings (e.g., of internal validity) and the criteria used for including or excluding studies. Eysenck (1984) and Rachman and Wilson (1980) contended that the conclusions of M. L. Smith et al.'s (1980) meta-analysis were flawed because important behavioral studies were omitted. The meta-analytic response is that critics are invited to define inclusion and exclusion criteria differently and see whether the conclusions are altered.

Clearly, the meta-analytic response to most criticisms is that issues can and should be addressed empirically. One cannot help but think that most of the criticism of meta-analysis was generated by a distaste for the results. For the most part, the critics were reluctant to empirically test their alternative hypotheses. However, two meta-analyses reanalyzed M. L. Smith and Glass's (1977) and the M. L. Smith et al. (1980) data in order to challenge some of the conclusions (Andrews & Harvey, 1981; Landman & Dawes, 1982). These challenges are considered next.

M. L. Smith and Glass's (1977) and M. L. Smith et al.'s (1980) Results Stand up Under Scrutiny

A frequent criticism of M. L. Smith and Glass's (1977; M. L. Smith et al.) meta-analyses was that many of the studies analyzed involved clients who were not clinically distressed and were not seeking treatment for some disorder, problem, or complaint. Indeed, only 46% of the studies analyzed by Smith, Glass, and Miller involved "patients with neuroses, true phobias, depressions, and emotional-somatic disorders—the type of patients who usually seek psychotherapy" and only 22% "concerned patients who had entered treatment themselves or by referral" (Andrews & Harvey, 1981, p. 1204). This is an apples-and-oranges argument. It contends that the effects produced by studies with clinically representative samples would be different from the effects produced by the nonclinically representative studies.

Andrews and Harvey (1981) addressed this criticism by analyzing the 81 studies from M. L. Smith et al.'s (1980) meta-analysis that involved clinically distressed participants who had sought treatment for their disorder, problem, or complaint. The average of the 292 effects produced by the 81 studies was .72, an effect size similarly produced by the two original meta-analyses, demonstrating that psychotherapy was beneficial to clinically distressed clients who sought treatment.

Landman and Dawes (1982) sought to address additional issues in M. L. Smith and Glass's (1977) meta-analysis. One of the criticisms discussed earlier was related to the quality of the studies reviewed, and Landman and Dawes addressed this criticism by analyzing only "studies of uniformly high methodological quality" (p. 507). Another problem alluded to in chapter 2 is related to independence of observations. Smith and Glass created dependent observations in many ways, but primarily by using multiple effect size measures derived from the multiple dependent measures in each study. Generally, dependent observations violate the assumptions of statistical tests, creating invalid conclusions. Whereas other violations of assumptions may have little effect on conclusions, nonindependence can have drastic effects, as is shown in chapter 8 when therapist effects are discussed.

Landman and Dawes (1982) examined 65 studies randomly selected from the studies in M. L. Smith and Glass (1977) as well as 93 additional ones, from which the two authors independently agreed that 42 contained a no-treatment control group and met the methodological rigor required for inclusion. Additionally, the study was used as the unit of analysis, rather than the individual outcome measure, eliminating dependent observations. On the bases of these 42 studies, the average effect size was found to be .90, considerably larger than Smith and Glass's initial estimate of .68, which was reflected in the subtitle of Landman and Dawes's article: "Smith and Glass' Conclusions Stand Up Under Scrutiny."

The impact of Smith and Glass's meta-analyses should not be underestimated. Until 1977, controversy reigned when it came to the issue of the benefits of psychotherapy. Many professionals as well as the lay public were lead to believe that psychotherapy was worthless. Although M. L. Smith and Glass's (1977) initial conclusion lead to much criticism, it was heralded in the popular press under the headline "Consensus Is Reached: Psycho-therapy Works" (Adams, 1979). Having withstood the challenges of the Andrews and Harvey (1981) and Landman and Dawes (1981) meta-analyses, the benefits of psychotherapy became accepted. Moreover, the meta-analysis method pioneered by Glass (1976) and used in the initial psychotherapy meta-analyses has been used in thousands of studies in education, psychology, and medicine (Hunt, 1997).

In the next section, the additional meta-analyses related to the efficacy of psychotherapy are summarized.

PRESENT STATUS OF THE ABSOLUTE EFFICACY OF PSYCHOTHERAPY

By 1993, there were more than 40 meta-analyses of psychotherapy in general or of particular psychotherapies for particular problems (Lipsey & Wilson, 1993). Generally, these meta-analyses showed that the treatment being studied was efficacious. Rather than review all of the meta-analyses, the reviews of meta-analyses are summarized.

In 1993, Lipsey and Wilson (1993) reviewed all meta-analyses related to the efficacy of psychological, educational, and behavioral treatments. Although they did not provide an aggregate effect size for psychotherapy, the effect sizes for meta-analyses for adults that compared treatments with no-treatment controls can be extracted from their tabular results (Lipsey & Wilson, 1993, p. 1183, Table 1, section 1.1). The mean effect size for these 13 meta-analyses was .81.

In 1994, Lambert and Bergin again reviewed all meta-analyses addressing the efficacy issue. After reviewing over 25 meta-analyses, they concluded that "the average effect associated with psychological treatment approaches one standard deviation unit" (i.e, an effect size of 1.00; Lambert & Bergin, 1994, p. 147). Using only studies that also contained a placebo group, Lambert and Bergin calculated an average effect size of .82 for psychotherapy versus no-treatment (see Lambert & Bergin, 1994, p. 150, Table 5.5).

In 1996, Grissom reviewed 68 meta-analyses that aggregated results from studies comparing psychotherapies with no-treatment controls. He used a *mean probability of superiority* measure to meta-meta-analyze the 68 meta-analyses. Converting to the more familiar effect size measure, Grissom found an aggregate effect size of .75 for the efficacy of psychotherapy.

From the various meta-analyses conducted over the years, the effect size related to absolute efficacy appears to fall within the range .75 to .85. A reasonable and defensible point estimate for the efficacy of psychotherapy would be .80, a value used in this book. This effect would be classified as a large effect in the social sciences, which means that the average client receiving therapy would be better off than 79% of untreated clients, that psychotherapy accounts for about 14% of the variance in outcomes, and that the success rate would change from 31% for the control group to 69% for the treatment group. Simply stated, *psychotherapy is remarkably efficacious*.

CONCLUSIONS

Absolute efficacy does not support either the contextual model or the medical model, but it does provide evidence that psychotherapy is efficacious and worth studying further. About 25 years ago, there was much controversy about whether psychotherapy produced outcomes that were better than the rate of spontaneous remission. Before the use of meta-analysis, opponents and advocates of psychotherapy were able to review and find support for their respective positions. Although the first meta-analyses were controversial, the results of the original and subsequent meta-analyses have converged on the conclusion that psychotherapy is remarkably efficacious. The history of the investigations of psychotherapy efficacy establishes meta-analysis as an objective and useful way to aggregate studies addressing the same hypothesis.

Having established the efficacy of psychotherapy, the focus now turns to whether the various psychotherapies are equally efficacious. Besides having immense practical importance, relative efficacy provides critical evidence relative to the contextual model versus the medical model debate.

4

Relative Efficacy: The Dodo Bird Was Smarter Than We Have Been Led to Believe

In 1936, Rosenzweig suggested that common factors were responsible for the apparent efficacy of existing psychotherapies. The logical inference was that psychological treatments that contained the common factors would produce beneficial outcomes, and consequently all psychotherapies would be roughly equivalent in terms of their benefits. The uniform efficacy of psychotherapies was emphasized in the subtitle of Rosenzweig's article by reference to the Dodo bird's conclusion at the end of a race in *Alice in Wonderland*: "At last the Dodo said, 'Everybody has won, and all must have prizes'" (Rosenzweig, 1936, p. 412). Since that time, uniform efficacy, which has been referred to as the Dodo bird effect, has been considered empirical support for those who believe that common factors are the efficacious aspect of psychotherapy. On the other hand, advocates of particular therapeutic approaches believe that some treatments (viz., those that they advocate) are more efficacious than others.

In this chapter, the evidence related to the relative efficacy of various psychotherapies will be explored. First, predictions of the contextual model and the medical model will be discussed. Then, research design considerations for determining relative efficacy will be presented. Finally, the empirical evidence, which is predominated by meta-analyses, will be reviewed.

MEDICAL AND CONTEXTUAL MODEL PREDICTIONS

The predictions of the medical model and contextual model relative to the uniformity of psychotherapy efficacy are straightforward. There are two possible results. The first is that treatments vary in their efficacy. That is, some treatments will be found to be immensely efficacious, some moderately efficacious, and some not efficacious at all. Presumably, the relative differences in outcomes are due to the specific ingredients of some treatments that are more potent than the specific ingredients of other treatments. Thus, variability in outcomes for various treatments provides evidence for the medical model of psychotherapy.

A second possible pattern of outcomes is that all treatments produce about the same outcome. If the factors that are both incidental to the treatments and common to all therapies were responsible for the efficacy of psychotherapy, rather than specific ingredients, then the particular treatment delivered would be irrelevant, and all treatments would produce equivalent outcomes. Of course, it could be argued that specific ingredients are indeed the causally important components, but that all specific ingredients are equally potent—a logically permissible hypothesis but one that seems implausible.

It is worth reiterating the differential hypothesis here. Important evidence relative to the medical–contextual model issue is produced by data about the relative efficacy of the various treatments that exist. If specific ingredients are responsible for outcomes, variation in efficacy of treatments is expected, whereas if the incidental aspects are responsible, homogeneity of effects (i.e., general equivalence of treatments) is expected.

RESEARCH METHODS FOR ESTABLISHING RELATIVE EFFICACY

Relative efficacy is typically investigated by comparing the outcomes of two treatments. However, there are inferential limitations of such designs. Many of the limitations can be addressed by meta-analytically aggregating the results of primary studies. In this section, research strategies for studying relative efficacy in primary and meta-analytic contexts will be presented.

Research Strategies for Studying Relative Efficacy at the Primary Study Level

The fundamental design for establishing relative efficacy is the comparative outcome strategy (Kazdin, 1994). In the comparative design, participants are randomly assigned to Treatments A and B, the treatments are delivered, and posttests are administered, rendering a design identical to the control-group design except that two treatments are administered (rather than one treatment and a control group). Comparative designs typically contain a control group as well so that it can be determined whether each of the treatments is superior to no treatment. However, the control group is not needed to answer the question, "Is Treatment A superior (or inferior) to Treatment B?"

There are two possible outcomes of comparative designs, both of which involve ambiguity of interpretation (see Wampold, 1997). One possible outcome is that the means of the outcome variables for the two treatments are not significantly different. Given the pervasive evidence for efficacy presented in chapter 3, assume that both treatments were superior to a no-treatment control group. Thus, as administered and assessed, the two treatments appear to be equally efficacious. However, there is ambiguity around interpretation of this result. Clearly, this result could be interpreted as support for the contextual model as both treatments presumably are intended to be therapeutic and conform to the conditions of the contextual model. However, it is difficult to rule out the possibility that the efficacy was due to the specific ingredients of the two treatments, where the specific ingredients have approximately equal potency. Moreover, it may be that one set of specific ingredients is more potent than the other, but that the statistical power to detect this difference was low, given that the effect is smaller than the treatment versus no-treatment effect (Kazdin & Bass, 1989).

It would appear that a less ambiguous conclusion could be reached by the second possible outcome of a comparative design, namely that the study yielded a superior outcome for one of the treatments compared. Presumably, if Treatment A was found to be superior to Treatment B, then the specific ingredients constituting Treatment A are active—that is, these ingredients were responsible for the superiority of Treatment A. However, an example of such a finding will demonstrate that ambiguity remains even when superiority of one treatment is found.

Snyder and Wills (1989) compared the efficacy of behavioral marital therapy (BMT) with the efficacy of insight-oriented marital therapy (IOMT). At posttest and 6-month follow-up, it was found that both BMT and IOMT were superior to no-treatment controls but equivalent to each other. The authors recognized that the finding could not disentangle the common factor–specific ingredient explanations: "Although treatments in the present study were relatively uncontaminated from interventions specific to the alternative approach, each treatment used nonspecific interventions common to both" (p. 45). Four years after termination of treatment, an important difference between the treatments was found: 38% of the BMT couples were divorced whereas only 3% of the IOMT were divorced (Snyder, Wills, & Grady-Fletcher, 1991). This result would seem to provide evidence for the specific ingredients of IOMT, but Jacobson (1991), a proponent of BMT, argued otherwise:

It seems obvious that the IOMT therapists were relying heavily on the nonspecific clinically sensitive interventions allowed in the IOMT manual but not mentioned in the BMT manual.... To me, the ... data suggest that *in this study* BMT was practiced with insufficient attention to nonspecifics. (p. 143)

Jacobson argued that the playing field was not level because there was an inequivalence in the potency of the aspects of treatment that were incidental to BMT and IOMT.

There is another problem with interpretations of statistically significant differences between the outcomes of two treatments. As discussed in chapter 2, statistical theory predicts that by chance some comparisons of treatments will produce statistically significant differences when there are no true differences (i.e., Type I errors). Although some comparative studies have produced differences between treatments (e.g., Butler, Fennell, Robson, & Gelder, 1991; Snyder et al., 1991), it may well be that these studies represent the few that would occur by chance. This problem is exacerbated by the fact that differences are often found only for a few of the dependent variables in a study (e.g., one variable, divorce rate, in Snyder et al.'s 1991 study).

The comparative treatment design is a valid experimental design to determine relative efficacy. Nevertheless, as is the case with any design, there are difficulties in making interpretations from a single comparative study, whether the results produce statistically significant differences or not. As was discussed theoretically in chapter 2 and illustrated in chapter 3, meta-analysis can address many of the issues raised by primary studies and can be used to estimate robustly an effect size for relative efficacy. Attention is now turned to the various meta-analytic strategies for determining relative efficacy.

Meta-Analytic Methods for Determining Relative Efficacy

Meta-analyses can be used to examine the relative efficacy of treatments over many studies, thus testing the hypothesis that treatments are uniformly effective versus the alternative that they vary in effectiveness. Meta-analysis provides a quantitative test of the hypotheses and avoids conclusions based on salient, but unrepresentative, studies. Persons and Silberschatz (1998) cited a number of studies that have shown the superiority of one treatment over another, but as discussed earlier, each of these studies may be flawed (e.g., due to allegiance) or contain Type I errors. In addition, studies that failed to show differences were not cited by Persons and Silberschatz (1998), leaving the questions about relative efficacy over the corpus of studies unanswered. Moreover, meta-analysis provides a quantitative index of the size of the effect that may be due to relative efficacy—if treatments are not equivalent in their effectiveness, then how different are they? Finally, meta-analysis can examine other hypotheses about relative effectiveness that cannot be answered easily by primary studies.

There are two primary meta-analytic means to examine relative efficacy. The first method reviews treatment package designs using no-treatment control-groups. According to this method, (a) treatments examined in studies are classified into categories (e.g., cognitive–behavioral therapy, or CBT, and systematic desensitization), (b) the effect size is computed for each treatment vis-à-vis the no-treatment control group, (c) the effect sizes within a category are averaged (e.g., the mean effect size for CBT is calculated across the studies that contain CBT and a no-treatment control group), and (d) the mean effect sizes for the categories are compared (e.g., CBT vs. systematic desensitization).

There is a fundamental flaw in making inferences based on the meta-analysis of no-treatment control group designs. The studies of treatments in a given category differ from the studies of treatments in other categories. For example, studies that compare CBT with a no-treatment control group and systematic desensitization with a no-treatment control group may differ on a number of dimensions other than treatment, such as outcome variables used, severity of disorder treated, presence of comorbidity of participants, treatment standardization, treatment length, and allegiance of the researcher.

One way to deal with the confounding variables is to meta-analytically model their mediating and moderating effects. Shadish and Sweeney (1991) for example, found that setting, measurement reactivity, measurement specificity, measurement manipulability, and number of participants moderated the relationship of treatment and effect size and that treatment standardization, treatment implementation, and behavioral dependent variables mediated the relationship of treatment and effect size. Modeling meta-analytic confounds post hoc is extremely difficult, with the same problems encountered in primary research, such as leaving out important variables, misspecification of models, unreliability of measurements, and lack of statistical power.

A second way to test relative efficacy meta-analytically is to review studies that directly compared two psychotherapies. For example, if one were interested in the relative efficacy of CBT and systematic desensitization, only those studies that directly compared these two treatments would be examined. This strategy avoids confounds due to aspects of the dependent variable, problem treated, setting, and the length of therapy, as these factors would be identical for each direct comparison (e.g., every direct comparison of CBT and systematic desensitization would use the same outcome measures). Shadish et al. (1993) noted that direct comparisons "have rarely been reported in past meta-analyses, and their value for controlling confounds seems to be underappreciated" (p. 998). It should be noted that some confounds, such as skill of therapist and allegiance remain in the direct comparison strategy. If therapist skill or allegiance are not well controlled in the primary study, then meta-analysis of such studies will similarly be confounded, although these confounds can be modeled, as discussed later in this chapter. There are a number of meta-analyses of direct comparisons in the area of psychotherapy outcome, some of which control or model remaining confounds.

Meta-analysis of direct comparisons of treatments raises an issue that must be resolved. In order to properly test the contextual model hypothesis, it is important that the treatments compared are instances of psychotherapy, as stipulated by the contextual model. That is, (a) both treatments would need to appear to the participants to be efficacious; (b) the therapists would have to have confidence in the treatment and believe, to some extent, that the treatment is legitimate; (c) the treatment would have to be delivered in a manner consistent with the rationale provided; (d) the participants would have to perceive the rationale as sensible; and (e) the treatment would have to be delivered in a healing context. Studies often include treatments that are not intended to be therapeutic and that, to any reasonably well-trained psychologist, would not be legitimate. Such treatments are often called "alternative" treatments or placebo controls (see chap. 5).

An example of a treatment that would not be intended to be therapeutic (and hence would not meet contextual model test) was used by Foa, Rothbaum, Riggs, and Murdock (1991) to establish empirical support for cognitive–behavioral treatments. The comparison treatment was supportive counseling for post-traumatic stress in women who had recently (within the previous year) been raped. In the supportive counseling treatment (a) clients were taught a general problem-solving technique, (b) therapists responded indirectly and were unconditionally supportive, and (c) clients "were immediately redirected to focus on current daily problems if discussions of the assault occurred" (Foa et al., 1991, p. 718). This counseling would not be seen as viable by therapists, in all likelihood, because it contains no particular theoretical rationale or established principles of change, and in the absence of other components, "few would accept deflecting women from discussing their recent rape in counseling as therapeutic" (Wampold, Mondin, Moody, & Ahn, 1997a, p. 227). Clearly, the supportive counseling treatment was not intended to be therapeutic, and therapists would not deliver the treatment with a sufficient sense of efficacy. To provide a fair test of the competing medical and contextual models, the comparisons of treatments must involve treatments that are intended to be therapeutic.

In the next section, the evidence bearing on the question of relative efficacy is reviewed. Additional problems with these analyses are noted, where appropriate.

EVIDENCE RELATED TO RELATIVE EFFICACY

Pre-Meta-Analytic Reviews and Studies—Chaos Revisited

As has been mentioned several times, Rosenzweig (1936) commented on the general equivalence of the various psychotherapeutic approaches, although, at the time, psychotherapy was predominantly psychodynamic. When behavior therapy came into existence, there was a concerted effort by advocates of this approach to show its superiority relative to "psychotherapy." In 1961, when Eysenck reviewed studies on the efficacy of psychotherapy, he also addressed the relative efficacy issue. In chapter 3, it was noted that he came to the conclusion that there was no evidence to support the efficacy of psychotherapy. However, on the basis of uncontrolled studies by Wolpe (1952a; 1952b; 1954; 1958), Phillips (1957), and Ellis (1957), Eysenck concluded that "neurotic patients treated by means of psychotherapeutic procedures based on learning theory, improve significantly more quickly than do patients treated by means of psychoanalytic or eclectic psychotherapy, or not treated by psychotherapy at all" (p. 720). On the basis of this evidence, Eysenck was quick to suggest that the specific ingredients of treatments based on learning theory were responsible for the superior outcomes:

> It would appear advisable, therefore, to discard the psychoanalytic model, which both on theoretical and practical plain fails to be useful in mediating verifiable predictions, and to adopt, provisionally at least, the learning theory model which, to date, appears to be much more promising theoretically and also with regard to application. (p. 721)

Interestingly, all three instances cited by Eysenck involved studies conducted by proponents of the method, which raises issues of allegiance (see chap. 7). Moreover, each of these treatments involved dubious applications of learning theory.[1] Eysenck's claims are interesting because they represents an early attempt to show that behavior therapy is more scientifically defensible than other therapies and that the benefits of such therapies are due to the specific ingredients, placing behavior therapy clearly in a medical model context.

At about the same time that Eysenck (1961) published his treatise on the superiority of learning theory treatments, Meltzoff and Kornreich (1970) also reviewed the research on the relative efficacy of various types of psycho-

---

[1]The reciprocal inhibition mechanisms proposed by Wolpe have been found to be flawed (see Kirsch, 1985). Phillips claimed that all behavior, pathological and normal, is the result of "assertions" made about oneself and relations with others, a claim that appears to be far afield from extant learning theories of the time. Although Ellis proposed no learning theory basis for his rational treatment, Eysenck commented that developing a learning theory explanation for it "would not be impossible" (Eysenck, 1961, p. 719).

therapy. Essentially, they had available the same literature as did Eysenck, yet they came to a very different conclusion:

> To summarize the present state of our knowledge, there is hardly any evidence that one traditional school of psychotherapy yields a better outcome than another. In fact, the question has hardly been put to a fair test. The whole issue remains at the level of polemic, professional public opinion, and whatever weight that can be brought to bear by authoritative presentation of illustrative cases. People may come out of different treatments with varied and identifiable philosophies of life or approaches to solving life's problems, but there is no current evidence that one traditional method is more successful than another in modifying psychopathology, alleviating symptoms, or improving general adjustment. (p. 200).

The early history of research summaries of relative efficacy mirrors that of absolute efficacy in that conclusions were idiosyncratic and influenced by the reviewers' preconceived notions.

In 1975, Luborsky et al. sought to conduct a comprehensive review of studies directly comparing different types of psychotherapy to address the relative efficacy question. Having realized the difficulty in locating and evaluating studies in past reviews, they commented that it was "not surprising that some previous reviewers have presented biased conclusions about the verdict of this research literature on the relative value of certain forms of psychotherapy" (Luborsky et al., 1975, p. 1000). Therefore, they systematically retrieved and evaluated studies. By reviewing only direct comparisons, they were able to rule out the confounds mentioned earlier in this chapter. However, meta-analytic procedures were unavailable to Luborsky et al. (1975), and they had to resort to box scores. Of 11 well-controlled studies comparing various traditional therapies (i.e., nonbehavioral), only 4 contained any significant differences. Only client-centered therapy had sufficient numbers of studies to examine relative efficacy of classes of traditional therapies; client-centered therapy was not significantly different from other traditional psychotherapies in 4 of 5 cases, and the remaining one favored another traditional therapy. There were 19 studies that compared behavior therapy with psychotherapy, and 13 found no differences. The remaining 6 favored behavior therapy, but 5 of the 6 received very low ratings for research quality. Luborsky et al. (1975) concluded that "*most comparative studies of different forms of psychotherapy found insignificant differences in proportions of patients who improved by the end of psychotherapy*" (p. 1003), although "behavior therapy may be especially suited for treatment of circumscribed phobias" (p. 1004).

In the same year Luborsky et al. (1975) published their review, Sloane et al. (1975) published the results of the most comprehensive study comparing analytically oriented psychotherapy (AOT) and behavior therapy (BT). The rigor used in this study was commendable, particularly given the period in which the study took place. Patients deemed appropriate for "talk" therapy, whose symptoms were not unduly severe, who desired psychological treatment, and who were between the ages of 18 and 45, were randomly assigned to the two treatments (viz., AOT and BT) and to a minimal contact control group ($n = 30$ in each group). The treatments lasted 4 months. Target symptoms were assessed before treatment, at the end of treatment, and 1 year after entering treatment. Two experienced behavior therapists and two experienced analytically oriented psychotherapists delivered the treatments. Although manuals were not used to guide treatment, the treatments were clearly distinguishable.

The general results of Sloane et al.'s (1975) study were that treated clients displayed superior outcomes to those untreated, but that AOT and BT were equally efficacious. The only differences found were that BT showed superior results vis-à-vis AOT on a social and work adjustment scale and an overall improvement rating scale at termination. An interesting aspect of this study was that a mix of disorders was included, such as anxiety, depression, character disorders, marital discord, adjustment disorder, and health-related complaints (e.g., obesity). At the time, BT was thought to be indicated for phobias and other problems with clear learning etiologies. So, Sloane et al. (1975) were impressed by the general effectiveness of BT:

> Behavior therapy is at least as effective, and possibly more effective than psychotherapy with the sort of moderately severe neuroses and personality disorders that are typical of clinic populations. This should dispel the impression that behavior therapy is useful only with phobias and restricted "unitary" problems.... Behavior therapy is clearly a *generally* useful treatment. (p. 224).

Although not noted by Sloane et al., the general effectiveness of BT in this study supported the notion that the efficacy of BT may be due to the incidental factors rather than the specific ingredients of BT.

As discussed, early reviews of outcome research diverged in terms of their conclusions. Advocates of BT found evidence that traditional psychotherapy was not efficacious, whereas BT was. On the other hand, other reviewers, having access to the same studies, came to the conclusions that traditional psychotherapy was efficacious. Toward the end of the pre-meta-analytic period, more rigorous reviews of controlled studies tended to find equivalence of outcomes for the various psychotherapies. As well, the best controlled and most rigorous comparative outcome study found few differences between traditional psychotherapy and behavior therapy. Nevertheless, the status of relative efficacy could not be examined critically until meta-analysis was applied to the outcome research.

General Meta-Analyses—Order Restored

There have been several meta-analyses that address the question of relative efficacy. They are presented in this section chronologically, with each correcting some problems of previous attempts and including current studies. Because the evidence has not been uniformly accepted by the psychotherapy community (e.g., Crits-Christoph, 1997; Howard et al., 1997; Wilson, 1982), the results of these meta-analyses are presented in some detail.

M. L. Smith and Glass (1977).   Although M. L. Smith and Glass's (1977) meta-analysis of psychotherapy outcomes is best known for the evidence that it produced relative to absolute efficacy, it also produced evidence about relative efficacy of various approaches to treatment. Smith and Glass classified over 800 effects from control group studies into 10 types of therapy and calculated the average effect size for each type along with the number of effect sizes and the percentile of the median treated person vis-à-vis the control group (see Table 4.1). On average, 60% of those treated with Gestalt therapy were better than the average untreated person, whereas 82% of those treated with systematic desensitization were better than the average untreated person. Overall, the type of therapy accounted for about 10% of the variance in effects, indicating that there appears to be a modest and significant amount of variance in outcome that is due to type of therapy. However, as discussed earlier, the effect sizes for the various types of therapy were derived from treatment versus no-treatment control group studies, and these studies differed on a number of variables, including duration, severity of problem, and type of outcome measure used. The effect sizes displayed in Table 4.1 are as invalid as Eysenck's (1952) comparison of recovery rates for psychotherapy and spontaneous remission derived from separate (and noncomparable) studies.

M. L. Smith and Glass (1977) adopted the following strategy to reduce the threats generated by these confounds. First, they created more general classes of therapy types by aggregating the 10 types into 4 super-classes: ego therapies (transactional analysis and rational emotive therapy), dynamic therapies (Freudian, psychodynamic, Adlerian), behavioral therapies (implosion, systematic desensitization, and behavior modification), and humanistic therapies (Gestalt and Rogerian). The 4 superclasses were determined using multidimensional scaling of experts' ratings of similarity of the types of therapy. Smith and Glass then compared the behavioral therapies superclass with the nonbehavioral therapies superclass (which consisted of all of the remaining therapies with the exception of Gestalt, which was omitted because there were too few studies and because it fell in the same plane as the behavioral therapies in the multidimensional scaling). The difference in the effect sizes for these two superclasses was 0.2 standard deviations, but this small difference was still confounded by such considerations as outcome variables and latency of measurement after termination. When only the studies that contained a behavioral and a

TABLE 4.1

Effect Sizes of 10 Types of Therapy on Any Outcome Measure
(From M. L. Smith and Glass, 1977)

Type of Therapy	Average Effect Size	No. of Effect Sizes	Median Treated Person's Percentile Status in Control Group
Psychodynamic	0.59	96	72
Adlerian	0.71	16	76
Eclectic	0.48	70	68
Transactional Analysis	0.58	25	72
Rational-Emotive	0.77	35	78
Gestalt	0.26	8	60
Client-Centered	0.63	94	74
Systematic Desensitization	0.91	223	82
Implosion	0.64	45	74
Behavior Modification	0.76	132	78

Note. From "Meta-Analysis of Psychotherapy Outcome Studies," by M. L. Smith and G. V Glass, 1977, *American Psychologist, 32*, p. 756. Copyright © 1977 by the American Psychological Association. Adapted with permission.

nonbehavioral treatment in the same study were compared (i.e., direct comparisons), the difference between the two superclasses shrunk to 0.07 standard deviations, which, given a standard error of 0.06, makes the difference between the behavioral and nonbehavioral treatments essentially zero (i.e., within 2 standard errors from zero).

M. L. Smith and Glass (1977) also modeled the confounds statistically. They regressed effect size onto study characteristics, including diagnosis, intelligence, age, the manner in which the client presented, latency to measurement of outcome, reactivity of outcome measure, as well as interactions, and found that about 25% of the variance in effects were due to study characteristics. Using these regressions, effect size for classes of treatments could be estimated (i.e., holding study characteristics constant). For example, for phobic clients, the following effects were found: psychodynamic = 0.92; systematic desensitization = 1.05; behavior modification = 1.12.

When study characteristics were considered, it appears that various types of therapy, broadly defined, produce generally equivalent outcomes, a conclusion reached by M. L. Smith and Glass (1977): "Despite volumes

devoted to the theoretical differences among different schools of psychotherapy, the results of research demonstrate negligible differences in the effects produced by different therapy types" (p. 760). Historically, it is
interesting to note that when Rosenzweig proposed in 1936 that common
factors were responsible for therapeutic change, he "assumed ... that all
methods of therapy when competently used are equally successful" (p.
413). Smith and Glass provided the first meta-analytic evidence that
Rosenzweig's conjecture was correct.

M. L. Smith and Glass's (1977) support for the Dodo bird effect un-
leashed a torrent of criticism. To those interested in the specific ingredients
of particular treatments, the Dodo bird effect was unacceptable:

> If the indiscriminate distribution of prizes argument carried true conviction ... we
> end up with the same advice for everyone—"Regardless of the nature of your
> problem seek any form of psychotherapy." This is absurd. We doubt whether
> even the strongest advocates of the Dodo bird argument dispense this advice.
> (Rachman & Wilson, 1980, p. 167)

The various issues raised seem to have been motivated by distaste for the result. Many of the issues were directed to the entire meta-analytic enterprise
rather than specific to the Dodo-bird conjecture and were discussed in chapter 3. Later in this chapter, the difficulty that some psychotherapy researchers
have in accepting the Dodo bird conjecture are discussed at length.

Nevertheless, there are a number of features of M. L. Smith and Glass's
(1977) analysis that create some caution in accepting the homogeneity of
outcome effects for the various types of counseling and therapy. First, all of
the studies reviewed appeared prior to 1977; hence, the findings may have
been time bound. Since that time, the cognitive therapies have proliferated,
treatments have been standardized with manuals, outcome measures have
been refined, and designs have become more sophisticated. Stiles et al.
(1986), in their thoughtful discussion of why true differences among therapies, if present, have not been detected, argued that true difference in treatment efficacy may have been obscured by poor research methods and that
as the methods and treatments improve, differences will be detected. This
argument implies that a conclusion made in 1977 should not be the last
word. Wampold, Mondin, Moody, Stich, et al. (1997) tested the improv-
ing-methods hypothesis, and this result is discussed later in this chapter.

A second issue is that to compare categories of treatments (such as cognitive–behavioral and psychodynamic), each treatment must be classified into
one and only one of the categories. However, defining the categories and
making classifications can be problematic. For instance, Crits-Christoph
(1997) classified an "emotionally focused therapy" (Goldman & Greenberg,
1992) as cognitive–behavioral, even though the treatment assumed that "psychological symptoms are seen as emanating from the deprivation of unmet

adult needs" and involved, in part, "identification with previously unacknowledged aspects of experience by enactment of redefined cycle" (p. 964). As mentioned earlier, Eysenck (1961) classified Ellis's (1957) rational psychotherapy as behavioral, even though Ellis did not articulate a learning theory basis for his treatment. The criteria for classification, in these cases, are not obvious. Moreover, classifying treatments assumes that the important differences are among classes of treatments, rather than among all treatments (Wampold, Mondin, Moody, Stich, et al., 1997). Often treatments within a category are compared in primary research studies to test hypotheses about the efficacy of specific ingredients. For example, a researcher interested in the specific ingredients of behavioral treatments for anxiety might compare in vivo with imaginal exposure. Ignoring within-category comparisons omits important information about the common factor–specific ingredient issue, as these comparisons typically are designed to demonstrate the efficacy of a particular ingredient. Finally, it appears that most direct comparisons of treatments are within-category comparisons (see, e.g., Shadish et al., 1993).

A final problem with Smith and Glass's (1977) analysis was that the statistical theory of meta-analysis was not fully developed at the time. As discussed previously, Smith and Glass's results are limited by the effect size measure used, the aggregation algorithm, the nonindependence of the effect sizes, and the statistical tests used.

M. L. Smith et al. (1980).   As indicated in chapter 3, M. L. Smith et al. (1980) extended M. L. Smith and Glass's (1997) meta-analysis by including additional studies and conducting further analysis. This extended analysis investigated relative efficacy.

M. L. Smith et al. (1980) investigated relative efficacy by categorizing treatments and comparing the effect sizes produced within categories and then aggregating effects within categories from treatment–no-treatment comparisons. The effects for six subclasses of treatments are shown in Table 4.2. As well, therapies were further classified into three broader classes: verbal (composed of dynamic, cognitive, and humanistic subclasses), behavioral (composed of behavioral and cognitive–behavioral subclasses), and developmental (developmental subclass). The effect sizes for these three classes also are shown in Table 4.2. As is evident in Table 4.2, there are clear differences among the effect sizes for the various subclasses and classes of treatments. However, there are problems with comparisons of subclasses or classes, the most serious of which is that the effects were derived from studies that differed in systematic ways. For example, cognitive–behavioral studies typically used outcome measures that were twice as reactive as those used in developmental therapies, and reactivity of measures was correlated strongly with effect size ($r = .18$), giving a decided advantage to cognitive–behavioral therapies.

TABLE 4.2

Effect Sizes for Various Psychotherapies
From M. L. Smith, Glass, & Miller (1980)

Therapy	Average Effect Size	Number of Effect Sizes
Subclass		
Dynamic	0.78	255
Cognitive	1.31	145
Humanistic	0.63	218
Developmental	0.42	157
Behavioral	0.91	646
Cognitive–behavioral	1.24	157
Class		
Verbal (dynamic, cognitive, and humanistic)	0.85	597
Behavioral (behavioral, cognitive–behavioral)	0.98	791
Developmental (developmental)	0.42	157

Note. Smith, Mary Lee, Gene V Glass, and Thomas I. Miller. *The Benefits of Psychotherapy.* Tables 5.4 and 5.7 © 1980. The Johns Hopkins University Press. Adapted with permission.

M. L. Smith et al. (1980) addressed the confounds inherent in comparing effect sizes from different studies in two ways. The first way was to use regression analysis to attempt to control for differences in various confounding variables. It turned out that the major confound was reactivity of outcome measure; when reactivity was taken into account, differences among subclasses were reduced dramatically. For example, the uncorrected difference between behavioral and dynamic therapies was 0.13, the corrected difference was 0.03.

With regard to the three classes of therapy, the relatively small difference between the behavioral class and the dynamic class (viz., effect size difference of 0.13) was virtually nonexistent when reactivity was considered (viz., difference of 0.03). M. L. Smith et al. (1980) made the following observation:

> In the original uncorrected data, the behavior therapies did enjoy an advantage in magnitude of effect because of more highly reactive measures. Once this ad-

vantage was corrected, reliable differences between the two classes disappeared. (p. 105)

It should be noted in these comparisons that the developmental subclass contained (a) vocational–personal developmental counseling, which involved providing skills to clients to facilitate adaptive development, and (b) undifferentiated counseling, which "refers to therapy or counseling that lacks descriptive information and references that would identify it with proponents of theory ... [and was] used as a foil against which a more highly valued therapy can be compared" (M. L. Smith et al., 1980, p. 73). Thus, developmental therapies, as operationalized by Smith et al., do not fit the definition of psychotherapy used in this book, as, for the most part, they were not intended to be therapeutic.

Statistically correcting differences among studies revealed that a single confounding variable, reactivity of the outcome measure, eliminated sizable differences among various classes and subclasses. However, M. L. Smith et al. (1980) recognized that examining studies that directly compare therapies (i.e., primary studies that used treatment comparison designs) provides a better estimate of differences among therapies. Because of the number of studies that compared treatments was relatively small, M. L. Smith et al. (1980) were restricted to comparing classes. Table 4.3 displays the results of these direct comparisons.

There are several important observations to make about the differences between therapy classes. First, as noted earlier, the developmental class does not contain treatments that are intended to be therapeutic and thus does not provide useful results for discriminating between the medical model and the contextual model. Second, although data were available in the primary study to calculate a between-treatments effect size (viz. the difference between means for the two treatments, respectively, divided by the standard deviation), M. L. Smith et al. (1980) chose to calculate the average effect sizes vis-à-vis the no-treatment control and then compare the size of the resulting average effect. This should not affect the results. However, Smith et al.'s effect sizes were based on slightly different numbers of outcome variables. This was presumably due to the fact that studies inconsistently reported summary statistics, but the effect on these results is unknown. The third observation is that the comparison between behavioral and verbal psychotherapies yielded a difference of 0.19, which is a small effect size (consult Table 2.4). Finally, even though direct comparisons control most confounds, some remain, the primary of which is allegiance (see chap. 7). The direct comparisons of behavioral and verbal therapies may have been conducted by researchers with allegiance to behavioral treatments, thus giving an edge to behavioral treatments. In Smith et al.'s meta-analysis, allegiance effects were relatively large (in the neighborhood of an effect size of 0.30), but Smith et al. did not control for allegiance. As we shall see later

TABLE 4.3

Results of Direct Comparisons Among Therapy Classes
From M. L. Smith, Glass, & Miller (1980)

Comparison	Average Effect Size	Difference	Number of Effect Sizes	Number of Studies
Verbal vs. Developmental		0.15		3
Verbal	0.51		4	
Developmental	0.36		4	
Behavioral vs. Developmental		0.56		13
Behavioral	0.95		52	
Developmental	0.39		34	
Verbal vs. Behavioral		0.19		56
Verbal	0.77		187	
Behavioral	0.96		178	

Note. Smith, Mary Lee, Gene V Glass, and Thomas I. Miller. *The Benefits of Psychotherapy.*
Table 5.14 © 1980. The Johns Hopkins University Press. Adapted with permission.

in this chapter (and in chap. 7), several apparent advantages for a particular therapy have been nullified by controlling for allegiance effects.

Although M. L. Smith et al. (1980) examined studies that directly compared treatments, D. A. Shapiro and Shapiro (1982) sought to directly assess relative efficacy through meta-analysis. Their meta-analysis is considered next.

D. A. Shapiro and Shapiro (1982).   In 1982, D. A. Shapiro and Shapiro addressed the problem related to confounds by conducting a meta-analysis of studies that directly compared two or more psychotherapies. Moreover, Shapiro and Shapiro included the behavioral studies that were omitted from previous meta-analyses, which invoked criticism (e.g., Rachman & Wilson, 1980). As well, Shapiro and Shapiro addressed several other criticisms leveled at previous meta-analyses.

D. A. Shapiro and Shapiro (1982) reviewed all studies published between 1975 and 1979 (inclusively) that contained two groups who received a psychological treatment and one group who received no treatment or minimal treatment (i.e., control groups); hence evidence about absolute as well as relative efficacy was obtained. Each treatment was classified into one of

15 categories, as shown in Table 4.4. It should be noted that minimal treatments were not treatments intended to be therapeutic and therefore do not provide evidence relative to discriminating between the medical and contextual models.

TABLE 4.4

Relative Advantage of Treatment Categories,
as Reported by D. A. Shapiro and Shapiro (1982)

Method	No. of Groups	No. of Studies	No. of Comparisons	Effect Size	Advantage
Behavioral	310	134	56	1.06	.32**
Rehearsal, self-control, and monitoring	38	21	16	1.01	.20
Biofeedback	9	9	9	.91	−.33
Covert behavioral	19	13	10	1.52	.22
Flooding	18	10	9	1.12	.11
Relaxation	42	31	27	.90	−.14
Systematic desensitization	77	55	50	.97	.04
Reinforcement	28	17	13	.97	.36
Modeling	11	8	6	1.43	.07
Social skills training	14	14	14	.85	.13
Study skills training	4	4	4	.26	−.75
Cognitive	35	22	20	1.00	.40***
Dynamic–humanistic	20	16	13	.40	−.53**
Mixed (mainly behavioral)	40	28	24	1.42	.52**
Unclassified (mainly behavioral)	18	14	14	.78	−.23*
Minimal	41	36	36	.71	−.56***

Note. Mixed treatments were those that contained features of more than one type of treatment; unclassified treatments were dissimilar to other types and were too infrequent to justify their own category; minimal treatments were treatments not indented to be therapeutic (e.g., placebo controls). From "Meta-Analysis of Comparative Therapy Outcome Studies: A Replication and Refinement," by D. A. Shapiro and D. Shapiro, 1982, *Psychological Bulletin, 92,* p. 584. Copyright © 1982 by the American Psychological Association. Adapted with permission.

*$p < .05$.
**$p < .01$.
***$p < .001$.

Overall, D. A. Shapiro and Shapiro (1982) found that the effect size for the treatments in comparison with control groups was between 0.72 and 0.98, a range that is consistent with the 0.80 value for absolute efficacy derived in chapter 3. The first set of results from D. A Shapiro and Shapiro (1982) that bear on the relative efficacy issue are found in Table 4.4. Clearly, there seems to be some variance in the effect size by category. Indeed, between 5 and 10% of the variance in effect size was due to treatment category (depending on how it was calculated). However, it must be kept in mind that the determination of variance due to treatment by this method does not take into account the confounds due to the fact that the studies differ in dependent variables, disorders treated, severity of disorder, skill of the therapists, and allegiance to the treatment, as discussed earlier. When some of these confounding variables were coded and analyzed, anywhere from 22 to 36% of the variance was accounted for by them.

The last column in Table 4.4 gives the effect sizes of each treatment type with the treatments with which it was compared. That is, for each comparison of a treatment type with some other treatment, the mean of the comparison group was subtracted from the mean of the designated treatment group, and the resulting difference was divided by the standard deviation. Thus, positive values in this column indicate that the designated treatment was superior to the treatments with which it was directly compared in the primary studies. For example, the value of .40 for cognitive indicates that cognitive therapy was superior to the treatments with which it was compared, and the average difference was .40 standard deviations. It appears that, according to this column, cognitive therapy and mixed therapies were superior to other therapies and that the same can be said of behavioral therapies as a superclass. As well, dynamic–humanistic, unclassified therapies, and (as expected) minimal therapies were inferior to other therapies. However, there are several issues to consider in interpreting these results. First, the comparison groups vary by category; for example, cognitive therapy comparisons were different than the comparisons for the dynamic–humanistic comparisons. Second, these comparisons included comparisons with minimal treatments, although Shapiro and Shapiro claimed that this did not affect the results greatly. Third, a preponderance of the dynamic–humanistic treatments contained no ingredients unique to the respective therapies and thus were not intended to be therapeutic, providing a poor test of the contextual model. Fourth, it should be realized that the significance levels of such comparisons are suspect because, at the time, the distributions of meta-analytic statistics had not been derived. Nevertheless, it is worth pointing out that the magnitude of the differences between treatments and comparisons (excluding minimal treatments) ranged from .04 to .53, significantly less than the .80 value related to absolute efficacy of psychological treatments.

TABLE 4.5

Pairwise Comparisons of Therapy Types by D. A. Shapiro and Shapiro (1982)

	Method B				
Method A	*Relaxation*	*Systematic Desensitization*	*Social Skills Training*	*Mixed*	*Minimal*
Rehearsal, self-control, and monitoring					.64** (6)
Biofeedback	−.20 (8)			−.72 (4)	
Covert behavioral					.54 (4)
Relaxation		−.24 (13)		−.59 (5)	.29 (4)
Systematic desensitization		.32 (5)		−.28* (7)	.50*** (15)
Reinforcement					.14 (5)
Social skills training		.06 (5)			.37* (4)
Cognitive		.53*** (9)	.28 (4)		.68* (7)
Dynamic/ humanistic			.35 (4)	−.93 (4)	
Unclassified	−.16 (4)	.02 (6)			.46* (6)

Note. All comparisons are Method A–Method B differences based on 1 difference score per study, *N*s of studies are given in parentheses. Mixed treatments were those that contained features of more than one type of treatment; unclassified treatments were dissimilar to other types and were too infrequent to justify their own category; minimal treatments were treatments not intended to be therapeutic (e.g., placebo controls). From "Meta-Analysis of Comparative Therapy Outcome Studies: A Replication and Refinement," by D. A. Shapiro and D. Shapiro, 1982, *Psychological Bulletin, 92,* p. 391. Copyright © 1982 by the American Psychological Association. Adapted with permission.

*$p < .05$.

**$p < .01$.

***$p < .001$.

D. A. Shapiro and Shapiro (1982) recognized the limitations of examining the relative advantage of therapies by the method represented in Table 4.4. The alternative used was to estimate the differences among the various pairwise comparisons of therapy types. Obviously, in the primary studies not all therapies were compared with all other therapies. Shapiro and Shapiro provided estimates of the pairwise comparisons of therapy types if the two types of therapies were compared in at least four studies and yielded at least 10 effect sizes. These pairwise comparisons are presented in Table 4.5. As expected, when treatments were compared with minimal treatments, they were generally superior to these controls. Of the 13 remaining comparisons, only 2 reached statistical significance ($p < .05$), although again one has to keep in mind that these significance levels were flawed. Nevertheless, only 2 of 13 comparisons demonstrated differences, which supports the homogeneity of treatment efficacy. As shown later in this chapter, the probability of obtaining a few statistically significant comparisons from multiple comparisons is extraordinarily large.

Further perusal of Table 4.5 reveals that several of the differences with the largest magnitude involved comparisons with mixed treatments, which were defined as "methods that defied classification into any one of the categories because they contained elements of more than one" (D. A. Shapiro & Shapiro, 1982, p. 584), which certainly makes interpretation of these differences difficult. If the purpose of direct comparisons of treatments is to establish the potency of a specific ingredient, then comparisons with a treatment that is a "cocktail" of many ingredients provides little evidence for the specificity of a particular ingredient.

In D.A. Shapiro and Shapiro's (1982) analysis, the only pairwise difference that was statistically significant and that did not involve minimal treatments or mixed treatments was the superiority of cognitive therapy to systematic desensitization, which could be construed as evidence of the efficacy of cognitive ingredients vis-à-vis the conditioning mechanisms of systematic desensitization. Although this appears to be the first meta-analytic evidence for specific ingredients, the advantage of cognitive therapy may have been due to the allegiance of the researchers to cognitive therapy in the studies reviewed by Shapiro and Shapiro. Berman, Miller, and Massman (1985) investigated the cognitive–systematic comparison further and found that the difference between these two therapies was only 0.06 and that the advantage for cognitive therapies found by Shapiro and Shapiro was due to the fact that the studies reviewed therein were conducted by advocates of cognitive therapy (see chap. 7 for a complete discussion of Berman et al., 1985).

The contribution made by D. A. Shapiro and Shapiro (1982) was that the focus was on studies that directly compared two treatments, eliminating the confounds discussed previously (e.g., dependent measures, disorder treated, severity). However, several other issues remain, including the need to classify treatments into categories (which eliminated analysis of direct comparisons within categories), unavailability of appropriate sampling theory for meta-analysis, and the date of the studies reviewed (viz., 1975 to 1980). These issues were addressed in the next meta-analysis reviewed.

Wampold, Mondin, Moody, Stich, et al. (1997).

Wampold, Mondin, Moody, Stich, et al. (1997) sought to address the issues in previous meta-analyses to provide an additional test of the Dodo bird effect. They included all studies from 1970 to 1995, in six journals that typically publish psychotherapy outcome research, and that directly compared two or more treatments intended to be therapeutic. Basing conclusions on direct comparisons eliminated many confounds, as discussed earlier. Treatments were restricted to those that were intended to be therapeutic (i.e., bona fide), so that treatments that were intended as control groups, or were not credible to therapists, were excluded. This restriction is important because the contextual model of psychotherapy stipulates that the efficacy of a treatment depends on therapist and client believing that the treatment is intended to be therapeutic. A treatment was determined to be bona fide provided (a) the therapist had at least a master's degree, developed a therapeutic relationship with the client, and tailored the treatment to the client; (b) the problem treated was representative of problems characteristic of clients, although severity was not considered (i.e., the diagnosis did not have to meet *DSM* criteria); and (c) the treatment satisfied two of the following four conditions: citation to an established treatment (e.g., a reference to Rogers, 1951, client-centered therapy), a description of the treatment was presented and contained reference to psychological mechanisms (e.g., operant conditioning), a manual was used to guide administration of the treatment, or the active ingredients of the treatment were specified and referenced. The retrieval strategy used resulted in 277 comparisons of psychotherapies that were intended to be therapeutic.

A unique feature of Wampold, Mondin, Moody, Stich, et al's (1997) meta-analysis was that treatments were not classified into therapy types. Classifying treatments into categories tests the hypothesis that there are no differences among therapy categories, whereas Wampold, Mondin, Moody, Stich, et al.'s (1997) meta-analysis tested the hypothesis that the differences among all comparisons of individual treatments is zero. Besides testing the more general Dodo bird conjecture, this strategy avoided several problems encountered by earlier meta-analyses. First, as demonstrated by D. A. Shapiro and Shapiro's (1982) meta-analysis, there are many pairwise comparisons of treatment categories that contain few or no studies. Second, classification of treatments is not as straightforward as one would believe (Wampold, Mondin, Moody, & Ahn, 1997). Third, comparison of treatment types eliminates from consideration all comparisons within treatment types, of which there are many and of which many were designed to test the efficacy of specific ingredients. Finally, and importantly, pairwise comparisons of treatment types obviates an omnibus test of the Dodo bird conjecture. For example, does the fact that 2 of 13 comparisons were significant in Shapiro and Shapiro's analysis indicate that there are few, but important differences, or that these 2 were due to chance?

Another feature of Wampold, Mondin, Moody, Stich, et al.'s (1997) meta-analysis was that all statistical tests relied on meta-analytic distribution theory (Hedges & Olkin, 1985), which provides more valid tests of the Dodo bird conjecture. The effect size used in this meta-analysis was based on the following equation:

$$g = (M_A - M_B)/s \; ,$$

where M_A and M_B were the means for the two treatments compared, and s was the pooled standard deviation. These effect sizes were corrected for bias, as described in chapter 2. However, before aggregating over studies, Wampold, Mondin, Moody, Stich, et al. (1997) aggregated over the various outcome measures, modeling the interdependence of these measures (see Wampold, Mondin, Moody, Stich, et al., 1997, Equations 4 and 5), thus eliminating the problems of nonindependent effect sizes that have plagued other meta-analyses.

The primary hypothesis tested in this meta-analysis was that the true differences among treatments intended to be therapeutic was zero. Two other hypotheses related to the Dodo bird conjecture were tested. Stiles et al. (1986) speculated that improving research methods, such as more sensitive outcome measures and manualized treatments, would detect true differences among treatments that had been obscured in the past. To test this hypothesis, Wampold, Mondin, Moody, Stich, et al. (1997) determined whether more recent studies, which presumably used better research methods, produced larger differences than did more dated studies. The second hypothesis was related to classification of studies. If specific ingredients were causal to treatment efficacy, then treatments within categories (such as cognitive–behavioral treatments) that contain similar ingredients would produce small differences, whereas treatments from different categories (cognitive behavioral and psychodynamic), which contain very different ingredients, would produce large differences. Wampold, Mondin, Moody, Stich, et al. (1997) tested this hypothesis by relating treatment similarity to the size of treatment differences. If the Dodo bird conjecture is not true (i.e., treatments differ in their efficacy), comparison of relatively dissimilar treatments would produce larger differences than comparisons of relatively similar treatments. On the other hand, if the Dodo bird conjecture was true, then treatment similarity would be irrelevant.

Avoiding classification of treatments into categories created a methodological problem. In previous meta-analyses of comparative outcome studies, treatments were classified into categories and then one category was (arbitrarily) classified as primary so that the algebraic sign of the effect size could be determined. For example, in D. A. Shapiro and Shapiro's (1982) comparison of various therapy types, cognitive therapy (vis-à-vis systematic desensitization) was classified as primary so that a positive effect size indicated that cognitive therapy was superior to systematic desensitization. Wampold, Mondin, Moody, Stich, et al. (1997), however, had to assign an algebraic sign to each comparison of treatments (i.e., for each primary study). There are two options, both of which were used. First, a positive sign could be assigned so that each comparison yielded a positive effect size. However, this strategy would overestimate the aggregated effect size; nevertheless, the aggregate of the positively signed effects provides an upper bound estimate for the difference in outcomes of bona fide treatments. The second option, which is to randomly assign the algebraic sign to the effect size for individual comparisons, creates a situation in which the aggregate effect size would be zero, as the plus- and minus-signed effects would cancel each other out. However, if there are true differences among treatments (i.e., the Dodo bird conjecture is false and specific ingredients are producing effects in some treatments), then comparisons should produce many large effects, creating thick tails in the distribution of effects whose signs have been randomly determined, as shown in Figure 4.1. On the other hand, if there are truly no differences among treatments (i.e., the Dodo bird conjecture is true), then most of the effect sizes will be near zero and those further out in the tails of the distribution would amount to what would be expected by chance. Wampold, Mondin, Moody, Stich, et al.'s (1997) meta-analysis tested whether the effects were homogeneously distributed around zero, as would be expected if the Dodo bird conjecture were true.

The evidence produced by Wampold, Mondin, Moody, Stich, et al.'s (1997) meta-analysis was consistent, in every respect, with the Dodo bird conjecture. First, the effects, with random signs, were homogeneously distributed about zero. That is, the preponderance of effects were near zero, and the frequency of larger effects was consistent with what would be produced by chance, given the sampling distribution of effect sizes. Second, even when positive signs were attached to each comparison, the aggregated effect size was roughly 0.20, which is a small effect (see Table 2.4 and discussion later in this section).

Wampold, Mondin, Moody, Stich, et al. (1997) found no evidence that the differences in outcome among treatments was related to either year in which the study was published or the similarity of the treatments. It does not appear that comparisons of treatments that are quite different produce larger effects than comparisons of treatments that are similar to each other,

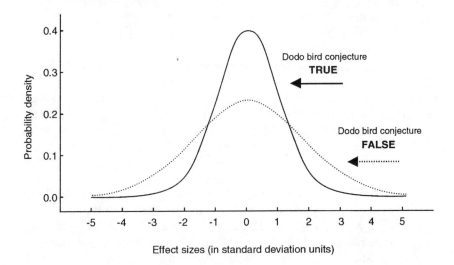

FIG. 4.1. A distribution of effect sizes (with signs determined randomly) when the Dodo bird conjecture is true and when it is false. Reprinted with permission, Figure 1, Wampold, B. E., Mondin, G. W., Moody, M., Stich, F., Benson, K., & Ahn, H. (1997). A meta-analysis of outcome studies comparing bona fide psychotherapies: Empirically, "All must have prizes." *Psychological Bulletin, 122,* 203–215.

a result consistent with the Dodo bird conjecture. The lack of relation between year and effect size indicates that improving research methods are not increasingly detecting differences among treatments.

Summary of General Meta-Analyses

The meta-analyses conducted to date have produced generally consistent results. The early meta-analyses (viz., M. L Smith & Glass, 1977; M. L. Smith et al., 1980) that did not rely on reviewing primary studies that directly compared psychotherapies found differences in efficacy among various classes of treatments. However, when confounds were statistically modeled, these differences were negligible. The early meta-analysis of direct comparisons among classes of treatments (viz., D. A. Shapiro & Shapiro, 1982) produced a few differences, but not more than expected by chance. Moreover, the one result that might have supported specific ingredients (viz., the superiority of cognitive treatments to systematic desensitization) was later shown to be nonexistent and most likely due to allegiance (see Berman et al., 1985). The most comprehensive meta-analysis (viz.,

Wampold, Mondin, Moody, Stich, et al., 1997) produced evidence entirely consistent with the Dodo bird conjecture of uniform efficacy.

Wampold, Mondin, Moody, Stich, et al. (1997) found that under the most liberal assumptions in which all differences between therapies was given a positive sign, the effect size for treatment differences was approximately 0.20. Grissom (1996) meta-meta-analyzed 32 meta-analyses that compared various psychotherapies, assigned positive signs to the differences, and calculated an effect size difference of 0.23, replicating the upper bound found by Wampold, Mondin, Moody, Stich, et al. (1997). Clearly, the upper bound on relative efficacy is in the neighborhood of 0.20. Although this is a liberal upper bound, the value of 0.20 is used when the variation in psychotherapy outcomes are summarized in chapter 9.

An effect size of 0.20 is a small effect in the social sciences (see Table 2.4), particularly so when contrasted with the effect size for the efficacy of psychotherapy (viz., 0.80). An effect size of 0.20 indicates that 42% of the people in the inferior treatment are "better" than the average person in the superior treatment. Moreover, an effect size of 0.20 indicates that only 1% of the variance in outcomes is due to the treatments. Finally, this effect size indicates that 45% of the people in the inferior treatment would be successfully treated, whereas 55% of the people in the superior treatment would be successfully treated. The point here is that even the most liberal estimate of differences among treatments is very small.

Criticisms of General Meta-Analytic Conclusion of Uniform Efficacy

A number of issues have been raised with regard to the general meta-analytic finding that psychotherapies intended to be therapeutic produce equivalent outcomes. These issues are addressed briefly in this section.

An ironic criticism of the meta-analytic findings was that the "indiscriminate distribution of prizes ... is absurd" (Rachman & Wilson, 1980, p. 167). The irony lies in the fact that such a claim would be made by the camp that was critical of the advocates of traditional psychotherapy, who were convinced of its effectiveness and were unwilling to consider the empirical evidence contrary to their opinion:

> An emotional feeling of considerable intensity has grown up in this field which makes many people regard the very questioning of its [psychotherapy's] effectiveness as an attack on psychotherapy; as Teuber and Powers (1953) point out; "To some of the counselors, the whole control group idea ... seemed slightly blasphemous, as if we were attempting a statistical test of the efficacy of prayer ..." (Eysenck, 1961, p. 697)

Yet when the empirical evidence supports a position contrary to the behaviorists, the conclusion is labeled "absurd." Moreover, the clinical expertise of the meta-analyst has been questioned: "All too often, the people who conduct these [meta-] analyses know more about the quantitative aspects of their task than about the substantive issues that need to be addressed" (Chambless & Hollon, 1998, p. 14). This last statement could just as well have been made by a psychoanalyst in 1960 with regard to the behaviorally oriented clinical scientists who used control group designs! Of course, it is unscientific to discount evidence because it cannot be brought into accord with one's underlying model, in this case the medical model of psychotherapy.

Another criticism of meta-analytic results that are consistent with the Dodo bird conjecture is that the conjecture cannot be true because there are counter examples—that is, there are studies that have found differences between treatments (Chambless & Hollon, 1998; Crits-Christoph, 1997). However, it is expected that a small proportion of studies will find a significant difference when the true difference between therapies is zero because the probability of a Type I error (falsely rejecting the null hypothesis of no differences) is typically set at 5%. Wampold, Mondin, Moody, Stich, et al. (1997) showed that the tails of the distribution of effect sizes for comparisons were consistent with a true effect size of zero—that is, the number of studies showing a significant difference for one treatment was exactly what would be expected by considering sampling error. Of course, the sampling error rate is exacerbated if counterexamples are selected on the basis of statistical significance on one or a few of many outcome measures. Crits-Christoph (1997) was able to locate 15 studies contained in Wampold, Mondin, Moody, Stich, et al.'s (1997) meta-analysis that compared cognitive–behavioral treatment to a noncognitive–behavioral treatment and for which one variable showed the superiority of the cognitive–behavioral treatment. Although there were numerous problems with the studies selected (e.g., the comparison group was not intended to be therapeutic; Wampold, Mondin, Moody, Stich, et al., 1997), the primary issue is that culling through a database to find instances of results (in this case 15 variables from a set of over 3000) that confirm one's notion will surely lead to confirmation of that notion. However, Crits-Christoph's attempt to find a trend in the data needs to be considered further. Suppose that there is a subset of treatments for which there are differences, but the size of the subset is insufficient to affect the overall conclusion of uniform efficacy. For example, suppose that uniform efficacy does not hold for depression, and if one were to examine only treatments of depression, systematic differences would appear. This is a possibility that needs to be examined and one that is taken up later in this chapter.

The implications drawn from the meta-analyses reviewed have been discounted by some because they represent the current state of outcome research but perhaps do not reflect the true state of relative efficacy or the future state of outcome research (Howard et al., 1997; Stiles et al., 1986).

One strand of this argument goes along the line that there are true differences among treatments, but limitations in research (e.g., poorly implemented treatments or insensitive outcome measures) mask the differences. Recall that Wampold, Mondin, Moody, Stich, et al. (1997) found no relation between publication date and the effect size for differences between treatments, indicating that improving research methods (e.g., use of manual-guided treatments) did not detect differences. Another strand of this argument is that although it may be true that there are no differences among currently available treatments, in the future more potent treatments might exist (Howard et al., 1997). As noted by Wampold, Mondin, Moody, and Ahn (1997):

> We would cherish the day that a treatment is developed that is dramatically more effective than the ones we use today. But until that day comes, the existing data suggest that whatever differences in treatment efficacy exist, they appear to be extremely small, at best. (p. 230)

In any case, until data are presented to the contrary, the scientific stance is to retain the null hypothesis, which in this case is that there are no differences in efficacy among treatments.

Another issue raised is that the psychotherapies compared in outcome research represent a limited subsample of all treatments mentioned in the literature or practiced (Crits-Christoph, 1997; Howard et al., 1997). Although this may be true, again, the null hypothesis should be retained until such time as evidence is found to the contrary. That is, until such time as additional treatments are included in primary studies, uniform efficacy fits the data better than any other model. But the issue here becomes more complex when it is realized that outcome research is expensive and consequently requires funding. Use of psychotherapy manuals, however, is a required element for research support (Kiesler, 1994), which then effectively limits outcome research to the subset of treatments compatible with manuals (Henry, 1998). If the criticism related to the limited inclusion of treatments is allowed to invalidate the uniform efficacy finding, then it would be impossible to ever conduct a meta-analytic test of the hypothesis.

A number of alternative hypotheses for the uniform efficacy result have been offered. For example, Crits-Christoph (1997) commented that including follow-up assessments in Wampold, Mondin, Moody, Stich, et al.'s (1997) meta-analysis attenuated differences because clients in the less efficacious treatment would seek other treatment for their disorder. Another alternative hypothesis is that differences will only be apparent for severe disorders: "With mild conditions, the nonspecific effects of treatments ... are likely to be powerful enough in themselves to affect ... outcomes leaving little room for the specific factors to play much of a role" (Crits-Christoph, 1997). These and several other alternative hypotheses could be true, but must be put to an empirical test in order to establish that some treatments are superior to other treatments (Wampold, Mondin, Moody, & Ahn, 1997). It should be noted that Wampold, Mondin, Moody, and Ahn (1997) reanalyzed their data and showed that when treatment outcomes were measured at termination only and disorders were limited to those that were severe (viz., *DSM–IV* disorders), the uniform efficacy result persisted.

Others have blamed the diagnostic system for the equivalence of outcomes. The argument is that *DSM* disorders are categories that contain multiple etiological pathways and that treatments specific to the pathways are needed (Follette & Houts, 1996). For example, cognitive–behavioral treatment would be indicated for those whose depression is caused by irrational cognitions, or social-skills training would be indicated for those whose depression is caused by loneliness resulting from a social-skills deficit that limits social relations. This conjecture, if true, would provide strong evidence for specific ingredients and would definitely support the medical model. However, as is shown in chapter 5, there is little evidence that the predictions of an interactive effect of treatment and etiological pathway exist.

It has been argued that the primary studies synthesized in meta-analysis are flawed due to problems with randomization, attrition, interactions with unknown causal variables, choice of outcome measures, and limited external validity (Howard, Krause, & Orlinsky, 1986; Howard et al., 1997) and consequently that meta-analyses are flawed as well. Howard et al. (1997) noted that meta-analysis "inherits all of the problems of these kinds of comparative experiments" (p. 224), which is true, to a certain extent, but does not invalidate the conclusion for the following reasons. If the outcome research conducted in psychotherapy is so flawed that the results transmit no information, then they should be abandoned altogether and decisions should not be based on results produced by such designs. Of course, it is the medical model that depends on such designs for legitimacy, so abandonment would be an admission of the failure of the medical model. However, no one is seriously recommending that such designs are totally invalid, only that there are threats to validity. Meta-analysis is advantageous because it can be used to determine whether results of such studies are consistently drawing the same conclusion (i.e., converge on a common estimation), in which case confidence is increased. This is exactly the case with uniform efficacy. There are flaws with all comparative studies, and making strong statements, either for practice or theory, from an individual study is risky. However, when 277 comparisons are homogeneously distributed about zero, as was the case in Wampold, Mondin, Moody, Stich, et al.'s (1997) meta-analysis, then it must be understood that the corpus of comparisons are consistent with a uniform efficacy conjecture, a conclusion that can be made with confidence.

A final criticism discussed herein is that the overall effect size for comparisons is the incorrect measure to establish uniform efficacy. Howard et al. (1997) recommended that treatments be scaled on the basis of efficacy:

> If we compare applications of psychotherapies by pairing the application of one with the application of another so as to calculate the difference between their outcomes, we are really looking, for practical purposes, to order a set of therapies on a common outcome metric. If therapy … 1 (T1) is D outcome units better than T2, T2 is D better than T3, and T3 is D better than T1, then the mean difference in outcome among the three therapies is D, but they cannot be ordered on a one-dimensional outcome metric; that is, the results of the three comparisons are inconsistent (the therapies' outcomes are not transitive). However, if we alter this scenario by having T1 2 D better than T3, we get a mean difference in outcome of 1.33 D and consistent results that order the three therapies as to outcome: T1 > T2 > T3. If each betters every other therapy in half their comparisons and is bettered in the other half, we have the inconsistent results of our first scenario. If the comparisons yield consistent results analogous to those of our second scenario, we get interpretable standings that order the set of therapies. The point is that we are not interested in awarding prizes contest by contest, comparison by comparison.… We need to scale the therapies on outcome, not to estimate a mean difference between all pairs of therapies. (Howard et al., 1997, p. 221–222)

Scaling therapies according to their efficacy, as recommended by Howard et al., is clearly desirable, provided that such a scaling is possible. If the contextual model is true, and all therapies produce generally equivalent outcomes, it is not possible to create an ordering that makes sense. As Howard et al. noted, if the true effect size for the difference between two treatments is zero, then half the studies would show an effect size favoring one treatment and the other half would show an effect size favoring the other (assuming the unlikely case that the sample means for the two groups are exactly equal). A true effect size for the difference of zero will result in many intransitive relationships, as differences obtained will be due to chance. Thus scaling therapies makes sense if and only if there are true differences among therapies. Given the consistent results of several meta-analyses indicating that uniform efficacy is pervasive, it does not make sense to attempt to scale therapies along an efficacy continuum. In a subsequent meta-analysis reviewed in this chapter, the intransitivity issue becomes apparent.

Meta-Analyses in Specific Areas

The possibility that there exists a subset of studies that show nonzero differences among treatments was discussed earlier. Briefly, meta-analyses in various areas are reviewed toward finding particular subsets that demonstrate consistent relative efficacy. Moreover, review of these meta-analyses will demonstrate issues related to (a) confounding due to variables such as allegiance, (b) lack of direct comparisons, and (c) classification and multiple comparisons.

Depression.   Because of the focus on depression in this book (see chap. 2), evidence in this area is reviewed first. In 1989, Dobson found meta-analytic evidence for the superiority of Beck's cognitive therapy vis-à-vis other treatments. However, that meta-analysis suffered from two problems. First, the primary studies were restricted to those that used the Beck Depression Inventory (BDI; Beck, Ward, Mendelson, & Erbaugh, 1961), a measure that consistently favors a cognitive approach.[2] Second, the allegiance of the investigators was not taken into account. Robinson, Berman, and Neimeyer (1990) attempted to correct these and other problems in earlier meta-analyses in the area of depression.

Robinson et al. (1990) located 58 controlled studies of psychotherapy treatments for depression that were published in 1986 or before. The treatments in these studies were classified as (a) cognitive, (b) behavioral, (c) cognitive–behavioral, and (d) general verbal therapy. The latter category was a collection of psychodynamic, client-centered, and interpersonal therapies. Although many analyses were reported in this meta-analysis, only the direct comparisons of these four types are discussed herein.

The meta-analysis of those studies that directly compared two types of therapy are reported in Table 4.6. Of the six pairwise comparisons, four were statistically significant and relatively large (viz., the magnitude of the significant comparisons ranged from .24 to .47). However, these differences could well be due to allegiance. Robinson et al. (1990) rated the allegiance, based on the nature of the report but also on prior publications of the investigators, and controlled for this variable. When allegiance was controlled, the estimate of the effect size disappeared, as shown in the last column of Table 4.6. Clearly, treatment class and allegiance are confounded and thus interpretation is difficult. Nevertheless, this meta-analysis indicated that there were no treatment differences that cannot be explained by the allegiance of the researcher (see chap. 7 for a more complete discussion of this meta-analysis).

---

[2]The bias of the BDI is suggested by an examination of the items, many of which refer to cognitions. However, empirical evidence is provided by D. A. Shapiro et al.'s (1994) study of cognitive–behavioral and psychodynamic–interpersonal therapies. Of the eight outcome measures, the *F* values for 6 of the differences were less than 1.00, indicating that there were absolutely no differences between the treatments. The BDI, however, produced a large effect in favor of the cognitive–behavioral treatment. Further evidence for the cognitive bias of the BDI is revealed in a meta-analysis that found that changes in cognitive style fostered by psychotherapy are related to decreases in depression, as measured by the BDI, but not by other measures of depression (Oei & Free, 1995).

TABLE 4.6

Direct Comparisons Between Different Types of Psychotherapy
for Depression as Determined by Robinson, Berman, and Neimeyer (1990)

		Effect Size[a]		
Comparison	N of Studies	M	SD	Estimate If No Allegiance
Cognitive vs. behavioral	12	0.12	0.33	0.12
Cognitive vs. cognitive–behavioral	4	−0.03	0.24	−0.03
Behavioral vs. cognitive–behavioral	8	−0.24*	0.20	−0.16
Cognitive vs. general verbal	7	0.47*	0.30	−0.15
Behavioral vs. general verbal	14	0.27*	0.33	0.15
Cognitive–behavioral vs. general verbal	8	0.37*	0.38	0.09

Note. Means, standard deviations, and standard errors are based on weighted least-squares analyses in which effect sizes were weighted by sample size. From "Psychotherapy for the Treatment of Depression: A Comprehensive Review of Controlled Outcome Research," by L. A. Robinson, J. S. Berman, and R. A. Neimeyer, 1990, *Psychological Bulletin, 108,* p. 35. Copyright © 1990 by the American Psychological Association. Adapted with permission.

[a]Positive numbers indicate that the first therapy in the comparison was more effective; negative numbers indicate that the second therapy in the comparison was more effective.

*$p < .05$.

In a later meta-analysis that investigated relative efficacy of treatments for depression and allegiance, Gaffan, Tsaousis, and Kemp-Wheeler (1995) reanalyzed the studies reviewed by Dobson (1989) and 35 additional studies published before 1995. All studies compared cognitive therapy for depression to another treatment. In keeping with Dobson (1989), only the BDI was analyzed. Although the decision to use only the BDI could be criticized as favoring cognitive therapy, as it is a measure heavily loaded with items related to thoughts, it does serve the purpose of eliminating dependencies among effect size measures within studies. Table 4.7 presents the results of Gaffan et al.'s analyses.

Before discussing the evidence with regard to relative efficacy presented by Gaffan et al. (1995), it should be noted that the effect sizes for the additional studies were nearly equal to values found generally for psychotherapy. For example, the comparison to waiting-list controls yielded an effect size of 0.89, compared with the global value of 0.80 determined in chapter 3. As shown in chapter 5, the value of 0.56 for comparison to attention controls is within the neighborhood for the value derived for such comparisons generally. Gaffan et al. (1995) speculated that the larger values for these two comparisons in Dobson's (1989) analysis might be due to the likelihood of submission for publication of large effects in earlier years, enthusiasm of pioneers of cognitive therapy, decreasing experience and expertise of cognitive therapists, and increasingly unpromising clients treated in primary studies.

The important effect sizes for the estimation of relative efficacy are the comparisons of cognitive therapy to behavioral therapy, other psychotherapy, and variants of cognitive therapy. Generally these comparisons yielded relatively small effects (magnitudes in the range of 0.03 to 0.34) and nonsignificant differences (only one of the six effect sizes was statistically significant). The effect sizes for the comparison to behavioral therapy for the two samples were in opposite directions (viz., 0.23 for the Dobson studies, indicating superiority of cognitive therapy, and −0.33 in the later studies, indicating superiority of behavioral therapy). Given that neither of these effects were significant, the most perspicuous explanation is that these values were random fluctuations. It should be noted that these differences are not adjusted for allegiance. Nevertheless, this meta-analysis showed nonsignificant advantages for cognitive therapy.

TABLE 4.7

Cognitive Therapy Versus Other Therapies for Depression
(Gaffan, Tsaousis, & Kemp-Wheeler, 1995)

	Dobson (1989) Studies		*Additional Studies*	
Comparison	*No. of Studies*	*Effect Size*	*No. of Studies*	*Effect Size*
Cognitive therapy vs.				
Waiting-list control	7	1.56**	11	0.89**
Attention control	6	0.72*	3	0.56*
Behavioral therapy	10	0.27	4	−0.33
Other psychotherapy	6	0.23	12	0.34*
Standard vs. variant cognitive therapy	8	−0.25	11	−0.03

Note. Effect size are aggregates for the comparison weighted by inverse of variance, as described in chapter 2. Positive effect sizes indicate that cognitive therapy is superior or that standard cognitive therapy is superior (when compared with variant; see last row). From "Researcher Allegiance and Meta-Analysis: The Case of Cognitive Therapy for Depression," by E. A. Gaffan, I. Tsaousis, and S. M. Kemp-Wheeler, 1995, *Journal of Consulting and Clinical Psychology, 63*, pp. 970, 974. Copyright © 1995 by the American Psychological Association. Adapted with permission.

*p < .05.

**p < .05.

The one statistically significant comparison between cognitive therapy and other psychotherapies in the additional studies needs further scrutiny. One of the essential features of the contextual model is that treatments are intended to be therapeutic and that they be based on psychological principles, as stipulated in the definition of psychotherapy given in chapter 1. Consider some of the 12 comparison therapies classified as "other psychotherapies." One psychotherapy was pastoral counseling, which was described as follows:

> Each session [included] approximately 75% of the time spent in nondirective listening and 25% of the time spent in discussing bible verses or religious themes that might relate to the patients' concerns. Parallel to the CBT treatments, homework was assigned. In the [pastoral counseling], however, this consisted of merely making a list of concerns to be discussed in the subsequent session. (Propst, Ostrom, Watkins, Dean, & Mashburn, 1992, p. 96)

Clearly, this treatment is not based on psychological principles and would not be considered a treatment intended to be therapeutic. Another treatment in this class was supportive, self-directive therapy, which was provided over the telephone by nonexperts, and involved bibliotherapy; therapists comments were restricted to "reflection of feelings, clarifications, and information seeking" (Beutler & Clarkin, 1990, p. 335). This therapy does not fit the definition of psychotherapy used in this book because there was no face-to-face interactions, the therapists were not trained, and the treatment was not based on psychological principles.[3] A third therapy classified as "other psychotherapy" was an exercise group. The point here is simple: It is meaningless to claim that the specific ingredients in cognitive therapy are responsible for the resultant benefits by showing that cognitive therapy is superior to pastoral counseling, supportive and self-directive therapy, exercise, or other treatments that plainly are not psychotherapy. Care must be exercised here because, as a general rule in this book, deleting studies from a meta-analysis because they do not support a position is discouraged. Nevertheless, comparisons of treatments intended to be therapeutic (e.g., cognitive therapy) to treatments that are not intended to be therapeutic and do not fit the definition of psychotherapy, particularly when the study is conducted by advocates of the former, cannot be used to establish the existence of specific effects.

The standard versus variants of cognitive therapy in Gaffan et al.'s (1995) meta-analysis is interesting because adding or removing components or changing the format of cognitive therapy does not seem to affect the efficacy of the treatment. This result is discussed further in chapter 5.

---

[3]Interestingly, for some types of patients, supportive, self-directed therapy was the most efficacious treatment.

A meta-analysis of cognitive therapy for depression by Gloaguen, Cottraux, Cucherat, and Blackburn (1998) is noteworthy because it is recent and because it used the state-of-the art meta-analytic procedures developed by Hedges and Olkin (1985, see also chap. 2). Gloaguen et al. reviewed all controlled clinical trials published from 1977 to 1996 that involved comparisons of cognitive therapy for the treatment of depression to other types of treatments for depression. All 48 studies that met the inclusion criteria used the BDI; to standardize the comparisons and to avoid nonindependent effect sizes, Gloaguen et al. restricted evaluation of outcome to this measure of depression. Moreover, effect sizes were computed from direct comparisons, eliminating many confounds. Effect sizes were adjusted for bias, aggregation was accomplished by weighting by the inverse of the estimated variance, and homogeneity of effect sizes was determined (see Hedges and Olkin, 1985; chap. 2). When compared with behavior therapies, the aggregate effect size was 0.05, which was not statistically significant. The 13 effect sizes derived from these comparison were homogenous, indicating a consistency that provides confidence in the conclusion that cognitive and behavior therapies of depression are equally effective, as there does not appear to be any moderating influences. However, cognitive therapy did appear to be superior to the class of "other therapies" (aggregate effect size for the 22 such comparisons was 0.24, which was significantly different from zero, $p < .01$), but the effects were still small (see chap. 2 and Table 2.4). However, the effect sizes were heterogenous, indicating that there was a moderating variable affecting the results.

The "other therapies" in Gloaguen et al.'s (1998) meta-analysis consisted of therapies that were not intended to therapeutic (e.g., supportive counseling, phone counseling) as well as therapies that were intended to be therapeutic. Wampold, Minami, Baskin, and Tierney (in press) hypothesized that the heterogeneity of the cognitive therapy–"other therapies" contrast was due to the fact that "other therapies" contained treatments intended to be therapeutic (i.e., bona fide therapies) and those not intended to be therapeutic (i.e., not bona fide) and that when cognitive therapy was compared with bona fide other therapies, the effect size would be zero, consistent with the Dodo bird conjecture. Indeed, when cognitive therapy was compared with bona fide therapies, the null hypothesis that the effect size was zero could not be rejected; when an outlier was eliminated, the aggregate effect size for this comparison was negligible (viz., 0.03). As expected, cognitive therapy was superior to treatments that were not bona fide (i.e., were essentially control groups). The results of Gloaguen et al.'s results and Wampold et al.'s re-analysis convincingly demonstrate that all treatments of depression that are intended to be therapeutic are uniformly efficacious.

CBT has been the established therapy for depression since 1979. The meta-analyses reviewed earlier indicate that, generally, cognitive therapies do not produce statistically different outcomes from other therapies, although in some cases the null results appeared only after allegiance was controlled. The most perspicuous difference appears to be between cognitive therapy and verbal therapies, although as was pointed out, the verbal therapies often contain treatments that do not fit the definition of psychotherapy (e.g., are not intended to be therapeutic). However, the verbal therapies that are intended to be the therapeutic appear to be as efficacious as cognitive therapy, the generally accepted standard. The question is thus, In a fair test between cognitive therapy and a bona fide verbal therapy, delivered by advocates of the respective therapies (i.e., controlling allegiance), would cognitive therapy be superior? This question was addressed directly in the National Institute of Mental Health Treatment of Depression Collaborative Research Program (NIMH TDCRP; Elkin, 1994), which was the first attempt in psychotherapy to conduct the analogue of the collaborative clinical trial used in medical studies.

The NIMH TDCRP compared four treatments for depression: CBT, interpersonal psychotherapy (IPT), imipramine plus clinical management, and pill-placebo plus clinical management. The contrast between CBT and IPT provided a good test of the relative efficacy of cognitive and verbal therapies. CBT was conducted according to the manual generally used for this treatment (Beck et al., 1979) and thus represents the prototypic cognitive therapy for depression. IPT, which is based on assisting the client to gain understanding of his or her interpersonal problems and to develop adaptive strategies for relating to others, was conducted according to the manual developed by Klerman, Weissman, Rounsaville, and Chevron (1984). IPT, which is a derivative of dynamic therapy, is an instance of a "dynamic therapy," "verbal therapy," or "other psychotherapy," depending on the type of classification scheme used. The specific ingredients of the two therapies were distinctive and readily discriminated (Hill, O'Grady, & Elkin, 1992).

The treatments were delivered at three sites (hence the classification as a *collaborative* study), thereby decreasing the possibility that the results were due to idiosyncracies of a particular site. The therapists, 8 in CBT and 10 in IPT, were experienced in their respective treatments, resulting in a design in which therapists are nested within treatments (see chap. 8). Moreover, therapists were trained and supervised by experts in the respective treatments. Finally, therapists adhered to the respective treatments. Given these therapist design aspects, it would appear that allegiance effects would be minimal.

The results for three overlapping samples of participants are considered in this section. The first sample was composed of the 84 clients who completed therapy (called the "completer" sample); the second sample was composed of the 105 participants who were exposed to the treatment for at least 3.5

weeks (called the "end point 204" sample because there were 204 participants in all four groups), and the third sample was composed of all 239 clients who entered treatment (called the "end point 239" sample because 239 participants entered the trial altogether). The relatively large number of participants provided good estimates of the relative efficacy of CBT and IPT. All participants met diagnostic criteria for a current episode of major depressive disorder. Outcome relative to depression was assessed with four measures: the Hamilton Rating Scale for Depression; the Global Assessment Scale; the BDI; and the Hopkins Symptom Checklist-90 Total Score.

The results for the three samples are provided in Table 4.8. In spite of the large samples, none of the differences between the treatments vaguely approached significance. Effect sizes for each variable and aggregate effect size[4] for each sample are presented in Table 4.8. The recovery rates for the completers, based on the Hamilton Rating Scale for Depression and the BDI are presented in Table 4.9.

The effect sizes for relative efficacy are minuscule by any standard; similarly, the difference between the recovery rates are small. Examining the effect sizes for this study can make a poignant point about relative efficacy. The aggregate effect size for the completers favored IPT by 0.13 standard deviation units; for individual variables the effect sizes ranged in magnitude from 0.02 to 0.29. These effect sizes translated into small and nonsignificant differences in recovery rates. In this study, effect sizes that ranged up to 0.29 were associated with nonsignificant and trivial differences in means as well as recovery rates. From that perspective, an upper bound in the neighborhood of 0.20 for the effect size for relative efficacy generally translates into differences that are inconsequential theoretically or clinically. In chapter 8, it will be shown that although the effects due to relative efficacy are small, they are inflated by therapist differences—that is, true treatment differences are even smaller than they appear.

Although there were criticisms of the NIMH TDCRP (e.g., Elkin et al., 1996; Jacobson & Hollon, 1996a, 1996b; Klein, 1996), it is the most comprehensive clinical trial ever conducted and one that provided a fair and valid test of relative efficacy of a cognitive and a verbal, dynamic therapy for depression. The meta-analyses and the NIMH TDCRP have provided convincing evidence that uniform efficacy exists in the area of depression. Given the prevalence of depression and the preponderance of treatments specific to depression, the Dodo bird effect in this area has important implications for delivery of services (see chap. 9) as well as providing evidence for differentiating the contextual and medical models.

---

[4]Aggregation was accomplished using the method developed by Hedges and Olkin (1985, pp. 212–213) and assuming that the correlation between pairs of measures was .50 (see Wampold, Mondin, Moody, Stich, et al., 1997).

TABLE 4.8

Comparison of Cognitive–Behavioral Treatment and Interpersonal
Psychotherapy for Depression—NIMH Treatment of Depression Collaborative
Research Program

Measure	Cognitive–Behavioral Treatment			Interpersonal Psychotherapy			Effect Size[a]
	N	M	SD	N	M	SD	
Completer Clients							
HRSD	37	7.6	5.8	47	6.9	5.8	−0.12
GAS	37	69.4	11.0	47	70.7	11.0	−0.12
BDI	37	10.2	8.7	47	7.7	8.6	−0.29
HSCL-90 T	37	0.47	0.43	47	0.48	0.43	0.02
Aggregate[b]							−0.13
End Point 204 Clients							
HRSD	50	9.0	7.0	55	9.1	7.0	0.01
GAS	50	66.5	12.6	55	67.2	12.6	−0.06
BDI	50	11.5	9.7	55	10.6	9.7	−0.09
HSCL-90 T	50	0.60	0.49	55	0.60	0.50	0.00
Aggregate[b]							−0.03
End Point 239 Clients							
HRSD	59	10.7	7.9	61	9.8	7.9	−0.11
GAS	59	64.4	12.4	61	66.3	12.4	−0.15
BDI	59	13.4	10.6	61	12.0	10.6	−0.13
HSCL-90 T	59	0.73	0.57	61	0.71	0.57	−0.03
Aggregate[b]							−0.11

Note. HRSD = Hamilton Rating Scale for Depression; GAS = Global Assessment Scale; BDI = Beck Depression Inventory; HSCL-90 T = Hopkins Symptom Checklist-90 Total Scores.

From "National Institute of Mental Health Treatment of Depression Collaborative Research Program: General Effectiveness of Treatments," by I. Elkin, T. Shea, J. T. Watkins, S. D. Imber, S. M. Sotsky, J. F. Collins, D. R. Glass, P. A. Pilkonis, W. R. Leber, J. P. Docherty, S. J. Fiester, and M. B. Parloff, 1989, *Archives of General Psychiatry, 46*, 971–982.

[a]Positive values indicate superiority of cognitive–behavioral treatment.

[b]Aggregate formed assuming correlations among dependent measures was .50 (see Wampold, Mondin, Moody, Stich, et al., 1997, for explanation).

TABLE 4.9

Comparison of Recovery Rates for Completers for Cognitive–Behavioral
Treatment and Interpersonal Psychotherapy for Depression—NIMH
Treatment of Depression Collaborative Research Program

Scale	Cognitive–Behavioral Treatment (N = 37)		Interpersonal Psychotherapy (N =47)	
	Number Recovered	*Percentage Recovered*	*Number Recovered*	*Percentage Recovered*
HRSD ≤ 6	19	51	26	55
BDI ≤ 9	24	65	33	70

Note. For HRSD, X^2 (1, N = 84) = 0.13, p = .72. For BDI, X^2 (1, N = 84) = 0.27, p = .60
HRSD = Hamilton Rating Scale for Depression; BDI = Beck Depression Inventory. From "The
NIMH Treatment of Depression Collaborative Research Program: Where We Began and Where We
Are," by I. Elkin. In A. E. Bergin, and S. L. Garfield (Eds.), *Handbook of Psychotherapy and Behavior
Change* (p. 121), 1994, New York: Wiley. Copyright © 1994 by John Wiley and Sons. Adapted by
permission of John Wiley & Sons, Inc.

Anxiety.   Since the demonstration that fear reactions in animals and
humans could be induced experimentally (see chap. 1), behavioral therapists have contended that various techniques imbedded in the classical
conditioning paradigm would be effective in the treatment of anxiety disorders. The most perspicuous therapeutic ingredient thought to lead to the
reduction of anxiety is exposure to the feared stimulus. Although there are
many variations of exposure techniques, exposure is a central component
of behavioral treatments of anxiety. Recently, however, cognitive treatments for anxiety have been developed; these treatments are based on the
notion that the appraisal of the reaction to the feared stimuli is critical and
that altering such appraisals is therapeutic. Cognitive–behavioral treatments combine techniques for altering cognitions with some behavioral
techniques. Outcome studies in the area of anxiety have focused primarily
on behavioral, cognitive, and cognitive–behavioral techniques.

Because behavioral and cognitive perspectives on anxiety rely on distinct
theoretical models, data on relative efficacy of outcomes in this area provides
important evidence about specific effects. A number of meta-analyses have
addressed relative efficacy of cognitive and behavioral treatments of anxiety,
as well as some other treatments (Abramowitz, 1996, 1997; Chambless &
Gillis, 1993; Clum, Clum, & Surls, 1993; Mattick, Andrews, Dusan, &
Christensen, 1990; Sherman, 1998; Taylor, 1996; van Balkom et al., 1994);
the results of these various meta-analyses are presented in Table 4.10.

Before reviewing the results of the various meta-analyses, several limitations should be noted. First, because many of the outcome studies of anxiety

TABLE 4.10

Summary of Meta-Analyses of the Relative Efficacy of Psychological Treatments of Anxiety

Author	Year	Direct Comparisons	Effect Size Type	Disorder	Treatments Compared	Results
Mattick, Andrews, Hadsi-Pavlovick, & Christensen	1990	No	Post vs. pre	Agoraphobia Panic	Various behavioral CT	Panic: EXP > no EXP Phobia: EXP > anxiety management + EXP No differences on anxiety or depression
Chambless & Gillis	1993	No	Post vs. pre or Tx vs. control (when control existed)	GAD Social phobia Agoraphobia Panic	CBT Behavioral	CBT = Behavioral (including EXP) in most instances
Clum, Clum, & Surls	1993	Some	Tx vs. control	Panic	Flooding Psychological coping Exposure Combination	No differences
van Balkom et al.	1994	No	Post vs. pre	OCD	CT Behavioral	No differences among various behavioral approaches Differences between CBT and behavioral not tested
Taylor	1996	No	Post vs. pre	Social phobia	EXP CT CT + EXP Social skills training	No differences

Abramowitz	1996	No	Post vs. pre	OCD	Various ERP	Some differences (see textual discussion)
Abramowitz	1997	Yes	Tx A vs. Tx B	OCD	ERP CT Components of ERP	No differences
Sherman	1998	No	Tx vs. control	PTSD	CBT CT EMDR Others	Treatments produce homogeneous outcomes (i.e., no treatment differences)

Note. Tx = Treatment; TxA = Treatment A; TxB = Treatment B; CBT = Cognitive behavioral treatment; EXP = Exposure; CT = Cognitive therapy; ERP = Exposure and response prevention; EMDR = Eye movement desensitization and reprocessing; GAD = Generalized anxiety disorder; OCD = Obsessive–compulsive disorder; PTSD = Posttraumatic stress disorder.

are uncontrolled (i.e., do not contain a control group), the effect sizes were typically calculated by comparing the posttest with the pretest; that is, (posttest mean–pretest mean)/standard deviation. Such effect sizes are inflated by regression toward the mean, as participants selected on the basis of extreme scores (as is the case with all studies of anxious individuals) will tend to score closer to the mean on the posttest in the absence of treatment (see Campbell & Kenny, 1999, for an excellent discussion of regression artifacts). More troublesome, however, is that only two of the meta-analyses examined direct comparisons of various treatments (viz., Abramowitz, 1997; Clum et al., 1993), leaving the conclusions of the other meta-analyses suspect because indirect comparisons are ubiquitously confounded with variables such as allegiance. None of the meta-analyses using indirect comparisons attempted to model allegiance or other confounds. Another problematic aspect is that the meta-analytic methods used did not take advantage of the statistical theory underlying the effect size statistics; few tests of homogeneity were conducted, and tests of average effect sizes and differences among treatments were not based on the sampling distributions of the statistics. Consequently, results from these meta-analyses must be interpreted cautiously. Finally, it should be noted that primary studies of various treatments, particularly those that directly compare two bona fide psychological treatments, are sparse. For example, one of the most recent meta-analyses presented in Table 4.10, the Abramowitz analysis (1997), examined direct comparisons of psychological treatment for obsessive–compulsive disorders, but was based on only six effect sizes derived from five studies.

Generally, as shown in Table 4.10, the meta-analyses yielded few differences among psychological treatments. The results of these meta-analyses are briefly discussed in this section, in chronological order.

Mattick et al. (1990), on the basis of a meta-analytic review of treatments for panic and agoraphobia, concluded that exposure treatments were superior to nonexposure treatments for panic disorder and that exposure treatments were superior to anxiety management combined with exposure for phobia. These conclusions, however, were not based on direct comparisons, but rather were derived from effect sizes based on posttests versus pretests, and they were either not tested statistically or were based on flawed statistical tests. Moreover, no differences were found on measures of anxiety or depression. Finally, the superiority of exposure treatments for panic disorder was not replicated in Chambless and Gillis's (1993) or Clum et al.'s (1993) reviews.

Chambless and Gillis (1993) examined the efficacy of cognitive therapy for a variety of anxiety disorders. Although effect sizes for cognitive therapy were calculated, comparisons of cognitive therapy with behavior therapy were made heuristically. Nevertheless, the authors made the following conclusions:

The findings from our review of studies on generalized anxiety disorder, panic disorder–agoraphobia, and social phobia demonstrate that CBT is an effective treatment for these disorders.... In general, CBT's effects equal and sometimes surpass those of behavior therapy without explicit cognitive components. The exception appears to be brief CBT excluding exposure instructions for highly avoidant clients with agoraphobia, for which there is a poor track record. (Chambless & Gillis, 1993, p. 256)

Clum et al.'s (1993) meta-analysis, which involved the use of direct comparisons among treatments, found no differences among psychological treatments of panic disorder. Moreover, when exposure was considered a control group, nonsignificant differences between psychological treatments and exposure were found.

van Balkom et al. (1994) meta-analyzed treatments of obsessive–compulsive disorder using effect sizes from posttests versus pretests. Unfortunately, there were very few effect sizes derived from cognitive treatments reviewed (three or less, depending on class of outcome measure); although effect sizes derived from behavioral treatments were generally larger than those for cognitive treatments, the authors did not test for differences. Behavioral treatments were classified as (a) self-controlled exposure in vivo, (b) therapist-controlled exposure in vivo, (c) spouse-controlled exposure in vivo, (d) thought stopping, or (e) miscellaneous (response prevention only, imaginal exposure, and modeling). No differences among the four classes of behavioral treatments were found.

Taylor (1996), using posttest–pretest effect sizes, compared the efficacy of treatments for social phobia. Treatments were classified as (a) exposure, (b) cognitive therapy, (c) cognitive therapy combined with exposure, and (d) social-skills training. No differences were found when the treatments were pairwise compared.

Abramowitz (1996) meta-analytically examined the efficacy of variation of exposure and response prevention treatments of obsessive–compulsive disorders using posttest–pretest effect sizes. It was found that for obsessive–compulsive symptoms, therapist-controlled exposure was superior to self-controlled exposure, and total response prevention was superior to partial response prevention, although there were no differences between in vivo and in vivo combined with imaginal exposure or between gradual exposure and flooding. For general anxiety symptoms, therapist-controlled exposure was again superior to self-controlled exposure; as well, in vivo plus imaginal exposure was superior to in vivo exposure. No differences were found for depression. Ambrowitz noted that the superiority of therapist-controlled exposure possibly provides evidence for general effects: "It is likely that a therapist's presence adds nonspecific effects to treatment in that coaching and support from a caring individual may put a person more at ease during exposure" (pp. 594–595).

Another meta-analysis reviewed herein examined direct comparisons of treatments for obsessive–compulsive disorder. Abramowitz (1997) reviewed comparisons among exposure and response prevention, cognitive therapy, and components of exposure and response prevention (i.e., either exposure alone or response prevention alone).[5] No differences among any pair of treatments were found.

The final meta-analysis examined is laudatory for its test of homogeneity. Sherman (1998) examined all controlled studies of treatments of posttraumatic stress disorder (PTSD). The predominant treatments were behavioral and cognitive behavioral, but also included psychodynamic, hypnotherapy, the Koach program, anger management, eye movement desensitization and reprogramming, adventure-based activities, psychodrama, and the Coatsville PTSD program. Effect sizes were calculated from treatment-versus-control contrasts and were derived from aggregating over the dependent variables in the individual studies and by aggregating within classes of dependent variables (viz., intrusion, avoidance, hyperarousal, anxiety, and depression). When one outlier, with an unrealistic effect size of 8.40, was eliminated, the remaining effect sizes derived from aggregating over all dependent variables within a study were found to be homogenous. The only target variable that showed heterogeneity was hyperarousal, which was attributed to the variety of methods used to assess this construct. The pervasive homogeneity across the various treatments demonstrated that treatments are producing consistent effects. Given the variety of treatments reviewed, the evidence produced by this meta-analysis is consistent with the hypothesis that treatments for PTSD are generally equivalent regardless of their specific ingredients. However, it should be noted that most of the treatments involved some type of exposure (broadly defined) to the traumatic event.

In total, it appears that there is little evidence that any one treatment for any one anxiety disorder is superior to any other. Exposure, a procedure imbedded in the classical conditioning paradigm, is often thought to be critical to the treatment of various anxiety disorders. However, the meta-analyses reviewed herein discovered little evidence that would suggest that this is the case. It appears that the cognitive therapies and exposure are equally effective. However, it should be noted that cognitive therapies and exposure therapies often contain overlapping elements. For example, if in cognitive therapy, clients discuss the feared stimulus, then the clients are experiencing an imaginal representation of the event, which could be interpreted as imaginal exposure.

Tarrier et al. (1999), recognizing that cognitive therapy and exposure are typically confounded, sought to compare cognitive therapy and exposure,

---

[5]Exposure-response prevention was also compared with relaxation, but relaxation in these studies was used as a control group and did not meet the definition of psychotherapy used in this book.

in which there were no overlapping aspects of the treatments, for the treatment of chronic PTSD. This study fits the evidentiary category of an exemplary study that addresses directly an important question relative to the contextual model–medical model question. In this study, participants were stratified on trauma category and randomly assigned to cognitive therapy or imaginal exposure. Cognitive therapy was "aimed to be emotion focused and to elicit patients' beliefs about the meaning of the event and the attributions patients made following it, taking into account their previous belief system, then to identify maladaptive cognitions and patterns of emotions and to modify these" (p. 14). Discussion of the trauma itself was avoided in order to distinguish the treatment from exposure. Imaginal exposure was "trauma focused and aimed to produce habituation of emotional response by instructing the patient to describe the event as if it was happening in the present tense while visualizing it" (p. 15). Treatments lasted 16 sessions. This study found that the patients' assessment of the credibility of the treatment and therapists' ratings of the motivation of the patients did not differ between the two treatments. Although patients generally improved from pretest to posttest, there were no significant differences between the two treatments on any of the seven outcome measures. The results of this study fail to support a specific-ingredient explanation for improvement in the area of posttraumatic stress disorder.

As was the case for depression, there is no convincing evidence that one treatment for any anxiety disorder is superior to another treatment. That is, there is insufficient evidence to reject the Dodo bird conjecture in the area of anxiety, which again supports a contextual model of psychotherapy.

Family and Marital Psychotherapies—The Problems With Multiple Comparisons.   The ubiquitous strategy for assessing relative efficacy is to classify treatments and compare the relative effect sizes for pairs of classes (Wampold, Mondin, Moody, Stich, et al., 1997, being the notable exception). One of the ambiguities that results from this strategy is that there are multiple tests of differences—one for each of the $J(J-1)/2$ comparisons, where J is the number of classes—which escalates the error rates. The typical meta-analysis has found a few of the $J(J-1)/2$ comparisons statistically significant. The question is, are the few significant differences due to chance or to true differences in efficacy?

The problems with multiple comparisons is illustrated by examining the results of a meta-analysis of family and marital psychotherapies conducted by Shadish et al. (1993). Shadish et al. (1993) retrieved 163 studies of family and marital psychotherapy, of which 105 contained comparisons of two or more treatments. The effect sizes for the comparisons among six marital and family orientations are presented in Table 4.11. Descriptions of the orientations are found in Shadish et al. (1993) and are consistent with generally accepted definitions of the orientations; the "unclassified orientation" contained bibliotherapies "as well as treatments that were not defined clearly enough to classify elsewhere" (p. 994).

Of the 15 comparisons, 3 were statistically significant. There are two problems that render interpretation of the three statistically significant results difficult, if not impossible. First, multiple comparisons escalate error rates. In this study, the criterion for statistical significance was set at .05; that is, α = Prob (Type I error) = 0.05 for each comparison of two therapies. However, the probability that there is one or more Type I errors in J independent comparisons is given by the following (see Hays, 1988):

$$\textbf{Prob (one or more Type I errors)} = 1 - (1 - \alpha)^J,$$

which, for the 15 comparisons of marital and family therapy orientations, is as follows:

$$\textbf{Prob (one or more Type I errors)} = 1 - (0.95)^{15} = 0.54.$$

However, the 15 comparisons are not independent, which escalates the error rate further. The upper bound for error rate of J nonindependent multiple comparisons is Ja (Hays, 1988), which in this case is $(15)(0.05) = 0.75$. Thus, in the 15 comparisons in Table 4.11,

TABLE 4.11

Relative Efficacy of Various Marital and Family Psychotherapeutic Orientations Expressed in Effect Size Units, as Reported by Shadish et al. (1993)

Orientation	1	2	3	4	5	6
Behavioral		−0.10	0.25	−0.10	0.25[a]	0.37[a]
Systemic			0.00	−0.05	−0.04	0.14
Humanistic				0.00	−0.12	−0.08
Psychodynamic					0.00	−0.02
Eclectic						−0.55[a]
Unclassified						

Note. Positive effect sizes indicate that the row orientation produced better posttest effects than the column orientation; negative effect sizes indicate the opposite. From "Effects of Family and Marital Psychotherapies: A Meta-Analysis," by W. R. Shadish, L. M. Montgomery, P. Wilson, M. R. Wilson, I. Bright, and M. R. Okwumabua, 1993, *Journal of Consulting and Clinical Psychology, 61*, p. 998. Copyright © 1993 by the American Psychological Association. Adapted with permission.

[a]Effect size significantly different from zero at $p < 0.05$.

0.54 ≤ Prob (One or more Type I errors) ≤ 0.75.

That is, in common language, one or more of the statistically significant comparisons likely was due to chance. This extraordinarily high error rate casts a pall over any interpretation of differences. No one would accept a medical treatment given the fact that the study that established its efficacy had up to a 75% chance of yielding an incorrect conclusion.

The second problem revolves around the consistency of the three specific comparisons that were statistically significant. Consider ordering the three orientations along an efficacy continuum, as suggested by Howard et al. (1997). This ordering can be accomplished with two anchors. If the behavioral orientation is the anchor, then the ordering is, from most efficacious to least efficacious, behavioral, eclectic, and unclassified, as shown in Figure 4.2. Behavioral treatments are 0.37 effect size units better than unclassified treatments and 0.25 effect size units better than eclectic treatments, making eclectic treatments 0.12 effect size units better than unclassified treatments. However, if eclectic treatments are the anchor, the ordering is different. Eclectic treatments are 0.25 effect size units worse than behavioral treatments and 0.55 effect size units worse than unclassified treatments, making unclassified treatments 0.30 effect size units better than behavioral. In one ordering, unclassified treatments are the least efficacious of the three, and in the other ordering they are the most efficacious. The three significant comparisons display intransitive relationships, casting doubt on the believability of the estimates of effect sizes for differences. The fact that the probability that one or more of these significant relationships occurred by chance provides an explanation for this intransitivity.

The comparisons of marital and family psychotherapies in Table 4.11 illustrate the problems inherent in trying to establish relative efficacy by classifying treatments and comparing classes. The typical outcome, seen over and over again in meta-analyses that use such a strategy, is that a few of the multiple comparisons were statistically significant. However, as has been illustrated, interpretation of these few statistically significant findings is perilous and should be avoided. Howard et al. (1997) have suggested ordering treatments by their relative efficacy. If the true difference between treatments is zero (i.e., the Dodo bird conjecture is true), as it appears to be, then occasionally significant differences will be found, either at the primary study or meta-analytic level, but these differences will be inconsistent.

CONCLUSIONS

In 1936, Rosenzweig speculated that "all methods of therapy when competently used are equally successful" (p. 413). In the 1970s and 1980s the evidence from initial meta-analyses were consistent with Rosenzweig's

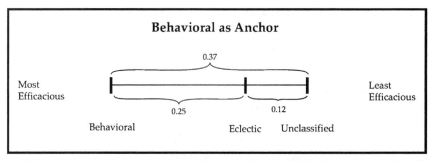

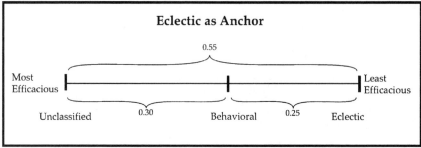

FIG. 4.2. Two orderings derived from multiple comparisons of marital and family psychotherapies.

conjecture. In the 1990s exemplary studies and methodologically sound meta-analyses unfailingly produced evidence that demonstrated that there were small, if not zero, differences among treatments. These results generalized to the subpopulations of treatments for depression and anxiety, two areas where behaviorally oriented treatments are thought to be particularly appropriate. The Dodo bird conjecture has survived many tests and must be considered "true" until such time as sufficient evidence for its rejection are produced.

The lack of differences among a variety of treatments casts doubt on the hypothesis that specific ingredients are responsible for the benefits of psychotherapy. One would expect that if specific ingredients were indeed remedial, then some of these ingredients would be relatively more beneficial than others. Uniform efficacy of treatments represents the first evidence that the medical model cannot explain the empirical findings in psychotherapy research.

5

Specific Effects: Weak Empirical Evidence That Benefits of Psychotherapy Are Derived From Specific Ingredients

The evidence presented in chapter 3 established that psychotherapy is a remarkably beneficial activity. Proponents of a particular treatment who believe that the specific ingredients of that treatment are necessary to produce client change attribute the success of the treatment primarily to its specific ingredients. In chapter 4, the evidence presented indicated that all bona fide therapies are uniformly efficacious, suggesting that specific ingredients are not critical to the outcomes of the treatments. Nevertheless, uniform efficacy of psychological treatments provides indirect evidence about specific ingredients; in this chapter evidence from research designed to examine directly the effects of specific ingredients is discussed.

Four research designs have been used to examine specific effects: (a) component designs, (b) comparative designs with placebo controls, (c) designs that examine mediating effects, and (d) Person × Treatment interactions. Component designs add or subtract a component containing specific ingredients purported theoretically to lead to beneficial outcomes in order to determine whether the ingredients are indeed efficacious. From an experimental design perspective, component designs are among the most rigorous tests of specificity. Nevertheless, a review of the component studies will show that the specific ingredients are not necessary to achieve the benefits of psychotherapy.

A second research strategy is to control for the incidental aspects of therapy by using placebo controls, which would ideally contain all the incidental aspects but none of the specific ingredients of a treatment. Unfortunately, in psychotherapy research it is impossible to design and implement such controls, as logically placebo controls cannot contain all the common factors of therapy. The logic as well as the results of comparisons with placebos are reviewed.

A third strategy involves testing whether treatments produce the hypothesized mediating effects. Each specific treatment provides an explanation for the disorder, complaint, or problem. If the treatment works through its hypothesized mechanism, then the treatment should affect a theoretically relevant intermediary variable. In turn, the mediating variable should remediate the disorder, complaint, or problem. Although establishment of mediating effects is experimentally difficult, the evidence for mediating processes is generally unconvincing that specific ingredients are operating as proposed by advocates of treatments.

The final strategy for establishing specificity is to examine the interactions of treatments with person characteristics that are theoretically relevant to the treatment. Essentially, if specificity is present, treatments for clients with deficits addressed by the treatment should improve more than clients without such deficits. For example, cognitive treatments should be indicated for clients with established maladaptive thoughts and disordered cognitive schemas, whereas interpersonal therapies should be indicated for clients with social deficits. That is, client deficits should moderate the efficacy of treatments. However, very few studies have produced the hypothesized moderation effects.

COMPONENT STUDIES

Design Issues

One of the most direct methods for identifying whether a given specific therapeutic ingredient leads to beneficial outcomes is to compare an entire treatment with that treatment minus the given specific ingredient, as shown in Figure 5.1. Presumably, the treatment has previously been shown to be efficacious. Therefore, the logic of the design is to "dismantle" the treatment in order to identify those ingredients that are critical to the success of the treatment. Studies that compare a treatment that has been shown to be efficacious with the same treatment minus one or a few critical components have been called *dismantling studies*. In a dismantling study, attenuation of the benefits when a critical specific ingredient is removed provides evidence that the specific ingredient is indeed therapeutic (see Fig. 5.1). Such a result would provide evidence for specific effects and thus be supportive of the medical model of psychotherapy. Borkovec (1990) described the advantages of the dismantling study:

> One crucial feature of the [dismantling] design is that more factors are ordinarily common among the various comparison conditions. In addition to representing equally the potential impact of history, maturation, and so on and the impact of nonspecific factors, a procedural component is held constant between the total package and the control condition containing only that particular element. Such a design approximates more closely the experimental ideal of holding everything but one element constant.... Therapists will usually have greater confidence in, and less hesitancy to administer, a component condition than a pure nonspecific condition. They will also be equivalently trained and have equal experience in the elements relative to the combination of elements in the total package.... At the theoretical level, such outcomes tell what elements of procedure are most actively involved in the change process.... At the applied level, determination of elements that do not contribute to outcome allows therapists to dispense with their use in therapy. (pp. 56–57).

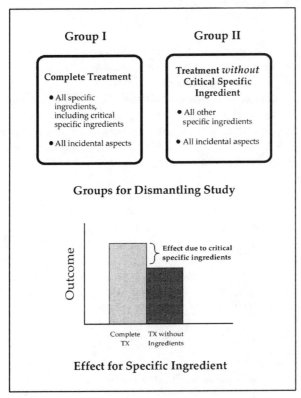

FIG. 5.1.   Dismantling study.

Dismantling studies are discussed thoroughly in clinically oriented research design texts (e.g., Heppner et al., 1999; Kazdin, 1998).

Another strategy to demonstrate specificity is to add an ingredient to an existing treatment package. In this design, which is called an *additive design* (Borkovec, 1990), there typically is a theoretical reason to believe that a specific ingredient will augment the benefits derived from the treatment:

> The goal is ordinarily to develop an even more potent therapy based on empirical or theoretical information that suggests that each therapy [or component] has reason to be partially effective, so that their combination may be superior to either procedure by itself. In terms of design, the [dismantling] and additive approaches are similar. It is partly the direction of reasoning of the investigator and the history of literature associated with the techniques and the diagnostic problem that determine which design strategy seems to be taking place. (Borkovec, 1990, p. 57)

The dismantling and additive designs have the goal of testing the efficacy of a given component or components of a treatment, and consequently they are referred to as component studies.[1] The component added or deleted may contain one or more ingredients, usually theoretically similar in their purported actions.

A prototypic component study was used by Jacobson et al. (1996) to determine what components of CBT are responsible for its established efficacy for the treatment of depression. Jacobson et al. separated CBT into three components: (a) behavioral activation, (b) coping strategies for dealing with depressing events and the automatic thoughts that occur concurrently, and (c) modification of core depressogenic cognitive schema. Participants were randomly assigned to (a) a behavioral activation treatment, (b) a behavioral activation plus coping skills related to automatic thoughts treatment, or (c) the complete cognitive treatment, which included behavioral activation, coping skills, and identification and modification of core dysfunctional schemas. Generally, the results showed equivalence in outcomes across the groups at termination and at follow-up, which casts doubt on the need for the cognitive components of CBT for depression. This study illustrates the logic of the component design; in this case, the evidence did not support the claim that the benefits of CBT for depression are derived from the cognitive components of the treatment, as would be expected in a medical model explanatory context.

---

[1] Some references use the term *component study* to refer specifically to dismantling studies (e.g., Borkovec, 1990). Here the term component study is used generically to include dismantling and additive designs.

Meta-Analytic Reviews of Component Studies

Ahn and Wampold (in press) conducted a meta-analysis of component studies of psychotherapeutic treatments that appeared in the literature between 1970 and 1998. They located 27 comparisons that attempted to isolate a specific component in order to test whether that component produced effects above those produced by the same treatment without the component. The 27 comparisons are shown in Table 5.1

For each study, an effect size was calculated by comparing the outcomes for the two groups (treatment vs. treatment without component) aggregated over the dependent variables within the study (see Wampold, Mondin, Moody, Stich, et al., 1997; also chap. 4). Then the aggregate effect size across the 27 studies was calculated using methods discussed by Hedges and Olkin (1985; see also chap. 2). The aggregate effect size was found to be equal to –0.20. Although the effect size was in the opposite direction of what was predicted, it was not statistically different from zero. Moreover, the effect sizes were homogeneous, suggesting that there were no moderating variables affecting the results. Thus, adding or removing a purportedly effective component does not increase the benefit of psychotherapeutic treatments as would be expected if the specific ingredients were remedial, as predicted by the medical model.

In a meta-analysis of allegiance effects in treatments of depression, Gaffan et al. (1995) found evidence related to the components of CBT for depression. Gaffan et al. compared the efficacy of standard CBT and variant CBT. Standard CBT was defined as "cognitive–behavioral therapy following the Beck et al. (1979) manual or closely similar techniques, given individually" (p. 967), and variant CBT was defined as " therapy described as 'cognitive' by the authors of the study, but deviating in one or more ways from the standard form … or having usual elements removed" (p. 967). Gaffan analyzed two sets of studies. In the first set of studies, retrieved from Dobson's (1989) meta-analysis of treatment for depression, eight comparisons of standard and variant CBT were aggregated, and it was found that the variant CBT outperformed the standard CBT ($d_+ = 0.25$), although the null hypothesis that the true effect size was zero could not be rejected. In a set of more recent studies (published between 1987 and 1994), 11 comparisons of variant and standard CBT were analyzed, and it was found that the two treatments were essentially equal in terms of their outcomes ($d_+ = 0.03$). This meta-analysis suggests that altering CBT does not attenuate the benefits of this treatment.

Component studies are proclaimed to be one of the most scientific designs for isolating components that are critical to the success of psychotherapy (Borkovec, 1990). However, Ahn and Wampold's (in press) meta-analysis indicated that over a corpus of component studies, there is

TABLE 5.1

Component Studies Reviewed by Ahn and Wampold (in press)

Author	Year	Disorder	More Components Tx Group	Fewer Components Tx Group	Component(s) Tested
Appelbaum et al.	1990	Tension headache	CT + PMR	PMR	Cognitive component
Barlow et al.	1992	Generalized anxiety disorder	CT + PMR	CT	Relaxation skills
Baucom et al.	1990	Marital discord	CT + PMR	PMR	Cognitive restructuring
			CR + BMT	BMT	Cognitive restructuring
			EET + BMT	BMT	Emotional expressiveness training
			EET + CR + BMT	BMT	Emotional expressiveness + Cognitive restructuring
Blanchard et al.	1990	Tension headache	CT + PMR	PMR	Cognitive component
Borkovec & Costello	1993	Generalized anxiety disorder	CBT	AR	Cognitive component + Self-control desensitization
Dadds & McHugh	1992	Child conduct problem	CMT + Ally	CMT	Social support
Deffenbacher & Stark	1992	General anger	CRCS	RCS	Cognitive component
Feske & Goldstein	1997	Panic disorder	EMDR	EFER	Eye movement
Halford et al.	1993	Marital discord	E-BMT	BMT	Cognitive restructuring + Generalized training + Affective exploration
Hope et al.	1995	Social phobia	CBT	Exposure only	Cognitive component
Jacobson et al.	1996	Depression	BA + AT	AT	Behavioral activation
			BA + AT	BA	Modifying automatic thoughts

Nicholas et al.	1991	Chronic low back pain	CT + PMR	CT	Relaxation skills
			BT + PMR	BT	Behavioral component
Ost et al.	1991	Blood phobia	Applied tension Package (BT)	Tension technique only	Exposure in vivo
			Applied tension package (BT)	Exposure in vivo only	Tension techniques
Porzelius et al.	1995	Eating disorder	OBET	CBT	Advanced CBT with a focus on coping skills & cognitive interventions
Propst, et al.	1992	Depression	CBT-Religious	CBT	Religious content modified to fit CBT
Radojevic et al.	1992	Rheumatoid arthritis	BT + Social support	BT	Family support
Rosen et al.	1990	Body image	CBT + Size perception training	CBT	Size perception training
Thackwray et al.	1993	Bulimia nervosa	CBT	BT	Cognitive component
Webster-Stratton	1994	Parenting effectiveness	GDVM + "ADVANCE"	GDVM	Cognitive social learning + Group discussion
Williams & Falbo	1996	Panic attack with agoraphobia	CBT	BT	Cognitive component
			CBT	CT	Behavioral component

Note. "ADVANCE" = cognitive training social learning program; AR = applied relaxation; AT = automatic thoughts; BA = behavioral activation; BMT = behavioral martial therapy; BT = behavioral therapy; CBT = cognitive–behavioral therapy; CMT = child management training; CR = cognitive restructuring; CRCS = cognitive and relaxation coping skills; CT = cognitive therapy; E-BMT = enhanced behavioral marital therapy; EET = emotional expressiveness training; EFER = eye fixation exposure and reprocessing; EMDR = eye movement desensitization and reprocessing; "GDVM" = videotape parent skills training program; OBET = obese binge-eating treatment; PMR = progressive muscle relaxation; RCS = relaxation coping skills; Tx = treatment.

From "Where oh where are the specific ingredients?: A meta-analysis of component studies in counseling and psychotherapy," by H. Ahn and B. E. Wampold, in press, *Journal of Counseling Psychology.* Copyright © 2001, by the American Psychological Association. Adapted with permission.

little evidence that components of treatments that contain purported specific and critical ingredients are indeed necessary to produce beneficial outcomes. In fact, the largest effect size for any of the 27 comparisons in Ahn and Wampold's data set was only 0.50, and more than one half of the effect sizes were negative (indicating that the component actually decreased the efficacy of the treatment). The results in the area of cognitive treatments for depression (Gaffan et al., 1995) were consistent with the general meta-analysis conducted by Ahn and Wampold. Clearly, there is little evidence that specific ingredients are necessary to produce psychotherapeutic change, as hypothesized by the medical model.

CONTROLLING FOR INCIDENTAL ASPECTS IN PSYCHOTHERAPY RESEARCH

Logic of Placebos in Medicine and in Psychotherapy

In psychotherapy research, research designs that use placebo control groups have been used to establish the specificity of various psychotherapeutic treatments. The logic of such designs is derived from the use of placebo treatments in medicine. Recall from chapter 1 that in the medical model in medicine, there are two types of effects. The first type consists of physicochemical effects due to specific medical procedures, and thus are called specific effects. The second type of effects are placebo effects, which are effects due to aspects of the medical treatment that are incidental to the treatment and nonphysicochemical. The field of medicine recognizes the presence of placebo effects but for the most part finds them of little interest.

In medicine, the existence of specific effects can be established by comparing a medical treatment with a placebo. To be valid, the placebo needs to be identical to the treatment in all respects, except that the placebo does not contain the specific ingredient of the medical treatment. For example, the efficacy and specificity of an ingested pharmacological pill is established by comparing its effects with a placebo pill that resembles the active pill in size, shape, color, taste, smell, and texture. The pill and the placebo are indistinguishable, except that the active pill contains a chemical compound which is purported, by theory, to be remedial for the disorder being treated; the placebo, however, contains no ingredients thought to be physicochemically remedial for the disorder. The placebo is the proverbial sugar pill. The equivalence of the drug and the placebo can be maintained only if the patient and the experimenter, as well as the evaluators, are unaware of the status of the pill administered to the patient. Consequently, medical placebo trials are double-blinded in that the patient, the experimenters, and the evaluators do not know whether a given patient is receiving the drug or the placebo. The field of medicine recognizes that expectations of the patient, experimenter, and evaluators have an effect on the measured effect of the treatment, and therefore maintaining the double-blind in medical research is critical to the integrity and validity of the research.

The logic of the placebo study in medicine is straightforward. If the drug condition is found to be superior to the placebo, then the efficacy of the specific ingredient is established because the only difference between the drug and the placebo is the specific ingredient. All other effects are controlled because they should logically be equivalent in the two conditions. Expectancy, for example, is controlled because neither the patient nor the experimenter knows whether or not the patient received the drug.[2]

Adherents of the medical model of psychotherapy use placebo psychotherapies in order to claim that the ingredients characteristic of a particular treatment are responsible for the benefits derived from the particular treatment. Unfortunately, using medical placebos as an analogue for psychotherapy placebos is problematic, and consequently the claim that psychotherapy placebos can be used to establish specificity is unjustified. Before discussing the problems with psychotherapy placebos, it should be noted that the popularity of the term placebo has waned and in lieu of it are the more vogue terms *alternate treatment, nonspecific treatment, attention control,* and *minimal treatment.* In addition, terms that reference particular approaches that are designed to exclude ingredients characteristic of the major approaches, such as *supportive counseling* and *nondirective counseling* are also used. The logic of all these treatments is the same in that the researcher attempts to control for the incidental aspects of treatments. In this section, the term placebo is used generically to include the various types of controls used by psychotherapy researchers.

It is difficult to define a psychotherapy placebo because the specific effects and the general effects are both derived through psychological processes (see Wilkins, 1983). In medicine, specific effects are physicochemically based, and placebo effects are psychologically based. The ingredients of the placebo are uncontroversial because there is general agreement about which ingredients have the potential to be remedial and which are inert physiochemically. For example, the lactose in a placebo pill used as a control for a drug indicated for HIV would not, by any reasonable physicochemical theory, be remedial for HIV; moreover lactose is not necessary for the treatment of HIV. Consequently, lactose is a an appropriate compound for the placebo and an inequivalence in the dosage of lactose in the drug and placebo would not be a threat to the validity of the study. On

---

[2]Whether double-blind placebo studies in medicine are truly blinded has been questioned. It appears that patients monitor themselves for the anticipated side-effects to determine whether they have been taking the drug. Furthermore, correctly guessing that one is taking the drug affects the outcome (Fisher & Greenberg, 1997).

the other hand, psychotherapy placebos must contain ingredients that are necessary for the delivery of the treatment and that are, according to many psychological theories, remedial for the disorder. The most perspicuous example of such an ingredient is the relationship between the therapist and the client. This relationship is technically necessary because psychotherapy by definition involves a relationship between therapist and client (see chap. 1). Moreover, most theories of change recognize the importance of the relationship; even strict behaviorists classify the relationship as necessary but not sufficient. Finally, the relationship is central to many change theories, including psychodynamic and client-centered theories.

Having to include ingredients in psychotherapy placebos that are necessary and remedial dictates that these ingredients must be comparable across the two conditions (treatment and placebo). To be valid logically, for example, the treatment and the placebo must involve comparable relationships between therapists and clients. However, the therapeutic relationship is only one such ingredient that must be equalized; others include the credibility of the treatment to the client, client expectation that the therapy is beneficial, the skill of the therapist, the preference of the client for the therapy, and the therapists' belief that the treatment is beneficial. Recall from chapter 4 that Jacobson (1991) claimed that BMT was at a disadvantage relative to IOMT because BMT contained fewer "nonspecific" elements than did IOMT. The same could be said for all placebos unless the equivalence of the treatment and the placebo vis-à-vis all nonspecific ingredients is established. It is logically and pragmatically impossible, however, to create psychotherapy placebos that contain, in terms of the quality and quantity, the same nonspecific ingredients contained in the psychotherapeutic treatment.

Many psychotherapy researchers have defined placebos in terms of a subset of the incidental aspects of psychotherapy treatments. For example, Bowers and Clum (1988) defined nonspecific treatments "as having two primary components: a discussion of the client's problems and the manipulation of the belief that one is getting an effective treatment" (p. 315). Borkovec (1990) argued that "perhaps the best description of the placebo condition, then, is that it involves contact with a therapist who engages in methods that the client believes will be helpful, even though the therapist (or investigator) believes that the method will be of only limited effectiveness relative to the therapy condition to which it is compared [and] whatever active ingredients it contains are common across many forms of psychosocial therapy" (p. 53). Others have defined placebos solely in terms of expectancy, the relationship, support, or other related factors. Clearly, defining and developing placebo control groups that are equivalent to treatment groups on all of the factors that are incidental to the theoretical approaches would be difficult, if not impossible, so researchers resort to making the treatment and placebo groups equivalent on one or a few common factors.

Not only is designing a placebo control group to control for all incidental aspects of treatment practically impossible, it is logically impossible. The logical problems in the development of placebo groups in psychotherapy research can be explicated by examining the double-blind in medical research. Recall, that the double-blind in medical research requires that neither the patient nor the administrator be aware of whether a given patient is receiving the treatment or the placebo. In psychotherapy research, one of the blinds will necessarily be absent. In psychotherapy research, it is obvious that therapists logically must be aware of the treatment being delivered; they have to be trained to deliver the active treatments as well as the placebo treatment in a manner consistent with the protocols for those treatments. As noted by Seligman (1995), "Whenever you hear someone demanding the double-blind study of psychotherapy, hold on to your wallet" (p. 965).

The fact that therapists are cognizant of whether they are delivering a treatment that was intended to be therapeutic or a placebo is critical to tests of the contextual model of psychotherapy. Recall that a required element of the contextual model is that the therapist believe that the therapy is beneficial. Placebos are designed by therapist–experimenters so that they are not intended to be therapeutic; trained therapists who deliver the placebos will also know that they are not intended to be therapeutic: "Therapist expectation, comfort, and enthusiasm [in placebo groups] are quite likely to vary considerably from those associated with active forms of treatment." (Borkovec, 1990, p. 54). The contextual model predicts that placebos will not be as therapeutic as bona fide treatments for the simple reason that the therapist is aware that he or she is delivering a treatment that is not intended to be therapeutic.

The failure to maintain blinds has been shown empirically to have considerable effects on assessed outcomes. Carroll, Rounsaville, and Nich (1994) conducted a study to assess how often psychotherapy and pharmacotherapy blinds are broken relative to evaluators of clinical functioning and how such breaks affect the assessment of clients. Cocaine-dependent participants were randomly assigned to four conditions: relapse prevention plus desipramine, clinical management (the psychotherapy placebo) plus desipramine, relapse prevention plus pill placebo, or clinical management and pill placebo. The clinical evaluators were unaware of assignments, and participants who informed the evaluators of their assignment were dropped from the study. The participant's true assignment was guessed correctly by the evaluator over half the time and greater than would be expected by chance; for those in the psychotherapy condition, the evaluators correctly guessed 77% of the time. For the subjective measures in the study, the pattern of ratings "worked in favor of the active psychotherapy condition" (p. 279), whereas no bias was detected for more objective measures. So, not only were evaluators able to guess the psychotherapy conditions with some regularity, subsequent subjective evaluations were biased in favor of active treatments.

A persuasive case that placebos have not controlled for the incidental factors of psychotherapy can be made by reviewing several studies that have used placebos. First, consider the placebo control group used by Borkovec and Costello (1993) to establish the efficacy of applied relaxation and CBT in the treatment of generalized anxiety disorder. The two treatments intended to be therapeutic, applied relaxation and CBT, contained many specific ingredients, whereas the placebo, labeled nondirective therapy (ND), did not contain these ingredients. In all three conditions, the rationale for the treatment was given to the clients. The initial rationale given to the ND clients was created to sound plausible and reasonable:

> Clients were told that therapy would involve exploration of life experiences in a quiet, relaxed atmosphere; the goal was to facilitate and deepen knowledge about self and anxiety. Therapy involved an inward journey that would change anxious experience and increase self-confidence. The therapist's role would be one of providing a safe environment for self-reflection and of helping to clarify and focus on feelings as the therapeutic vehicle to facilitate change. The clients' role was described to emphasize their unique efforts to discover new strengths through introspection and affective experiencing. (Borkovec & Costello, 1993, p. 613)

Therapists were instructed to create an "accepting, nonjudgmental, empathic environment, to continuously direct client attention to primary feelings, and to facilitate allowing and accepting of affective experience using supportive statements, reflective listening, and empathic communications" (Borkovec & Costello, 1993, p. 613). However, any direct suggestions, advice, or coping methods were not allowed.

At the end of the first session, the researchers assessed clients' perceptions of the credibility of the treatment and their expectancy of their improvement. No significant differences between the treatments were found on these variables. They also assessed relationship constructs at several points during therapy; again there were no significant differences. In addition they measured experiencing, for which the ND participants experienced deeper emotional processing.

ND in this study was superior to most other placebos in the literature, but nonetheless was deficient on a number of dimensions. To begin with, the therapists were trained in the laboratory of the researcher, an advocate of the two treatments in the study. Furthermore these therapists delivered all of the treatments, were certainly aware that ND was not intended to be therapeutic, and knew that the laboratory in which the study was conducted had an allegiance to the active treatments (see chap. 7). Moreover, the authors recognized that the treatment was not intended to be therapeutic: "We chose a simple, reflective listening ND only to provide a nonspecific condition for control purposes: our intention was not to do a comparative outcome study contrasting the best available experiential therapy with cognitive–behavioral therapy" (p. 612). So, the therapists were forbidden to use methods that most nondirective therapists would use and could not give any suggestions, advice, or discuss how the clients might cope with their anxiety. While credibility and expectancy may have been comparable at the end of the first session, it is not clear that such ratings would be maintained throughout the therapy, given the proscriptions on the ND therapists. The placebo ND condition did not resemble either of the other two treatments with their active ingredients removed; rather it was a degraded form of a different therapy, experiential therapy, conducted by therapists who knew it was not intended to be therapeutic and who had allegiance to the treatments with which it was compared.

In spite of these problems, Borkovec and Costello concluded that "from these results, we have drawn the conclusion that the behavioral therapy [viz., applied relaxation] and the CBT contain active ingredients in the treatment of GAD, independent of nonspecific factors" (p. 617). However, there are issues in addition to the placebo group that make this conclusion tenuous. First, expectancy ratings at the end of the first session correlated, on average, .43 with outcome.[3] That is, almost 20% of the variance in outcome was accounted for by one simple common factor (viz., expectancy) measured at the first session. The average effect size for AR versus ND was 0.50, which indicates that treatment accounts for about 6% of the variance in outcome (see Table 2.4). This indicates, assuming that the ND did control for all incidental aspects of applied relaxation and CBT, that a single common factor, measured very early on, accounts for more than three times the sum total of the variance accounted for by all specific ingredients! There is another anomaly in these findings that casts doubt on the necessity of the specific ingredients. CBT contained all of the ingredients of AR as well as cognitive ingredients, but the results showed that AR and CBT were equivalent, which is a clear indication that the ingredients in CBT are not necessary to produce benefits. Yet the frequency of practicing relaxation and relaxation-induced anxiety during treatment showed no relationship with outcome, discounting the specific ingredients in AR. Finally, at the end of 12 months, the three therapies were equivalent in their outcomes, even when clients who sought additional treatment were eliminated from

---

[3]It should be noted that the authors of this study did not attempt to examine how the nonsignificant difference in expectancy affected the outcomes in the three groups. The authors reported that the expectancy and credibility ratings were not significant, $p > .20$. However, given 55 participants and a p value of .20, this translates into a correlation coefficient of .27 (Rosenthal, 1994, Equations 16–23), which is large enough to account for the differences in outcomes between the active treatments and ND, particularly because the expectancy rating was so highly correlated with outcome. It is well know that covariates with nonsignificant relationships with outcome can, nonetheless, have dramatic effects (Porter & Raudenbush, 1987).

the analysis. So, this study, which has an exemplary placebo group, has provided only very weak evidence for specific effects.

If Borkovec and Costello's (1993) study was a commendable attempt at constructing a placebo that, although equal to the active treatments minus the specific ingredients, contained factors incidental to the active treatments, then consider the following ill-advised attempt. In this case, the placebo was labeled "supportive psychotherapy" and was compared with interpersonal psychotherapy for the treatment of depression among individuals with HIV (Markowitz et al., 1995):

> Supportive psychotherapy, defined as noninterpersonal psychotherapy and noncognitive behavioral therapy, resembles the client-centered therapy of Rogers, with added psychoeducation about depression and HIV. Unlike interpersonal psychotherapists, supportive psychotherapists offered patients *no explicit explanatory mechanism for treatment effect and did not focus treatment on specific themes* [italics added]. Although supportive psychotherapy may have been hampered by the proscription of interpersonal and cognitive techniques, it was by no means a nontreatment, particularly as delivered by empathic, skillful, experienced, and dedicated therapists. Sixteen 50 minute sessions of interpersonal therapy were scheduled within a 17-week period. The supportive psychotherapy condition had between eight and 16 sessions, determined by patient need, of 30–50 minute duration. (p. 1505)

Here the treatments explicitly differ along the dimensions of (a) whether rationale for treatment was provided, (b) the structure of treatment, (c) the length of treatment, and (d) the duration of treatment. Not surprisingly, it was found that the supportive psychotherapy was less beneficial than the interpersonal psychotherapy. These differences were attributed to the specific ingredients: "Our findings follow clinical intuition in showing an advantage for a treatment that targets depression over a nonspecific alternative" (Markowitz et al., 1995, p. 1508).

A placebo control group used by Foa et al. (1991) falls between the commendable placebo designed by Borkovec and Costello (1993) and the ill-designed placebo of Markowitz et al. (1995). Foa et al. compared stress-inoculation training, prolonged exposure, and supportive counseling (the placebo), for the treatment of PTSD resulting from a recent rape. Supportive counseling consisted of the following:

> Supportive counseling followed the nine-session format [as in the other treatments], gathering information through the initial interview in the first session and presenting the rationale for treatment in the second session. During the remaining sessions, patients were taught a general problem-solving technique. Therapists played an indirect and unconditionally supportive role. Homework consisted of the patients keeping a diary of daily problems and her attempts [sic] at problem solving. Patients were immediately redirected to focus on current daily problems if discussions of the assault occurred. No instructions for exposure or anxiety management were included. (pp. 717–718)

Clearly, supportive counseling was not intended to be therapeutic, as "in the absence of other components, few would accept deflecting women from discussing their recent rape in counseling as therapeutic" (Wampold, Mondin, Moody, & Ahn, 1997, p. 227). Moreover, the therapists were supervised by Foa, whose allegiance was to the stress-inoculation training and prolonged exposure. Finally, no attempt was made to determine whether the participants found supportive counseling credible or whether they expected it to be beneficial. Nevertheless, Foa et al. (1991) included supportive counseling "to control for nonspecific therapy effects" (p. 716).

The basic problems with psychotherapy placebos have been discussed in this section. Logically and pragmatically, psychotherapy placebos cannot control for the incidental aspects of psychological treatments. More complete discussions of the problems with placebos are found in the literature (Brody, 1980; Critelli & Neumann, 1984; Grünbaum, 1981; P. Horvath, 1988; A. K. Shapiro & Morris, 1978; Shepherd, 1993; Wilkins, 1983, 1984).

For all their problems, it should be recognized that placebo treatments do contain one or more of the aspects of psychotherapy that are incidental to various psychotherapies. Placebos are sufficiently credible to clients that they continue in treatment. Although the therapists know that they are delivering a treatment not intended to be therapeutic, they create and maintain some degree of therapeutic relationship with the clients. Being naturally desirous to help those in distress, the therapists likely take an empathic stance toward their clients in the placebo treatments. Thus, according to the contextual model, it is reasonable to expect that placebo treatments will be more beneficial than no treatment, although clearly less beneficial than a treatment fully intended to be therapeutic. Consequently, both the medical model and the contextual model posit that placebos treatments will be more beneficial than no treatment but less beneficial that treatments intended to be therapeutic.

Meta-Analyses

Many of the early meta-analyses examined the effects of placebos. However, because the results of meta-analyses of placebos have been relatively consistent, two particularly informative meta-analyses published in 1988 are reviewed. Bowers and Clum (1988) reviewed 69 studies published from 1977 to 1986 that contained at least one behavioral psychotherapy intended to be therapeutic as well as groups designated as placebo, attention, or nonspecific control. Each placebo was rated as to its credibility vis-à-vis the active treatment. The overall efficacy of the treatments versus no-treatments was 0.76, consistent with absolute efficacy meta-analyses reviewed in chapter 3. The comparison of treatment and placebo yielded an effect size of 0.55, indicating that the placebo was 0.21 effect size units superior to no treatment. Generally, the credibility ratings of the placebo conditions was unrelated to the treatment–placebo effect size, although those studies with the highest credibility ratings produced smaller effect sizes than those that were rated second highest. Interpretation of the difference between these two credibility groups is not clear. Moreover, the lack of a relationship between credibility of treatment and outcome would tend to indicate that credibility is not a perspicuous common factor, although a plethora of assessment issues relative to credibility can be raised. Nevertheless, this meta-analysis found clear evidence that treatments intended to be therapeutic are superior to placebos and that placebos are superior, albeit by a small margin, to no treatment.

In another meta-analysis of placebo effects, Barker, Funk, and Houston (1988) reviewed only studies in which the placebo treatments generated a reasonable expectation for change. Criteria for inclusion were that (a) the study compared a psychological treatment with a placebo that involved psychological–behavioral components (i.e., not pill placebos), (b) expectancy was assessed for the treatment and the control, and (c) there were no statistical differences in expectancy ratings between the treatment and the placebo conditions. A total of 17 studies containing 31 treatments were retrieved. The comparison of a treatment with the placebo produced an effect size of 0.549, and the comparison of placebo to no treatment was 0.472, indicating that treatments were clearly superior to placebos with adequate expectation for change and that such placebos were also superior to no treatment.

Interestingly, both Barker et al. (1988) and Bowers and Clum (1988) chose to define placebos in terms of one factor, either credibility or expectancy, respectively. On the basis of the superiority of the treatment to the placebo, the authors of both studies concluded that benefits of psychotherapy were due, in large part, to specific ingredients. However, as discussed earlier, placebos are inevitably deficient; stipulating equivalence on one dimension is insufficient to claim that all common factors are controlled.

In 1994, Lambert and Bergin reviewed 15 meta-analyses and arrived at the following effect sizes:

psychotherapy versus no-treatment	=	**0.82**
psychotherapy versus placebo	=	**0.48**
placebo versus no-treatment	=	**0.42**

This pattern of effect sizes is exactly what both the medical model and the contextual model predict. Interpretation of the placebo versus no-treatment control group effect size is made by consulting Table 2.4. An effect size in the neighborhood of 0.42 indicates that 66% of people in the placebo group are better at the end of treatment than those who receive no treatment, that about 4% of the variability in outcome is due to assignment to placebo versus no-treatment, and that receiving the placebo raises the success rate from about 40% to 60%.

An interpretation of the placebo versus no-treatment comparison provides an estimate of the proportion of variance in psychotherapy outcomes that is due to common factors. Recall that no placebo can adequately control for all elements of the contextual model, as therapist belief in the efficacy of treatment is a necessary common component of all treatments, but typically is absent for placebos. Moreover, as discussed earlier, all placebos are deficient in several additional ways. That is, placebo treatments contain some, but not nearly all, common factors. The effect produced by placebos (vis-à-vis no treatments), thus, is due to one or more common factors that are contained in the placebo. Consequently, the placebo versus no-treatment comparison provides a lower bound for the effect produced by common factors. That placebos account for about 4% of the variance in outcomes indicates that a small set of common factors, maybe not delivered with enthusiasm or belief, can be relatively effective. Recall from chapter 4 that treatments accounted for at most 1% of the variance in outcome (i.e., the proportion of variance due to specific factors is at most 1%). Consequently, a conservative estimate of the ratio of general effects to specific effects is 4 to 1. Thus it appears that general effects are much more explanatory than are specific effects.

MEDIATING PROCESSES

Specificity can be demonstrated by examining the causal pathways of a treatment. It is expected that the benefits of a given treatment will be mediated by a predictable psychological process. For example, according to the traditional precepts of cognitive therapy (e.g., Beck et al., 1979), depression is characterized by negative automatic thoughts, negative beliefs, and negative attributions about the self and others; consequently, depression is reduced by challenging the negative thoughts and replacing the negative beliefs with more benign or positive ones. Diagrammatically, the hypothesized mediating process of cognitions is shown in the top of Figure 5.2. Statistically, a variable m is said to mediate the relationship between an independent variable x and a dependent variable y provided (a) x and y are correlated, (b) x and m are correlated, and (c) when m is accounted for, the relationship between x and y is null or, in the case of partial mediation, significantly decreased (Baron & Kenny, 1986).

Establishment of cognitions as a mediating variable for the relationship between cognitive therapy and depression would provide evidence for the specific ingredients in cognitive therapy. With regard to the first condition for mediation, the relationship between cognitive therapy (the independent variable x) and depression (the dependent variable y) is clearly established, as cognitive therapy has been shown unequivocally to be an efficacious treatment for depression (see chap. 4). The veridicality of the mediational model for cognitive therapy is examined by considering various alternatives explanations for the efficacy of cognitive therapy, which are presented in Figure 5.2.[4]

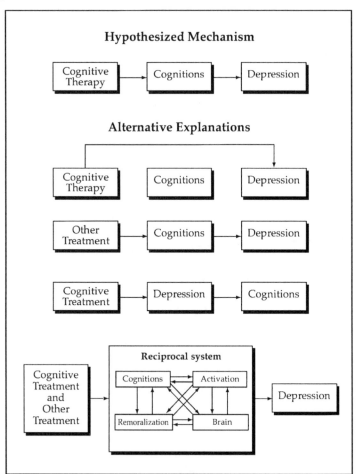

FIG. 5.2.   Causal models for cognitive therapy for depression.

[4]The various models presented here overlap with the various causal models systematically developed and presented by Hollon et al.(1987). As discussed later, regardless of the form of the alternative, specificity requires that a given therapy affects mediating constructs differently than therapies hypothesized to work through alternative mediating constructs.

The first alternative is that the effects of cognitive therapy are not mediated by changing cognitions. That is, cognitive therapy does not modify cognitions but decreases depression through some other mechanism. This alternative was convincingly ruled out by a meta-analysis of the role of cognitions in cognitive therapy conducted by Oei and Free (1995). Oei and Free retrieved 43 studies of various treatments of depression that included measures of cognitive style. The most common cognitive measures used in the studies were the Dysfunctional Attitude Scale and the Automatic Thoughts Questionnaire, two measures developed to assess the cognitions hypothesized to be targeted by cognitive therapy. In this meta-analysis, it was found that there was a relationship between change in cognitions and cognitive therapy, strengthening the case for the specificity of cognitive therapy. There is no question that cognitive therapy, cognitions, and depression are interrelated; the issue is to understand the nature of the interrelationships.

The second explanation that mitigates against the specific ingredients of cognitive therapy would be the discovery of a relationship between therapies that do not contain ingredients intended to modify cognitions and subsequent changes in cognitions. Oei and Free (1995) also meta-analytically tested the relationship of noncognitive psychological therapies and change in cognitions. It was found that cognitive therapy and other therapies did not differ significantly in terms of their effect on cognitions. Moreover, drug therapies produced changes in cognitions equivalent to the two classes of psychological treatments. The fact that noncognitive psychological treatments and drug treatments change cognitions in a manner indistinguishable from cognitive therapy clearly detracts from a specific ingredient argument for the efficacy of cognitive therapy.

Another challenge to the specificity of cognitive treatments for depression comes from the component study conducted by Jacobson et al. (1996) discussed earlier in this chapter. This study provides compelling evidence that cognitive interventions are not needed to effect changes in cognition. Recall that there were three interventions: (a) behavioral activation; (b) behavioral activation plus coping skills related to automatic thoughts; and (c) complete cognitive treatment, which included behavioral activation, coping skills, and identification and modification of core dysfunctional schemas. Behavioral activation contained no cognitive ingredients, whereas the latter two did contain cognitive ingredients, although only the full treatment was intended to alter core dysfunctional schemas. Nevertheless, behavioral activation altered negative thinking and dysfunctional attributional styles as well as either of the two cognitive treatments, contrary to predictions. In conjunction with the results that all three treatments were equally efficacious, the evidence from this study convincingly suggests that ingredients designed specifically to alter cognitions are not necessary in order to alter cognitions and reduce depression.

A third alternative explanation is that cognitive therapy is an efficacious treatment for depression, but that change in cognitions is a result of decreased depression, not a cause (see Figure 5.2). Ilardi and Craighead (1994) conducted a review of CBT for depression that investigated the timing of changes in CBT. They made the following conclusion:

> Taken together, the eight studies reviewed herein provide compelling evidence that rapid improvement in depressive symptomatology typically occurs with the first few weeks of treatment with CBT. It appears that the majority of total symptomatic improvement occurs *within the first three weeks of treatment* … with 60–80% of the total decrease in depression severity typically occurring by Week 4…. The hypothesized mechanism of cognitive mediation, on the other hand, would probably not be expected to account for any substantial improvement observed in the earliest weeks of CBT, since the specific techniques designed to facilitate a reduction in depressive thoughts are not formally introduced until several sessions into the treatment. According to the CBT manual …, the initial cognitive restructuring techniques—challenging "automatic thoughts" and generating alternative interpretations—typically are not introduced until the fourth therapy session; and, of course, one would not expect patients to apply such procedures without a bit of practice. (pp. 140, 142)

One explanation for the rapid response to cognitive therapy is that it decreases depression quickly through means other than the modification of thoughts and that reducing depression results in a modification of maladaptive thoughts. This explanation is bolstered by other findings from Oei and Free's (1995) meta-analysis. They found that depression and cognitions were related only when depression was measured by the BDI and only for psychological treatments. These findings suggest that the cognition–depression link is not fundamental to the change process. However, it should be noted that in two well-conducted studies, DeRubeis and colleagues (DeRubeis & Feeley, 1990; Feeley, DeRubeis, & Gelfand, 1999) found that change in depression occurs subsequent to therapist administration of problem-focused, specific aspects of cognitive therapy, a result that is contrary to Ilardi and Craighead's conclusion (these studies are examined more closely in chap. 7). On the other hand, Simons, Garfield, and Murphy (1984), in another well-conducted study, found that cognitive and pharmacological treatments had similar effects on cognitions and that, in both conditions, cognitions had similar effects on depression.

The final alternative explanation considered herein is that various treatments influence a reciprocal system that, in turn, affects depression. There are several variations of the reciprocal system explanation for the efficacy of cognitive therapy. In one variation, Free and Oei (1989) hypothesized that cognitive therapy induces an adaptive cognitive style, which then affects the catecholine balance in the brain, whereas pharmacological treatments restores the catecholine balance, which in turn changes maladaptive cognitions. Ilardi and Craighead (1994), on the basis of their review of the timing of changes in cognitive therapy, contended that cognitive therapy (as well as other therapies) produced rapid change in depression as a result of the remoralization of the client:

> The mediational role of nonspecific processes in CBT (or any other therapeutic treatment, for that matter) might be expected to be especially prominent in the very early, as opposed to middle and later, stages of treatment. As Frank observed, "indirect support for the hypothesis [that nonspecific processes mediate clinical improvement] is that many patients improve very quickly in therapy, suggesting that their favorable response is due to the reassuring aspects of the therapeutic situation itself rather than to the specific procedure." (Ilardi & Craighead, 1994, p. 140)

Moreover, clients who are sufficiently remoralized in the early stages in therapy, according to Illardi and Craighead, are able to successfully apply the cognitive techniques taught in CBT and consequently complete their recovery. Another reciprocal process could involve behavioral activation, as Jacobson et al. (1996) found that the activation component of CBT was sufficient to induce change in depression.

A final variation of the reciprocal system explanation is one in which various causal factors are fused. A fusion model, as well the logical issues inherent in such a model, were well explicated by Hollon, DeRubeis, and Evans (1987) in a discussion of Beck's perspective on cognitions in CBT:

> Whether Beck would endorse a model based on mutual reciprocal causality between the separate components is not clear. He might argue for the correspondence between the cognitive processes and depression or between either and biological processes. In a recent monograph, Beck (1984b) suggested, "Thoughts do not cause the neurochemical changes and the neurochemical changes do not cause the thoughts. Neurochemical changes and cognitions are the *same processes* (italics added) examined from different perspectives" (p. 4). Although in arguing for an identity between these processes he appears to rule out causal mediation, he went on to say, "The cognitive approach, expressed in terms of the verbal and nonverbal behavior of the therapist, produces *cognitive-neurochemical* changes" (Beck, 1984b, p. 118).... In such a model, any change in depression, no matter how it was caused, would invariably be associated with comparable and correlated change in cognitive processes.... Beck's revised unitary model may well reject the notion of separation of components, obviating any causal mediation, because Beck sees those components as merely different perspectives on the same phenomenon (A. T. Beck, personal communication, March 27, 1986). (Hollon et al., 1987, pp 144–145)

The implications of a fusion model for specificity are profound, because the causal mechanism of change would be identical regardless of the treatment. That is, any efficacious treatment would ipso facto affect the unitary system composed of the fused components related to depression. It would not be possible to demonstrate that a given treatment, say cognitive therapy, affects clients differently than any other treatment. Adopting a fused model would preclude demonstrating the specificity of any therapeutic action.

Establishment of specificity for cognitive therapy depends on the finding that cognitive therapy affects a particular mediating construct differently than does a treatment that is hypothesized to operate through different mediating constructs. Consequently, studies that examine solely the process of one therapy cannot establish that the change mechanisms are unique to that therapy. The most informative study would be one that examines various treatments and assessed the hypothesized mediating constructs of each treatment. The most comprehensive of such studies was the NIMH TDCRP, which compared CBT, IPT, psychopharmacological treatment (viz., imipramine; IMI), and clinical management (CM; see chap. 4 for a more complete description of this study). In this study, instruments were administered to assess the hypothesized causal mechanisms and were reported by Imber et al. (1990). As discussed in this chapter, cognitive treatments for depression are based on changing distorted cognitions. In the NIMH TDCRP, the Dysfunctional Attitude Scale (DAS) was used to measure the hypothesized mediating construct for cognitive therapy. IPT, which presumes a relation between interpersonal relations and depression, focuses on interpersonal conflict, role transitions, and social deficits. The Social Adjustment Scale (SAS) was used to assess social processes that are hypothesized to be critical to the efficacy of IPT. IMI is hypothesized to influence brain chemistry (neurotransmitter and receptor sensitivity) and consequently affect neurovegetative and somatic symptoms, which were measured with the Endogenous scale from the Schedule for Affective Disorders and Schizophrenia (SADS). Specificity of therapeutic action predicts that each of the treatments would affect the mediating constructs uniquely; that is, CBT, IPT, and IMI-CM would change scores on the DAS, SAS, and SADS, respectively. Using data only from those clients who completed treatment, few of the predicted relationships were verified:

> Despite different theoretical rationales, distinctive therapeutic procedures, and presumed differences in treatment processes, none of the therapies produced clear and consistent effects at termination of acute treatment on measures related to its theoretical origins. This conclusion applies, somewhat surprisingly, not only to the two psychotherapies but also to pharmacotherapy as practiced in the TDCRP. (Imber et al., 1990, p. 357)

A limitation of this study is that the mediating constructs were assessed at the end of treatment and thus cannot rule out a reciprocal process whereby each treatment affected its hypothesized construct, which in turn affected the other constructs. Nevertheless, the TDCRP, the most comprehensive clinical trial for the treatment of depression to date, did not provide evidence to support the specificity of the three treatments.

Although the detection of mediating effects would be construed as evidence for a medical model explanation of psychotherapy, little evidence has been found for such effects. The evidence relative to cognitive–behavioral treatment of depression was examined, and the absence of the hypothesized mediating processes was conspicuous. Indeed, no mediating relationship in any area of psychotherapy has been unambiguously detected. In medicine, mediating processes are well established in the preponderance of treatments. For example, the efficacy of antibiotics is bolstered by the documented reduction of bacteria as well as the disappearance of symptoms. That no such corresponding mediating process has ever been unambiguously demonstrated in psychotherapy casts doubts on a medical model interpretation of psychotherapy.

INTERACTION WITH TREATMENTS

The medical model posits that there are specific treatments for specific disorders. Nevertheless, the results reviewed in chapter 4 indicate that there is little evidence that any particular treatment that is intended to be therapeutic is superior to any other. If the medical model is indeed adequate to explain the benefits of psychotherapy, then the uniform efficacy of treatments for particular disorders must require a modification of the medical model. One modification of the medical model involves flaws in the system for identifying specific disorders:

> Treatment outcome studies based on selecting subjects using *DSM*-like criteria consistently fail to show significantly large treatment differences that would help us understand etiology and inform treatment selection. Take, for example, the results of the NIMH Treatment of Depression Collaborative Research Program (Elkin, Parloff, Hadley, & Autry, 1985). The results of this multimillion dollar study suggest that it makes relatively little difference what treatment depressed clients receive (Elkin et al., 1989). This is hardly a surprise. A syndromal classification system assumes that a depressive is a depressive is a depressive. However, there are several well-developed accounts for how depression might come about (e.g., biological, behavioral, cognitive–behavioral, and interpersonal theories, etc.). If one assumed that depressive symptoms were one possible endpoint from a number of etiological pathways and that any group of persons with depression contained a number from each pathway, then comparative outcome studies are forever doomed to get equivalent results because those who have had a biological cause might respond to medication but not those who were interpersonally unskilled, and so on. So far there is little evidence that there are common etiological pathways that describe a uniform course or response to treatment for any reasonable proportion of the *DSM–IV* categories. Even the notion of uniqueness of symptoms clustering to reveal an underlying problem finds little support. In the National Comorbidity Study (Kessler et al., 1994), over half of the participants who received one diagnosis over the course of a lifetime had at least one other diagnosable disorder as well. (Follette & Houts, 1996, p. 1128)

The thesis here is clear: The commonly used diagnostic categories do not correspond to entities with uniform psychological–biological etiologies, and consequently various treatments for disorders that have multiple determinants will produce similar outcomes. That is, clients within disorders are heterogeneous with regard to the causal factors creating the disorder and therefore would respond differentially to various treatments.

The heterogeneity of clients with regard to etiology premise is that a specific treatment (say Tx A) that targets a particular causal process A' will have superior outcomes for those clients for whom it can be demonstrated that the disorder is caused by A' than will other treatments targeted toward other causal processes. This is a causal process moderation hypothesis, as shown in Figure 5.3. If the medical model is correct, then the interaction presented in Figure 5.3 should be found in studies that match treatment to clients on the basis of theoretical grounds.

It should be noted that there are other interaction effects that should not be construed as being supportive of the medical model and might even be supportive of the contextual model. Recall that one of the elements of the contextual model is the client's belief that the treatment is beneficial. Therefore, clients who find the rationale for Tx A convincing will have better outcomes with Tx A, whereas clients who find the rationale for Tx B convincing will have better outcomes with Tx B. In this case, the interaction between a person characteristic (viz., belief in rationale of treatment) and treatment supports the contextual model.

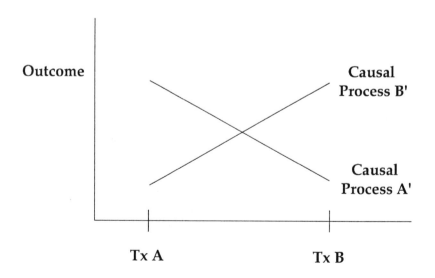

FIG. 5.3.   Causal process moderation hypothesis.

Evidence for Interaction With Treatment Effects

Although no meta-analyses have been conducted relative to person characteristic–treatment interactions, a number of narrative reviews have been published and are informative. In 1988, Dance and Neufeld examined interactions relative to a variety of disorders, including anxiety, depression, pain management, smoking, and weight reduction, and they came to the following conclusion:

> It is apparent that attempts to identify client variables predictive of differential treatment responsiveness have been disappointing. There are no well-documented client characteristics that can serve as a basis for treatment selection. (p. 209)

Although Dance and Neufeld found several constructs that showed some promise to moderate treatment efficacy (e.g., active vs. passive coping styles), none involved causal processes of the disorders.

In 1991, B. Smith and Sechrest discussed methodological considerations in person characteristic–treatment interactions and attempted to find instances in which theoretically predicted interactions were present. They concluded that the evidence for such interactions was "discouraging" and suggested that the theoretical underpinnings of psychotherapies may be flawed:

> To a meta-scientist the movement toward [person characteristic–treatment interaction] research might be viewed as a symptom of a degenerating program of research. Programs can be said to be degenerating if they (a) fail to yield new predictions or empirical success and/or (b) deal with empirical anomalies through ad hoc maneuvers that over complicate rather than clarify the problem of interest (Gholson & Barker, 1985). Perhaps psychotherapy researchers should be seriously and dispassionately reconsidering the core assumptions of their theories rather than building an elaborate [person characteristic–treatment interactional model] on a crumbling theoretical foundation. (Smith & Sechrest, 1991, p. 237).

In a thorough review of client variables in psychotherapy, Garfield (1994) failed to report any support for causal moderation, as predicted by the medical model. Considering that Garfield culled from the literature over one hundred studies related to how characteristics of the client influence outcome, the fact that no study was found that displayed an interaction between the nature of the psychological process related to the disorder and outcome suggests that there is sparse evidence, if any, to support causal moderation.

Although reviews of interactions between client characteristics and treatment have failed to produce evidence to support causal moderation, there are a number of well-conducted individual studies that bear on the issue and deserve review. First, the studies related to depression are reviewed, followed by studies of other disorders.

As discussed earlier, moderational proponents believe that cognitive therapy should be indicated for clients with demonstrated deficits related to irrational and distorted cognitions as well as dysfunctional attributions about events. To test this hypothesis, Simons, Lustman, Wetzel, and Murphy (1985) investigated whether cognitive therapy would have particular efficacy with clients with demonstrated deficits in cognitive coping strategies. In this study, data were analyzed for participants who were randomly assigned to a cognitive therapy group or to a nortriptyline group. The predicted cognitive deficits were assessed with three instruments: the Automatic Thoughts Questionnaire, the Dysfunctional Attitudes Scale, and the Hopelessness Scale. Strengths in cognitive coping were also assessed (via the Self-Control Schedule). For each treatment modality, response to treatment was investigated by regressing the BDI onto variables related to cognitive deficits and strengths after accounting for pretreatment BDI scores. For the cognitive group, only the Self-Control Schedule accounted for a significant proportion of the variance, implying that the hypothesized cognitive deficits did not predict outcome. For the pharmacological treatment, none of the cognitive variables predicted outcome, although the Self-Control Schedule did account for relatively large, but nonsignificant ($p = .08$), proportion of the variance. These results suggest that cognitive deficits do not differentially predict responsiveness to the two treatments as predicted by the medical model.

The results for the Self-Control Schedule are complicated to interpret. First, the researchers did not test for the differences in the regression coefficients, but rather chose to dichotomize scores on this variable. When examined in this way, it appears that participants with high learned resourcefulness do better with cognitive therapy, whereas those with low learned resourcefulness do better with pharmacotherapy.[5] Various explanations were given for this result, but one has particular relevance to the contextual model versus medical model differentiation:

> Cognitive therapy relies on a specific explanation for the development and treatment of depressive symptoms. The model is based on the belief that the thoughts, attitudes, and interpretations mediate feelings and behavior. The cognitive therapist offers this set of assumptions to the patient and helps the behaviors. Examination of the [Self-Control Schedule] items reveals that in order to achieve a high score, a patient must already endorse this explanatory model.... The congruence between the patient's and the therapist's conceptualization of the problems and how they are best approached may be a powerful facilitator of treatment response (Frank, 1971; Garfield, 1973). In contrast, patients with low

---

[5]Dichotomizing continuous variables to test for interactions can be problematic (Maxwell & Delaney, 1993).

[Self-Control Schedule] scores may find it difficult to accept the self-help quality of cognitive therapy. Rather they may prefer a therapeutic situation in which they assume a more passive role and leave the therapy to the therapist. (Simons et al., 1985, p. 86)

Clearly, this interpretation emanates from the contextual model prediction that belief in the rationale for treatment leads to beneficial outcomes. Thus, the results of this study provide no evidence for causal moderation, as predicted by the medical model. Instead, it provides some evidence for the need for belief in the rationale of a treatment, as predicted by the contextual model.

Theoretically, psychological treatments should not be particularly effective with depressions whose etiology is biological. More specifically, the medical model predicts that clients with biologically caused depressions would benefit relatively more from drug treatments whereas clients with depressions caused by psychological factors would benefit more from a psychologically based treatment such as cognitive therapy. McKnight, Nelson-Gray, and Barnhill (1992) investigated this hypothesis by randomly assigning participants to a cognitive therapy condition or to a medication condition. The biological basis of depression was determined by whether an abnormal response to the Dexamethasone Suppression Test (DST) was obtained, a method that has strong indirect support (see McKnight et al., 1992). Half of the abnormal responders (i.e., those with biological etiology) and half of the normal responders were randomly assigned to the cognitive therapy and to the medication conditions. Pretreatment levels of dysfunctional thoughts were also assessed. The results showed that although both treatments were efficacious, response to DST did not differentially predict outcome. The prediction that abnormal responders would benefit relatively more from medication was not corroborated, a result that fails to support the specific ingredient conjecture. However, those in the cognitive therapy group did show greater reduction in dysfunctional thoughts, a result that does support specific ingredients, although the authors recognized it might be possible that " dysfunctional thoughts are a correlate rather than a causal antecedent to depression" (McKnight et al., 1992, p. 108; also see previous section).

Client characteristics and treatment interactions were investigated in the NIMH TDCRP. Using the NIMH TDCRP data, Barber and Muenz (1996) investigated the "theory of opposites," which suggests that effective therapists react to clients in ways that are contrary to the client's typical patterns, either in terms of interpersonal dynamics, personality, or behavior. Consequently, Barber and Muenz (1996) hypothesized that avoidant clients would benefit from IPT, whereas obsessive clients would benefit from cognitive therapy, a hypothesis that was verified. A brief examination of "theory of opposites" will show, however, that support for this theory is not evidence for the medical model. A medical model of psychotherapy posits specific causes of depression and specific therapeutic actions that will remediate the depression by addressing the causal factors. The "theory of opposites," however, proposes a general therapeutic stance that is independent from particular disorders, their causes, and the therapeutic actions specific to the causes of the disorder. In this study, the interaction effect is related to personality styles (avoidant and obsessive) that might dispose a client to be more compatible with one treatment than another, but it is not an instance of causal moderation, as predicted by the medical model.

In another anlaysis of the NIMH TDCRP data, Barber and Muenz (1996) found that nonmarried clients benefited more from IPT than from cognitive therapy and that married people benefited more from cognitive therapy than from IPT. This interaction was not predicted and does not flow straightforwardly from the theoretical underpinnings of the respective treatments. Furthermore, Barber and Muenz (1996) reported no interactions between causal pathways and treatment, and none have been reported elsewhere.

The evidence related to an interaction between etiological pathways of depression and treatment does not support specific effects, as posited by the medical model. In fact, within studies investigating causal moderation, evidence has been found for interactions that support a contextual model. Attention is now turned to studies of substance abuse.

For many years, there has been speculation that client characteristic–treatment interactions would exist in the area of substance abuse, as the treatments are conceptually diverse, encompassing such approaches as 12-step programs, cognitive therapies, and motivation enhancement. To test various hypotheses about such interactions, Project MATCH, a collaborative clinical trial, was sponsored by the National Institute on Alcohol Abuse and Alcoholism (Project MATCH Research Group, 1997). In this study, 16 matching (i.e., client–treatment interaction) hypotheses were developed on the basis of theory and research. Participants, in an "outpatient" arm and in an "aftercare" arm, were assigned to cognitive–behavioral coping skills therapy, motivational enhancement (MET), and 12-step facilitation therapy (TSF). Client characteristics studied included alcohol involvement, cognitive impairment, conceptual level, gender, meaning seeking, motivation, psychiatric severity, sociopathy, support for drinking, and type of drinking. Some of these hypotheses were clear instances of causal moderation; for example, responsiveness to the cognitive therapy would be predicted by cognitive impairment. Whether other hypotheses could be construed as evidence for causal moderation was ambiguous. Because the study was designed to test matching effects, special attention was given to design issues related to interactions. For example, because the power to detect interactions typically is small (compared with main effects), Project MATCH used over 1500 clients in order to detect small but theoretically important effects.

The results of Project MATCH indicated that the three treatments were, for the most part, equally effective in both the aftercare and outpatient arms of the study. Of the 16 matching hypotheses in each arm, only one significant result was detected: For outpatients, clients whose psychiatric severity was relatively low had more abstinent days in the TSF condition than in the CBT condition. Clearly, the limited support for theoretically relevant interactions must be interpreted as lack of support for the premise that the specific ingredients of alcohol treatments are differentially active with various types of clients. Project MATCH involved an enormous effort to detect theoretically derived interactions, yet very limited evidence for the hypothesized interactions was found.

It should be noted that interactions have been found in other well-conducted substance abuse studies. Maude-Griffin et al. (1998) found that, contrary to many previous studies, CBT was superior to a 12-step program for cocaine abusers. They also found one robust interaction effect: High abstract reasoners were significantly more likely to be abstinent in the CBT treatment than were low abstract reasoners, whereas the opposite was found for the 12-step program. Again, the lack of support for four other hypotheses and the fact that the abstract reasoning hypothesis was not related to specific causal mechanism fails to provide significant evidence for the specific ingredients argument.

Interactions between treatments and characteristics of the clients that support the specificity of treatments has been a cornerstone of the medical model of psychotherapy since 1969, when Paul asked the question, "What treatment, by whom, is most effective for this individual with that specific problem, under which set of circumstances, and how does it come about?" (p. 111) In the subsequent thirty years, not one interaction theoretically derived from hypothesized client deficits has been documented robustly, casting doubt on the specificity of psychological treatments.

CONCLUSIONS

In chapter 4, the uniform efficacy of treatments provided indirect evidence that specific ingredients were not responsible for the benefits of psychotherapy. In this chapter, research designed particularly to detect the presence of specificity were reviewed. The results of studies using component designs, placebo control groups, mediating constructs, and moderating constructs consistently failed to find evidence for specificity. The history of psychological treatments is littered with examples of treatments that are beneficial to clients but whose psychological explanation for the benefits have failed to be verified (e.g., systematic desensitization and biofeedback). In this chapter it was found that the ingredients of the most conspicuous treatment on the landscape, cognitive–behavioral treatment, are apparently not responsible for the benefits of this treatment.

If specific ingredients are not remedial in and of themselves, then the alternative hypothesis that the commonalities of treatment are responsible for the benefits must be entertained. In the next chapters, evidence is presented that shows that many common factors are indeed related to outcome, as hypothesized in the contextual model.

6

General Effects: The Alliance as a Case in Point

In chapter 4, when the Dodo bird declared, with regard to psychotherapy, that "All must have prizes," the evidence that specific ingredients were not crucial components of psychological treatments began to accumulate. In chapter 5, the search for the efficacy of particular specific ingredients revealed little evidence that any one ingredient was necessary to produce therapeutic results. Examination of the efficacy of placebo treatments, which contain some but not all common factors, revealed that common factors are indeed related to outcome. Thus far, the evidence seems to indicate that specific ingredients account for little of the variance in outcomes, whereas common factors appear to account for at least a modest amount of variance. If this is the case, then there should be one or more common factors that can consistently be shown to be necessary to produce beneficial outcomes. In this chapter, the size of the general effects produced by the therapeutic alliance will be estimated. If the general effects for this one common factor are relatively large, particularly in comparison with specific effects, then evidence is found to support the contextual model of psychotherapy rather than the medical model of psychotherapy.

The alliance between the client and the therapist is the most frequently mentioned common factor in the psychotherapy literature (Grencavage & Norcross, 1990). The concept of the alliance between therapist and client originated in the psychoanalytic tradition and was conceptualized as the healthy, affectionate, and trusting feelings toward the therapist, as differentiated from the neurotic component (i.e., transference) of the relationship.

149

Over the years, the concept of the alliance has been defined pantheoretically to include other aspects of the relationship, including (a) the client's affective relationship with the therapist, (b) the client's motivation and ability to accomplish work collaboratively with the therapist, (c) the therapist's empathic responding to and involvement with the client, and (d) client and therapist agreement about the goals and tasks of therapy. (For a succinct discussion of the alliance, see Gaston, 1990; A. O. Horvath & Luborsky, 1993.)

There are a number of reasons for selecting the alliance as a common factor to examine. First, the alliance is mentioned prominently in the psychotherapy literature and draws attention from theorists across many disparate approaches. Indeed, the alliance has been described as the "quintessential integrative variable" of psychotherapy (Wolfe & Goldfried, 1988, p. 449). Second, there are a sufficient number of studies that have investigated the association between alliance and outcome using a variety of well-developed and accepted measures. Third, the alliance is theorized to contain a component that encompasses agreement between client and therapist on the goals and tasks of the therapy. Belief in the therapy and conviction that the course of therapy will be helpful is a critical component of the contextual model, as described herein. Of course, there are other common factors, such as the provision of treatment rationale or client expectation for change, that could be reviewed as well. However, presentation of the entire literature on all of the common factors is beyond the scope of this book. Nevertheless, the establishment of a robust connection between one common factor and outcome provides compelling evidence for the contextual model of psychotherapy, particularly in light of the fact that there is a paucity of research establishing the efficacy of any specific ingredient (see chap. 5).

In this chapter, two meta-analyses examining the relationship between the alliance and outcome as well as several well-conducted studies are reviewed. The goal is to estimate the general effects produced by the alliance, should an association between alliance and outcome be found. In these reviews, several methodological issues will be discussed.

META-ANALYTIC STUDIES

By 1990, many st⬚⬚⬚⬚⬚ the relation between the strength of the a⬚⬚⬚⬚⬚herapy. In 1991, A. O. Horvath and Sym⬚⬚⬚⬚⬚lysis to examine the alliance–outcome r⬚⬚⬚⬚⬚ter publication of additional studies, M⬚⬚⬚⬚⬚0) conducted another meta-analysis to ⬚⬚⬚⬚⬚ne.

Horvath and Symonds—Evidence for a Strong Alliance–Outcome Relationship

A. O. Horvath and Symonds (1991) retrieved 20 studies that (a) assessed the alliance, as rated by the client, therapist, or observers; (b) assessed outcome; and (c) reported a quantitative measure of the relationship between the alliance and the outcome of psychotherapy. The relationship between alliance and outcome in these 20 studies was typically reported as a Pearson product–moment correlation, which is an appropriate statistic to index the association between two continuously measured variables. Consequently, A. O. Horvath and Symonds (1991) used meta-analytic methods to aggregate correlation coefficients across studies (see Hedges & Olkin, 1985, chap. 11). Moreover, they avoided issues of dependent effects by aggregating within studies before conducting the meta-analysis.

The 20 studies were published between 1978 and 1990, contained an average of 40 participants, involved treatments that lasted an average of 21 sessions, and used therapists with an average of 8 years of experience. The aggregated correlation coefficient for the 20 studies was .26, which is sufficiently large to reject the null hypothesis that the population correlation of alliance and outcome was 0 ($z = 8.48$, $p < .001$). Thus, there appears to be a robust relationship between the alliance formed by therapist and client and the outcomes that are produced by the therapy. For comparison purposes, it is useful to convert the aggregated correlation coefficient to a d statistic, which is typically used to report effect size for group differences, as described in chapter 2. A correlation of .26 is equivalent to a d of 0.54 (see Table 2.4), which is a medium-sized effect and can be interpreted as saying that about 7 % of the outcome is associated with the alliance. Keep in mind that in chapter 3, differences among treatments produced, at most, an effect size of 0.20, which indicates that about 1% of outcome was due to treatment ████████████████████ actor, alliance, accounted for at least sever ███████████████████ treatment differences.

A. ████████████████████ determined that the aggregate correlation ██████████████████ idicating that the studies were not estimat ████████████████ tion. Accordingly, they searched for sourc ████████████████ ossible source of heterogeneity involve ████████████████ the alliance and outcome. Table 6.1 prese ████████████████ pective. One of the striking results is that c ████████████████ icipants (i.e., therapist and client), it is the clients' perspective of the alliance that is most strongly related to outcome. In addition, observers' ratings of the alliance tended to converge with the clients' perspective, which is consistent with pervious research (e.g., Tichenor & Hill, 1989). The significance of the clients' perspective is important, as discussed in chapter 9.

TABLE 6.1

Aggregate Correlation Coefficients of Alliance and Outcome
by Rater Perspective

	Alliance Rater			
Outcome Rater	Client	Therapist	Observer	Row Aggregate
Client	.31	.13	.20	.21
Therapist	.22	−.20	.31	.17
Observer	.29	−.17	.18	.10
Column Aggregate	.27	−.03	.23	.20

Note. From "Relation Between Working Alliance and Outcome in Psychotherapy: A Meta-Analysis," by A. O. Horvath and B. D. Symonds, 1991, *Journal of Counseling Psychology, 38,* p. 144. Copyright © 1991 by the American Psychological Association. Adapted with permission.

One of the problems with interpreting the strong correlational relationship between the alliance and outcome is that, as any elementary statistics student knows, "correlation does not imply causation." One alternative explanation for the correlation is that a third variable might be causing both the alliance and the outcome. The results in Table 6.1 help to rule out one third-variable threat to the validity of the alliance–outcome correlations. A typical problem that plagues process–outcome correlations is that when a single rater rates both targets (i.e., process and outcome), a method variance, or "halo effect," is present and may be responsible for the correlation (Hoyt, 2000; Hoyt & Kerns, 1999). For example, if a client is generally pleased by therapy, he or she will likely rate both the process and the outcome of therapy favorably, thereby inflating the correlation between the two. In Table 6.1, the main diagonal represent the correlations produced by common raters (e.g., client rating both alliance and outcome). In the present case, if halo effects were present, then the correlations of the main diagonal of Table 6.1 would be larger than the off-diagonal correlations, which was not the case. Moreover, Hoyt (Hoyt, 2000; Hoyt & Kerns, 1999) has shown that it is unlikely that this method variance is greater than the attenuation of correlations due to rater error. Thus it appears that the correlations of alliance and outcome in this meta-analysis were not spuriously due to method variance.

Another problem with correlations is that the causality can be in either direction; that is, positive outcomes may produce better alliances rather than the alliance causing better outcomes. There is evidence from the A. O. Horvath and Symonds (1991) meta-analysis that the alliance is responsible for the outcome of therapy rather than vice-versa. It may well be that clients who experience progress in therapy form a better alliance with the therapist than clients who do not have a beneficial experience (i.e., outcome causes the alliance). If such were the case, then the correlation between alliance and outcome would be small when measured in early sessions before therapeutic progress had been achieved. Horvath and Symonds reported the alliance–outcome correlations for early and late phases of therapy; the correlations were virtually identical. The correlation based on the assessment of the alliance early in therapy was .31, whereas the correlation based on the assessment of the alliance late in therapy was .30. However, when alliance was based on averaging the alliance over multiple sessions, the alliance–outcome correlation dropped to .17, a pattern that fits theoretically with conceptualizations of the alliance:

> The comparatively weak relation between averaged alliance and outcome may be due to these ratings capturing the relatively large between-session fluctuations of the alliance that are typical of the middle phase of therapy (Horvath, 1986). These variations are thought to occur as a consequence of the breaks and subsequent repair of the relationship (Horvath & Marx, 1988; Safran et al. 1990). It has been suggested that the degree of success in resolving the disruption of the interpersonal process is more predictive at this time in therapy than the quantitative aspects of the alliance. (A. O. Horvath & Luborsky, 1993, p. 145)

Thus, the evidence presented by Horvath and Symonds does not support the contention that progress in therapy causes the alliance or that halo effects are artifactually causing both the alliance and outcome.

Some would contend that the alliance is not a common factor in that it is particularly strategic in some therapies (e.g., psychodynamic and client-centered), necessary but not sufficient for others (e.g., CBT), and irrelevant for others (e.g., systematic desensitization or rational–emotive therapy). A. O. Horvath and Symonds (1991) investigated this hypothesis by segregating studies into three classes. They found that the alliance–outcome correlations were .17 for psychodynamic treatments, .28 for mixed–eclectic, and .26 for cognitive therapies, differences that were not statistically significant. However, only two studies in the database investigated cognitive therapy. Thus, the question of whether the alliance is equally potent across therapies cannot be considered settled by this meta-analysis.

Martin et al. (2000)—Confirming the Alliance–Outcome Relationship

Given that approximately 60 studies examining the relationship between alliance and outcome had been published since the A. O. Horvath and Symonds (1991) meta-analysis, Martin et al. (2000) undertook to examine this relationship. The additional studies allowed the meta-analytic examination of additional factors that bear on the alliance issue, including whether the relationship is a function of the particular instrument used to assess the alliance.

The authors located 79 studies that contained quantitative indices of the alliance–outcome association, focused on clinical populations, involved individual therapy, and appeared between 1977 and 1997. Estimation of effect size was accomplished by aggregating correlation coefficients. To eliminate the dependence of effect sizes within studies, the correlations were averaged within each study. Aggregation across studies was accomplished by weighting the correlations by sample size.

The overall alliance–outcome correlation was .22, which is slightly smaller than A. O. Horvath and Symonds' (1991) estimate of .26, but still in the medium-sized effect range ($r = .22$ is equivalent to $d = .45$ and indicates that 5% of the variance in outcomes is associated with the alliance). The correlations were homogeneous, obviating the need to disaggregate them by examining moderator variables. Moreover, the standard error of the alliance–outcome correlation was very small (i.e., near zero), generating confidence in the estimate of .22. Thus, for the purpose of the this chapter, an alliance–outcome correlation of .22 is used as a viable estimate for the general effects due to the alliance.

In a strategy with dubious justification, Martin et al. (2000) conducted an additional analysis in which the correlations within studies were treated as though they were independent. Not unexpectedly, these correlations were heterogenous. In a search for the source of heterogeneity, further analysis showed that six of the seven scales used to measure the alliance showed a statistically significant relationship to outcome, whereas a seventh did not. However, the scale that did not produce a significant alliance–outcome correlation was used infrequently (11 times out of 260 nonindependent correlations). This analysis provides evidence that the strong relationship between alliance and outcome is not dependent on the particular scale used to measure the alliance.

Martin et al. (2000) came to the following conclusion:

> The relation of the alliance and outcome appears to be consistent, regardless of many of the variables that have been posited to influence the relationship.... In sum, the present meta-analysis indicates that the overall alliance–outcome correlation represents a single population of effects that cannot be reduced by a moderator variable into a more explanatory model of the relation of the alliance and outcome. (p. 446)

The meta-analyses (viz., A. O. Horvath & Symonds, 1991; Martin et al., 2000) have produced evidence that there is a moderately strong relationship between the alliance and outcome in psychotherapy. Attention is now turned to well-conducted individual studies that have investigated the role of the alliance in therapy. These studies are useful for examining the role of the alliance in particular treatments (e.g., CBT for depression) as well as across various treatments. Moreover, particular threats to validity were addressed in these studies.

INDIVIDUAL STUDIES OF THE ALLIANCE

In this section, individual studies of the alliance and outcome will be reviewed. In several of these studies, examination of the relationship between alliance and outcome was made in the context of a well-designed randomized comparative design, which rules out threats to validity and allows comparison of the alliance across types of treatments.

Alliance and Outcome in CBT for Depression

Burns and Nolen-Hoeksema (1992) used structural equation modeling to examine the role of therapeutic empathy, one component of the alliance, in the treatment of depression with CBT. From the origins of CBT for depression, the alliance has been recognized as a necessary but not sufficient condition for change (see Beck et al., 1979). Although many studies have examined empathy and outcome, this study sophisticatedly modeled the effects of therapist and client characteristics in order to rule out these confounding sources of the empathy–outcome relationship in a large sample ($N = 187$).

One particular difficulty in modeling the relationship between empathy and depression is their reciprocal influences. For example, level of depression may be related to a client's perceptions of empathy in that the therapist may be less empathic toward a more depressed client, or a depressed client may not recognize and respond to the therapist's empathy. In the first stage of Burns and Nolen-Hoeksemas's (1992) analysis, they removed the effects of concurrent depression (as measured by the BDI) from empathy (as measured by the Empathy Scale, or ES, a scale completed by clients). Similarly, they removed the effects of empathy from depression as measured by the 12-week BDI scores. These residualized scores were then used for subsequent analyses.

To rule out other possible confounding variables, in the second stage of analysis the relationship between empathy (after removing the effects of concurrent depression) and recovery was modeled accounting for these confounding variables. For example, in one structural equation, the 12-week BDI was predicted from initial BDI, empathy, therapist experience, income, homework compliance, presence of borderline personality disorder, medication status, number of sessions completed, sex, age, and education. In a second structural equation, empathy was predicted from

12-week BDI, the therapists' general level of empathy, and borderline personality disorder. Various models were compared by excluding various predictor variables, thereby identifying the important sources of variance.

For all of the models tested, therapeutic empathy predicted depression, indicating that high levels of therapist empathy lead to clinical improvement. This relationship was robust in that it was present in models that controlled for various spurious relationships. On the other hand, depression had a very small effect on empathy. The authors made the following conclusion:

> The patients of therapists who were the warmest and most empathic improved significantly more than the patients of the therapists with the lowest empathy ratings, when controlling for initial depression severity, homework compliance, and other factors. This indicates that even in a highly technical form of therapy such as CBT, the quality of the therapeutic relationship has a substantial impact on the degree of recovery. This is the first report we are aware of that has documented the causal effect of therapeutic empathy on recovery when controlling for the simultaneous causal effect of depression on therapeutic empathy. However, the reciprocal causal effect of therapeutic empathy on depression was negligible, indicating that a depressed mood may not greatly bias patients' perceptions of the therapeutic alliance. (Burns & Nolen-Hoeksema, 1992, p. 447)

The results of this study caused the authors to alter their clinical practice:

> All patients are now required to complete the therapeutic empathy forms after every session and to return these forms to their therapists at subsequent visits. Thus, difficulties in the therapeutic alliance can be more rapidly identified and addressed. It is our clinical impression that this frequently leads to improvements in the therapeutic empathy scores and to rapid reductions in BDI scores. (Burns & Nolen-Hoeksema, 1992, p. 445)

Alliance and Outcome Across Treatments— The NIMH TDCRP

An important issue with regard to the alliance as a common factor is whether its effect on outcomes is similar across disparate therapies. Two studies have examined the relationship of alliance to outcome for the four treatments in the NIMH TDCRP (see chap. 4 for a complete description of this study). Recall that in this study there were four treatments for depression: CBT, IPT, IMI-CM, and pill placebo plus clinical management.

In one of the two studies related to the NIMH TDCRP, Krupnick et al. (1996) investigated the relationship of observer-rated alliance using an early session (usually Session 3) and the average observer-rated alliance over all the sessions. The therapeutic alliance was assessed by using a version of the Vanderbilt Therapeutic Alliance Scale (VTAS), which was modified to apply to all four treatments. As used, the VTAS was composed of a Patient scale and a Therapist scale. Analysis involved predicting Hamilton

Rating Scale for Depression (HRSD) and BDI scores using multiple regression and remission status with logistic regression. All analyses partialled out pretreatment severity and treatment and focused on (a) the alliance and (b) the alliance–treatment interaction. The latter interaction tests whether the alliance was related to outcome differentially for the four treatments.

The results of this study showed a consistency of alliance–outcome relationship across treatments. First, there were no statistically significant differences among the mean alliance ratings for the four treatments. Using the early sessions, the Patient scale accounted for about 8% of the variance in HRSD and BDI scores. The mean therapeutic alliance scores were more highly related to outcome, accounting for up to 21%. On the other hand, the treatment variable (i.e., differences among the four groups) accounted for at most 2% of the variance (which takes into account that one of the treatments, CM, was a placebo condition). The early alliance was related to remission as well; a unit increase in alliance score increased the estimated odds of remission threefold. There was only one significant treatment–alliance interaction, which involved the early alliance for the BDI; here, CBT showed a relatively lower relationship between alliance and outcome than did the other treatments. The authors made the following conclusion:

> The results also showed a significant relationship between total therapeutic alliance ratings and treatment outcome across modalities, with more of the variance in outcome attributed to alliance than to treatment method. There were virtually no significant treatment group differences in the relationship between therapeutic alliance and outcome in interpersonal psychotherapy, cognitive behavior therapy, and active and placebo pharmacotherapy with clinical management. (Krupnick et al., 1996, p. 536)

The results of the this study diverged from those of A. O. Horvath and Symonds's (1991) meta-analysis in that the average alliance ratings were more highly related to outcome than were the early ratings. Nevertheless, the early ratings of alliance, which are presumably less affected by therapeutic progress, remained highly correlated with outcome.

Another analysis of the alliance–outcome relationship in the NIMH TDCRP was conducted by Blatt, Zuroff, Quinlan, and Pilkonis (1996). In this study, alliance was assessed by patients' responses to the Barrett-Lennard Relationship Inventory (B-L RI), which was administered as part of the NIMH TDCRP protocol. To avoid confounding alliance with therapeutic progress, Blatt et. al. used the B-L RI scores that were obtained at the end of the second session. In this study the authors also examined the Perfectionism and the Need for Approval subscales, which were derived from the DAS. Using planned comparisons, the alliance was significantly lower in the two pharmacological conditions (i.e., IMI-CM and pill placebo plus clinical management) than in the two psychotherapies (i.e., CBT and

IPT), but there were no statistically significant differences between the two psychotherapies. As well, alliance was unrelated to pretherapy DAS scores, suggesting that perceptions of the alliance were independent from perfectionism and need for approval.

In terms of outcome, the alliance scores were correlated with five continuous outcome measures, after partialling out pretest scores on the measures (i.e., residualized gain scores). Three of the five correlations were statistically significant, and the correlations ranged from –.11 to –.26, where negative correlations indicate that higher levels of the alliance were related to lower levels of depression. As well, the B-L RI was significantly related to dropout from treatment. Thus, patients who experienced a positive alliance very early in treatment were less likely to drop out of treatment and to have greater amelioration of depression.

CONCLUSIONS

In chapter 5, many different designs failed to find sufficient evidence that any specific ingredient was responsible for the benefits of psychotherapy. Examination of a single common factor, the working alliance, convincingly demonstrated that this factor is a key component of psychotherapy. The alliance appears to be a necessary aspect of therapy, regardless of the nature of the therapy. Proponents of most treatments recognize that the relationship between the therapist and the client is critical but not sufficient. However, it appears that the relationship accounts for dramatically more of the variability in outcomes than does the totality of specific ingredients.

7

Allegiance and Adherence: Further Evidence for the Contextual Model

Allegiance to a treatment approach and adherence to the respective protocol are important concepts that differentiate the meaning model and the contextual model of psychotherapy. Allegiance refers to the degree to which the therapist delivering the treatment believes that the therapy is efficacious. One of the sacrosanct assumptions of a client is that their therapist believes in the treatment being delivered. Because psychotherapy is an endeavor based on trust, violation of this assumption would appear to undermine the tenets of the profession. For the most part, practicing therapists choose the approach to psychotherapy that is compatible with their understanding and conceptualization of psychological distress and health, the process of change, and the nature of the client and his or her issues.[1] Consequently clients can rest assured that their therapist is committed to and believes in the therapy being delivered. Conceived in this way, therapist allegiance is a common factor that exists across therapies as they are typically delivered.

Adherence is defined as the "extent to which a therapist used interventions and approaches prescribed by the treatment manual, and avoided the use of interventions and procedures proscribed by the manual" (Waltz et al.,

---

[1]It is fully recognized that managed care limits the freedom that therapists have to deliver treatments that they deem to be optimal. In a sense, such limitations result from the imposition of a medical model onto the practice of psychotherapy.

1993, p. 620). Thus, adherence is a measure of the degree to which the specific ingredients of a treatment are present and the specific ingredients of other treatments are absent.

It appears, at first glance, that allegiance is a common factor, whereas adherence is related to the delivery of specific ingredients. Nevertheless, medical and contextual model predictions for allegiance and adherence are complex and need elaboration.

PREDICTIONS FOR ALLEGIANCE AND ADHERENCE

In the contextual model, therapist allegiance is a critical component necessary for the efficacious delivery of a psychotherapeutic treatment. Although allegiance may be universal in practice settings, there is reason to believe that allegiance varies considerably in clinical trials of psychotherapy. Consider, for example, a clinical trial comparing cognitive–behavioral and interpersonal treatments for depression in which a crossed design (see chap. 8) is used. In such a design, each therapist would provide all of the treatments but might have allegiance to only one of the treatments. When clinical trials are conducted by proponents of a particular treatment, the therapists may be graduate students of the proponent or otherwise affiliated with the proponent's research laboratory. Consequently these therapists would have greater allegiance to the treatment affiliated with the laboratory than with the other treatment being delivered in the study. In drug studies in medicine, allegiance effects are controlled because the persons administering the treatment do not know which treatment they are delivering; similar blinding is impossible in psychotherapy studies because the therapist is always cognizant of the treatment being provided (see chap. 5). In psychotherapy studies, allegiance can therefore be confounded with the treatment (i.e., some treatments use therapists with more allegiance than other treatments); also, because allegiance varies, the effects of allegiance on outcome can be investigated.

Because therapist belief in the treatment is a critical component of the contextual model, this model predicts that allegiance will be related to outcome—the greater the allegiance, the better the outcome. Proponents of the medical model might recognize that allegiance is consequential but would not consider allegiance to be central to treatment. The relative unimportance of allegiance in the medical model is demonstrated by the fact that allegiance is not considered when control groups (placebos or alternative treatments) are designed. That is, clinical scientists seem to be unconcerned that therapists do not have allegiance to placebo treatments or alternative treatments, thus making the assumption that allegiance effects are nonexistent.

Allegiance to treatment provides a test of the medical model versus the contextual model: Allegiance is a critical factor in the contextual model but relatively unimportant in the medical model.

With regard to adherence, medical model predictions are relatively straightforward. If specific ingredients are responsible for psychotherapeutic benefit, then adherence to the manual should be related to outcome. That is, therapists who provide the ingredients that are purportedly necessary for change would have better outcomes than therapists who do not provide such ingredients. On the other hand, adherence to a treatment for which the specific ingredients are inert should have no relation to outcome. If a treatment is composed of specific ingredients that are not remedial for the disorder, then adherence to the treatment would not provide any benefit to the clients. This interaction, which is shown in Figure 7.1, demonstrates the prototypical pattern of results that should be present if the medical model is explanatory for the benefits of psychotherapy.

The contextual model requires the delivery of ingredients consistent with a rationale for treatment. Yet the contextual model clearly is less dogmatic about the ingredients and certainly allows eclecticism, so long as there is a rationale that underlies the treatment and that the rationale is cogent, coherent, and psychologically based. Sol Garfield (1992), a prominent proponent of a common factors approach, discussing the results of a survey of eclectic therapists, described the role of adherence in a contextual model context:

> These eclectic clinicians tended to emphasize that they used the theory or methods they thought were best for the client. In essence, procedures were selected for a given patient in terms of that client's problems instead of trying to make the client adhere to a particular form of therapy. An eclectic therapy thus allows the

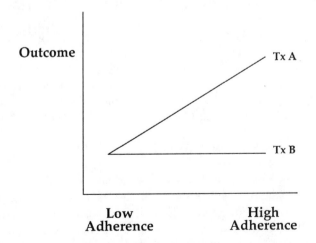

FIG. 7.1.   Medical model prediction for adherence. Tx A contains ingredients remedial for disorder, and Tx B contains ingredients that are not remedial for disorder.

therapist potentially to use a wide range of techniques, a view similar to my own in most respects.... This approach is clearly opposite to the emphasis on using psychotherapy manuals to train psychotherapists to adhere strictly to a specific form of therapy in order to ensure the integrity of the type of psychotherapy being evaluated. (p. 172)

Thus, according to the contextual model, adherence to a manualized treatment is not required and is not thought to be related to outcome. Nevertheless, therapists working from a contextual model perspective will necessarily have a cogent rationale for the treatment, and consequently the therapeutic actions will be consistent with that rationale. Consider the case of a therapist with a phobic client who has little psychological mindedness, who approaches the world from a scientific perspective, and who conceives of the therapist as a doctor who will provide a cure. Although there are many approaches that the therapist could use, the therapist believes that systematic desensitization would be well received by this client and is efficacious in this instance and consequently administers the treatment in a manner consistent with the rationale. However, this therapist, who ascribes to a contextual model of psychotherapy, presumes that the efficacy of the treatment is due to many factors unrelated to the specific ingredients of systematic desensitization (he or she has read the literature related to active ingredients and systematic desensitization; see, e.g., Kirsch, 1985). So, although this therapist would not be concerned about precisely following the procedures of systematic desensitization, the treatment would be consistent with such a protocol; for example, the therapist would avoid making interpretations or seeking insights. Thus, the contextual model suggests that treatments should be coherent and consistent, but it does not require technical adherence to a protocol.

In the next sections, the research evidence related to allegiance and adherence is presented. Because the predictions emanating from the two models are complex, care is needed in making conclusions. In several areas the research evidence is consistent with the contextual model predictions, whereas in others areas the evidence is ambiguous. However, precious little evidence exists to bolster the case of the medical model of psychotherapy.

EVIDENCE RELATED TO ALLEGIANCE

In the years when there was a "tendentious and adversarial" (M. L. Smith, Glass, & Miller, 1980, p. 7) debate about whether psychotherapy was beneficial, allegiance effects were ignored. Recall that Eysenck (1961) claimed that therapies based on learning theories (i.e., behavior therapies) were superior to other therapies or to no treatment (see chap. 4). This claim was based on studies conducted by advocates of behavior therapy, and thus allegiance may well have played a part in the demonstrated superiority of behavior therapies in the studies cited by Eysenck. One of the studies cited by Eysenck, which was conducted by Albert Ellis (1957) provides a historical perspective from which to examine the research evidence related to allegiance.

Ellis had been trained to conduct orthodox psychoanalysis and for 3 years practiced using "the sofa, free association, extensive dream analysis, and resolution of the transference neurosis" (Ellis, 1957, p. 350). Gradually he abandoned this approach in favor of an active, face-to-face approach that relied more heavily on interpretations. Around 1955, Ellis departed dramatically from the psychodynamic tradition and developed a method he called rational psychotherapy (now called rational emotive therapy; Ellis, 1993). Ellis described the basis of the treatment as follows:

> It is an application of the theory that much of what we call emotion is nothing more than a certain kind—a biased, prejudiced kind—of thought, and that human beings can be taught to control their feelings by controlling their thoughts—or by changing the internalized sentences, or self-talk, with which they largely created these feeling in the first place. The main emphasis of the therapist who employs rational techniques is on analyzing the client's current problems—especially his negative feelings of anger, depression, anxiety, and guilt—and concretely showing him that these emotions arise not from past events or external situations but from his present irrational attitudes toward or illogical fears about these events and situations. (Ellis, 1957, p. 344)

Ellis's (1957) study involved a comparison of "three techniques of psychotherapy": orthodox psychoanalysis, psychoanalytically oriented psychotherapy, and rational psychotherapy. Ellis wanted to eliminate "the important factor of the therapist's experience and skill" and at the same time use a therapist who was "equally enthused and open-minded" toward the therapies. Choice of a therapist meeting those qualifications was solved by "fortunate accident," as Ellis determined that he was such a therapist!

To compare the three therapies, Ellis (1957) used 78 cases of clients he treated with rational psychotherapy for at least 10 sessions, matched them with 78 cases from his files when he practiced psychoanalytic psychotherapy, and used 12 cases from his files when he practiced psychoanalysis. Outcome was assessed by Ellis, who determined shortly after completion of the treatment whether the client had made little or no progress, had some distinct improvement, or had made considerable improvement. The results showed that clients treated by rational therapy had better outcomes than those treated by the other therapies. Not much training in research design is needed to realize that there are multiple threats to the validity of this study. Particularly troublesome, however, in spite of Ellis's claim that he was "equally enthused and open-minded" (p. 345) to all therapies, was the issue of allegiance. That he gradually became dissatisfied first with orthodox psychoanalysis and then with psychoanalytically oriented psychotherapy and that he was the developer and vociferous proponent of rational psychotherapy were not a concern for him (or for those who cited this study as supporting the relative superiority of behavior therapies). It is reasonable to believe that his advocacy of the rational psychotherapy and his gradual discontent with the other two therapies affected the delivery of the treatments as well as the evaluation of client outcomes.

Design Issues

Given the perspective of Ellis's (1957) study, attention is now turned toward the empirical evidence related to allegiance. In Ellis's study, treatment and allegiance were completely confounded in that he was the only therapist. Apparently, allegiance to treatment is not sufficiently interesting to researchers that primary studies are conducted to determine effects due to allegiance. Nevertheless, conclusions about allegiance can be made indirectly, as described in this section.

Although primary studies do not assess individual therapists' allegiance to treatment, the allegiance of the therapists in outcome studies often can be inferred. As discussed earlier, if the researcher is a proponent of one of the treatments administered in the study, and the therapists are trained by the researcher, then it can be inferred that the therapists have allegiance to that treatment. Consider, for example, a study of cognitive therapy and applied relaxation (as well as a psychopharmacology condition) for the treatment of panic disorder, conducted by Clark et al. (1994).[2] David M. Clark, the lead author of the study, was clearly a proponent of cognitive therapy. The introduction of the article predominately discussed cognitive therapy and clearly identified applied relaxation as an established alternative that was selected in order to validate cognitive therapy. In the method section, two articles were cited as the basis for cognitive therapy, and both were authored by Clark, whereas the alternative therapy was devised and advocated by another group of researchers. Additionally, the two therapists used in the study were coauthors (viz., Salkovskis & Hackman) of the research. Finally, Clark, the first author of the study and a proponent of cognitive therapy, served as the clinical supervisor. The allegiance of the authors of this study is unambiguous; moreover, the inference that the therapists were committed to the cognitive therapy and had less loyalty to applied relaxation appears to be supported, as well. This example demonstrates how researcher advocacy for a treatment translates into therapist allegiance. Although researcher advocacy can lead to multiple biases (e.g., nonblind and biased evaluations, nonrandom data entry errors), it is clear that thera-

---

[2]This study is cited as evidence to classify cognitive therapy for panic disorder as an empirically supported treatment and as evidence for the specificity of cognitive therapy (DeRubeis & Crits-Christoph, 1998).

pist allegiance in clinical trials is present when the researcher–treatment advocate trains and supervises the therapists, and the therapists have loyalty to the researcher and the treatment approach.

Studies can be designed and undertaken that reduce or eliminate allegiance. A good example of a study that minimized allegiance effects is the NIMH TDCRP (Elkin, 1994, see also chap. 4). The authors of the study were not proponents of the two psychological treatments administered (viz., CBT and IPT), and the design of the study was developed through various committees of experts. The sites at which CBT and IPT were administered were selected from applications from groups using CBT and IPT. Consequently the treatments were delivered by therapists trained and supervised by proponents of the respective treatments.

The effects of allegiance can be investigated by comparing results across studies. That is, comparisons of the size of effects obtained when allegiance is present to the size of effects when allegiance is neutral or to another treatment in the study indexes the degree to which allegiance is influencing outcome. In the next section, several meta-analyses that have examined allegiance are reviewed.

Meta-Analytic Evidence Relative to Allegiance

Examination of allegiance effects have been scattered throughout various meta-analyses of outcome in psychotherapy. The earliest attempt to identify allegiance effects appeared in M. L. Smith et al.'s (1980) meta-analysis. Recall from chapter 3 that Smith et al. conducted an extensive search of all published and unpublished controlled studies of counseling psychotherapy through 1977. In all, 475 studies were found, which produced an average effect size (treatment versus control) of 0.85, which is a large effect. Allegiance in each study in this meta-analysis was determined by the "direction of stated research hypotheses, favorable results of previous research uncritically accepted, rationalizations after failure to find significant effects for the favored treatment, and outright praise and promotion of a point of view" (Smith et al., 1980, p. 119). Often the alternative treatments against which the favored treatment was compared would "be treated with obvious disdain, and would not be given much opportunity for success" (Smith et al., 1980, p. 119). Unequivocal allegiance effects were detected. When compared with control groups, treatments for which the experimenter had allegiance produced an average effect size of 0.95, whereas treatments for which the experimenter had an allegiance against the treatment produced an effect size of 0.66. The difference between these two effect sizes (viz., an effect size of 0.29) is a rough estimate of allegiance effects.

A few years later, an interesting allegiance effect for a particular researcher appeared when Dush, Hirt, and Schroeder (1983) meta-analyzed studies that investigated self-statement modification (SSM). At the time, cognitive therapies were experiencing a wave of popularity. Three approaches predominated: Ellis's rational–emotive therapy (as discussed earlier in this chapter), Beck's cognitive therapy, and Meichenbaum's SSM. Dush et al. retrieved 69 studies that compared SSM with a no-treatment control group or with a placebo control group. As shown in Table 7.1, the average of the effect sizes for SSM vis-à-vis no-treatment controls and placebo controls were 0.74 and 0.53, respectively. These values are in accordance with treatment efficacy values found across meta-analyses (see chaps. 3 and 5). However, when studies were segregated on the basis of whether the studies were authored or coauthored by Meichenbaum, dramatic differences in effect sizes emerged. The effect sizes produced by studies authored or coauthored by Meichenbaum were nearly twice as large as the other studies when comparisons were made with no-treatment controls and more than twice as large when comparisons were made with placebo controls (see Table 7.1). More telling is that the placebo controls appear to be markedly deficient in those studies conducted by Meichenbaum, as the effect size using placebo controls and no-treatment controls produced almost identical effect sizes (i.e., placebo controls appeared to be essentially no-treatment controls). Using the difference between Meichenbaum's effect sizes and the other study effect sizes, allegiance effects in the range of 0.60 to 0.70 were obtained. These SSM studies clearly show an allegiance effect for Meichenbaum, the developer and primary advocate for SSM treatments.

Dramatic allegiance effects have also been found for comparisons between cognitive therapy and systematic desensitization (SD). From chapter 4 recall that D. A. Shapiro and Shapiro (1982) found one of the few

TABLE 7.1

Effect Sizes for Self-Statement Modification by Whether
(Co-) Authored by Meichenbaum (From Dush, Hirt, & Schroeder, 1983).

Study Allegiance	No-Treatment Controls		Placebo Controls	
	M	No.	M	No.
Meichenbaum (co-authored)	1.23	95	1.24	41
Meichenbaum referenced	0.62	398	0.48	255
Other	0.74	276	0.44	196
Total	0.74	768	0.53	492

Note. From "Self-Statement Modification With Adults: A Meta-Analysis," by D. M. Dush, M L. Hirt, and H. Schroeder, 1983, *Psychological Bulletin, 94,* p. 414. Copyright © 1983 by the American Psychological Association. Adapted with permission.

meta-analytic differences between classes of treatments intended to be therapeutic. Specifically, they retrieved nine studies that compared cognitive therapy with SD and found that cognitive therapy was superior by 0.53 effect size units. This is a large difference, particularly given that the nine studies involved direct comparisons of these two treatments, thereby ruling out many confounds (see chap. 4). However, a year later, Miller and Berman (1983) reviewed studies that compared cognitive therapy and SD and found nonsignificant differences. Berman et al. (1985), sought to resolve the discrepancies between Shapiro and Shapiro (1982) and Miller and Berman (1983) by including all the studies reviewed by these two prior reviews as well as more recent studies that were not contained in either of the previous reviews. Berman et al. were able to identify 20 studies that compared cognitive therapy and SD. This meta-analysis was laudatory in that effect sizes were adjusted for bias, weighted by sample size, and averaged across dependent measures in each study.

The results of Berman et al.'s (1985) meta-analysis showed that cognitive therapy and SD were essentially equivalent. For the 20 studies of direct comparisons, the effect size was 0.06, where a positive effect size indicated that cognitive therapy was superior to SD. Clearly, the difference between cognitive therapy and SD was negligible and inconsistent with D. A. Shapiro and Shapiro's (1982) result. Berman et al. hypothesized that the discrepancy was due to allegiance effects; they classified studies on the basis of whether the researcher had allegiance to cognitive therapy, to SD, or to neither. For the 10 studies for which there was allegiance to cognitive therapy, those treatments were superior to SD (average effect size = 0.27); on the other hand, for the 5 studies in which there was allegiance to SD, the SD treatments were superior to cognitive therapy (average effect size = –0.38). Thus, allegiance effects were 0.65—that is, $0.27 - (-0.38)$. Again, the presence of strong allegiance effects was detected.

Another meta-analysis that found strong allegiance effects is Robinson et al.'s (1990) review of treatments for depression. This meta-analysis was summarized in chapter 4 (see Table 4.6). Although Robinson et al. found differences in the efficacy of various treatments of depression, these differences were accounted for by differences in allegiance to the various treatments. Further examination of the allegiance effects in this meta-analysis demonstrate the strength of such effects. In this meta-analysis, allegiance was rated on a 5-point scale, using the cues discussed previously (e.g., direction of hypotheses, degree of detail provided about treatments). The two raters used in this meta-analysis showed remarkable consistency in their ratings of allegiance (intraclass correlation of .95). After the corpus of studies was reviewed, the correlation between the allegiance ratings and the effects produced by the study was .58, which is remarkably large. That is, about one third $[(.58)^2 = 0.34]$ of the variance in effect sizes produced in the studies reviewed was due to the allegiance of the researcher. Because study outcomes may have influenced the writing of the introductions of the articles in the meta-analysis, Robinson et al. identified a subset of studies for which the allegiance of the researcher could be established by previous publications of the author; for these studies, the relation between allegiance and outcome remained high ($r = .51$). All told, Robinson et al. found large allegiance effects in an area of established psychotherapy outcome research.

Although Robinson et al. (1990) found strong allegiance effects for treatments of depression, Gaffan et al. (1995) produced evidence that allegiance effects may be decreasing over time. Gaffan et al. examined two sets of studies that compared cognitive therapy and other therapies. The first set contained 28 studies reviewed in Dobson (1989) and published between 1976 and 1987. The second set contained 37 studies published between 1987 and 1994. For the first set, there was an advantage for cognitive therapy relative to control groups or alternate treatments (see chap. 4 and Table 4.7). In addition, there were relatively strong allegiance effects, and allegiance effects were related to the effect sizes obtained from comparisons of cognitive therapy and the other groups. For the second set of studies, the comparative effect sizes were generally smaller (see Table 4.7); allegiance effects were also smaller. Moreover, allegiance effects were not related to effect sizes. The authors made the following conclusion:

> The relationship is present in Dobson's set of studies partly because comparisons with large [effect sizes] favoring [cognitive therapy] CT were associated with strong allegiance toward CT, especially before 1985, and partly because [effect size] and allegiance declined together from the late 1970s to the 1980s. By the 1990s, both these associations had disappeared. (Gaffan et al., 1995, p. 978)

Conclusions Related to Allegiance

Meta-analyses investigating allegiance have generally found allegiance effects, with the exception of Gaffan et al. (1995). The magnitude of allegiance effects ranged up to 0.65. Given that the upper bound for specific effects was approximately 0.20, it is clear that allegiance to the therapy is a very strong determinant of outcome in clinical trials. That the effects due to the allegiance accounts for dramatically more of the variance in outcome than does the particular type of treatment implies that therapist attitudes toward therapy is a critical component of effective therapy, consistent with the contextual model of psychotherapy.

EVIDENCE RELATED TO ADHERENCE

Recall that adherence is defined as the "extent to which a therapist used interventions and approaches prescribed by the treatment manual, and avoided the use of intervention procedures proscribed by the manual" (Waltz et al., 1993, p. 620). Adherence is a meaningless concept in the absence of a manual that specifies the therapeutic actions that are prescribed and proscribed. As explained in chapter 1, there are ingredients of each treatment that are unique and purportedly essential, which have been labeled in this book as specific ingredients.

Research Issues

There are some issues related to adherence and its measurement that need further clarification. First, adherence needs to be distinguished from competence. Competence refers to the "level of skill in delivering the treatment, [where] skill [is] the extent to which their therapists conducting interventions took the relevant aspects of the therapeutic context into account and responded to these contextual variables appropriately" (Waltz et al., 1993, p. 620). However, competence can be applied to both the specific ingredients as well as the ingredients that various treatments have in common. For example, a psychodynamic therapist should be skilled at delivering interpretations as well as in forming a strong working alliance with the client.[3] In this chapter the focus is on adherence to the treatment protocol and not on competence; competence is considered in chapter 8.

A second issue is that adherence to a manual may be affected by the client. A compliant and motivated client will participate enthusiastically in a treatment, whereas the recalcitrant client will resist therapeutic interventions. The therapist of a motivated client will find it relatively easy to adhere to the treatment protocols. Although treatment manuals specify therapeutic actions for resistant clients, there will inevitably be a tendency to abandon therapeutic actions that are resisted and are unsuccessful. Indeed, Barber et al. (1996) found that the degree to which clients improved in the first three sessions predicted the degree to which the therapist adhered to the treatment protocol in a subsequent session. Therefore, as the literature on adherence is reviewed, it will be important to realize that a relationship between outcome and adherence may be the result of a compliant and motivated client.

Three types of studies are examined to determine the degree to which adherence to a manual produces beneficial outcomes. The first type of study addresses whether two treatments, each guided by manuals, can be discriminated. For example, are there observable differences between cognitive–behavioral treatment and interpersonal psychotherapy for depression, and if so, are the differences those that would be expected theoretically? Although such studies do not produce evidence that adherence is related to

---

[3]Waltz et al. (1993) proposed a contextual definition of competence that is restricted to a specified treatment: "We do not assume that any therapist behaviors represent universal expressions of competence across treatments" (p. 620).

outcome, discrimination of treatments is a necessary condition for establishing an adherence–outcome connection. The second type of study examines whether treatments that are guided by manuals result in superior outcomes to treatments conducted without manuals. The presumption here is that for a given type of treatment, therapists using a manual will adhere to the treatment protocol to a greater extent than would be the case for therapists who are not bound by a manual. The third type of study examines the relationship between adherence to a manual and outcome.

Discrimination of Treatments

Although there are no meta-analyses related to discrimination of treatments, well- conducted studies in a number of areas indicate that treatments can be discriminated on the basis of their respective theoretical frameworks. There has been a long history of examining observed differences among various types of therapies (e.g., Auerbach, 1963; Brunink & Schroeder, 1979; Sloane et al., 1975; Strupp, 1958). In this section, a few of the more recent studies that involve treatments delivered with manuals are reviewed briefly.

In 1982, shortly after the advent of manuals, Luborsky, Woody, McLellan, O'Brien, and Rosenzweig investigated whether judges could recognize three treatments for drug abuse: (a) drug counseling, (b) supportive–expressive therapy, and (c) CBT. Besides being guided by the manual, the therapists were supervised by experts in the respective treatments. The specific ingredients of each of the manuals were used to compose rating scales that assessed the degree to which 15-min segments of randomly selected sessions contained these specific ingredients. Two independent raters were used in each of two studies. In the first study, the raters were able, on the basis of the rating scales, to identify correctly 70% of the treatments. After revising the scales slightly for a second study, raters were able to identify correctly 80% of the treatments. With one notable exception, the ingredients characteristic of each treatment were rated to be present more often for that treatment than for the other treatments. However, "giving support," which was theoretically characteristic of supportive–expressive therapy, was present in approximately equal amounts in each of the treatments, suggesting that this ingredient may be a common factor rather than a specific ingredient. This study provided convincing evidence that treatments delivered with manuals were differentiable on the basis of their specific ingredients.

Hill et al. (1992) examined adherence to manuals in the NIMH TDCRP (see chap. 4 for a more complete description of this study). Adherence to the three treatments was assessed with the Collaborative Study Psychotherapy Rating Scale (CSPRS), which was developed through consultation with the trainers of the treatments as well as an examination of the ingredients specified in the manuals for three treatments, CBT, IPT, and CM. The

CSPRS contained three modality-specific scales. The CBT, IPT, and CM scales contained 28, 28, and 20 items, respectively, that assessed whether the specific ingredients of the three treatments were absent or present to varying degrees. In addition, the CSPRS included two non-modality-specific scales, which measured facilitative conditions (FC; eight items) and explicit directiveness (ED; four items). The CSPRS was used to rate Sessions 1, 4, 7 or 8, and 14 or 15 for each client.

The results of adherence for the TDCRP indicated that the therapists in all conditions adhered to the treatment protocol. Variance components were calculated for (a) modality (i.e., CBT v. IPT v. CM), (b) site, (c) Modality × Site, (d) therapist (within Modality × Site), (e) client (within therapist), (f) session, (g) Modality × Session, (h) Site × Session, (i) Modality × Site × Session, (j) Therapist × Session, and (f) rater. For the modality-specific scales, the largest proportion of variance was accounted for by modality, as expected. About 70% of the variance was due to modality, whereas the other factors accounted for negligible amounts of variance. In all cases, the variance components reflected the predicted relationship: The scores for the CBT scale was highest for CBT sessions, the scores for the IPT scale were highest for IPT sessions, and the scores for the CM scale were highest for the CM sessions. As expected, the ED scale was highest for the CBT and CM sessions, as these treatments were more directive than IPT. On the FC scale "cognitive–behavioral therapists and interpersonal therapists were equivalent, indicating that both groups were viewed as supportive, competent, involved, warm, and empathic" (p. 78). As with Luborsky et al.'s (1982) study, it appears that there were distinct differences among treatments along the lines of the specific ingredients as well as a conspicuous common factor related to support that was present in all of the treatments.

There are many other studies that have found the expected theoretical differences as well as commonalities, among various treatments (e.g., Goldfried, Castonguay, Hayes, Drozd, & Shapiro, 1997; Jones & Pulos, 1993; Stiles, Shapiro, & Firth-Cozens, 1989; Wiser & Goldfried, 1993). Moreover, there is compelling evidence that training therapists to deliver manualized treatments increases adherence to the manual (see Binder, 1993; Crits-Christoph et al., 1991; Henry, Schacht, Strupp, Butler, & Binder, 1993; Henry, Strupp, Butler, Schacht, & Binder, 1993). Because treatments differ along the expected theoretical dimensions, and therapists can be trained to adhere to manuals, the evidence related to adherence and outcome can now be critically reviewed.

Manuals and Outcome

As discussed previously (see chap. 1), manuals allow "researchers to demonstrate the theoretically required procedural differences between alternative treatments in comparative outcome studies" (Wilson, 1996, p. 295). According to the medical model, adherence to the manual is vital as the specific ingredients contained in the manual are purportedly remedial for the disorder being treated. Consequently, treatments delivered with manuals should be more beneficial to clients than are treatments delivered without manuals. The meta-analyses that bear on this question are now reviewed to show that this is not the case; the use of manuals does not appear to offer any particular benefits to clients.

An opportune domain in which to examine the effects of using a manual is in the area of depression, because manuals for the treatment of depression have been in existence since the late 1970s (e.g., Beck et al., 1979). In 1990, Robinson et al.'s meta-analysis of treatments for depression contained approximately equal numbers of treatments conducted with manuals and without manuals (see chap. 4 for a discussion of this meta-analysis). They found the following:

> When treatments were directly compared with one another, however, the absolute magnitude of effect sizes from 11 studies that used formal manuals ($M = 0.28$, $SD = 0.30$) did not differ reliably from the absolute magnitude of effect sizes from 14 studies in which no manuals were used ($M = 0.34$, $SD = 0.18$), $t(23) = .55$, $p = .6$. Similar results were observed when we examined studies comparing treated groups with wait-list controls. The effect sizes of 14 studies using manual-driven therapies ($M = 0.82$, $SD = 0.64$) did not differ systematically from the effect sizes of 17 studies for which no manual was developed ($M = 0.84$, $SD = 0.74$), $t(29) = 0.07$, $p = .9$. Although the use of treatment manuals has increased in recent years, these data provide no indication that their use either increases therapeutic efficacy or allows for a finer differentiation of the relative effectiveness of treatments. (Robinson et al., 1990, p. 36)

The effects of manuals can be investigated by examining comparisons of the efficacy of treatments delivered in controlled clinical trials with the efficacy of treatments delivered in clinically representative situations. Typically, in clinical trials, treatments are standardized, and therapists are trained and supervised to deliver the treatments being studied; that is, adherence to a manual is expected. On the other hand, in practice settings, therapists have greater latitude to deviate from standard protocols. One of the bases of the empirically supported therapy movement is that treatments shown to be efficacious for a particular disorder and for a particular population should be transported to practice settings. Shadish, Matt, Navarro, and Phillips (2000) made the following observation:

> The literature on practice guidelines (e.g., Nathan, 1998) is based partly on the assumption that therapy under clinically representative conditions is less effective than it could be if therapists used empirically supported psychological therapies that have been found efficacious in controlled research with a delineated population (Chambless & Hollon, 1998; Kendall, 1998). (Shadish et al., 2000, p. 512)

At this point, it is useful to review the terminology used to refer to outcomes of controlled experiments and the outcomes of therapy as practiced. In clinical trials, treatments are delivered in a standard fashion (typically guided by a treatment manual), within a time limit, by therapists who are trained specifically for the study and are closely monitored and supervised. The term *efficacy* has been used to describe positive results of clinical trials, which have become "the 'gold standard' for measuring whether a treatment works" (Seligman, 1995, p. 966). Seligman (1995) suggested that the term *effectiveness* be used to refer to the outcomes of counseling and psychotherapy as practiced in real-life clinical settings.

Effectiveness was directly investigated by Seligman (1995) on the basis of a survey conducted by *Consumer Reports*. Approximately 180,000 readers of *Consumer Reports* were asked to complete the survey if they had experienced stress or emotional problems for which they had sought help from "friends, relatives, or a member of the clergy; a mental health professional like a psychologist or a psychiatrist; your family doctor; or a support group" (Seligman, 1995, p. 967). Approximately 7,000 readers responded, of which 2,900 saw a mental health professional. Overall, the conclusion was that counseling and psychotherapy was effective:

> Treatment by a mental health professional usually worked. Most respondents got a lot better. Averaged over all mental health professionals, of the 426 people who were feeling *very poor* when they began therapy, 87% were feeling *very good, good,* or at least *so-so* by the time of the survey. Of the 786 people who were feeling *fairly poor* at the outset, 92% were feeling *very good, good,* or at least *so-so* by the time of the survey. These findings converge with meta-analyses of efficacy. (Seligman, 1995, p. 968)

Clearly, the *Consumer Reports* study is flawed from the perspective of internal validity; not unexpectedly, it has been criticized for all of the obvious (and some not-so-obvious) reasons, such as lack of a control group, self-report of clients, and selection biases (see e.g., Brock, Green, Reich, & Evans, 1996; Hunt, 1996; Kotkin, Daviet, & Gurin, 1996; Mintz, Drake, & Crits-Christoph, 1996). Nevertheless, it suggests that psychotherapy delivered in practice is beneficial, but leaves open the question of the comparative benefits of treatments delivered in the context of clinical trials and clinically representative treatments.

In 1997, Shadish et al. meta-analytically investigated the clinical trial–practice question by examining studies that were contained in 15 previous meta-analyses. They categorized treatments in the studies contained in the meta-analyses according to their clinical representativeness. Shadish et al. found that of the total corpus of studies in the original meta-analyses (in excess of 1000 studies), only 56 studies contained treatments that met criteria for being "somewhat similar" to clinic therapy, which was defined as treatments that (a) were conducted outside a university, (b) involved clients referred through the usual clinical routes, and (c) used experienced professional therapists with regular caseloads. Only 15 studies from these meta-anlayses contained treatments that met the additional criteria that the treatment did not rely on a manual or was not monitored, and only 1 study contained a treatment that passed the complete set of criteria for clinical representativeness. Several analyses were conducted on these data, yielding a general conclusion that those studies conducted in clinical settings did not produce smaller effects than those produced by the original meta-analyses. Clearly, the outcomes of clinic therapy were not demonstrably inferior to the outcomes of therapy conducted in clinical trials, although this conclusion must be tempered by the extremely small number of studies that contained treatments similar to clinical therapy.

Shadish et al.'s (1997) conclusions about clinically representative treatments are tempered by the meta-analytic findings of Weisz and colleagues (Weisz, Weiss, & Donenberg, 1992; Weisz, Weiss, Han, Granger, & Morton, 1995) that child and adolescent psychotherapy delivered in clinics is either not effective or is less effective than comparable laboratory therapy. However, Weisz's analyses were plagued by problems, in that the clinic therapy studies examined were conducted many years ago, contained clients who were more severely disordered than typical clients in clinical trials, and contained clients with multiple disorders.

To address multiple problems with earlier meta-analyses related to clinically representative treatments, Shadish et al. (2000) conducted a comprehensive meta-analytic investigation of clinically representative treatments. In the previous meta-analysis, Shadish et al. (1997) relied on coding from previous meta-analyses, a problem rectified in Shadish et al. (2000) by using a standardized coding scheme for all studies. Moreover, the latter study refined the criteria used for clinical representativeness, allowing for greater range and continuity in this variable.

Shadish et al. (2000) retrieved 90 studies that spanned the range of clinical representativeness, including clinically representative studies from Weisz et al. (1995). Clinical representativeness was determined by coding 11 criteria: (a) clinically representative problems, (b) clinically representative setting, (c) clinically representative referrals, (d) clinically representative therapists, (e) clinically representative structure, (f) clinically representative monitoring, (g) demographic heterogeneity, (h) problem heterogeneity, (i) pretherapy training of therapists, (j) therapy freedom, and (k) flexible number of sessions. Clearly, some of these criteria were related to adherence (e.g., structure, pretherapy training, therapy freedom), whereas others were not. The meta-analysis found that clinical representativeness was confounded with other variables, but when the confounding variables were controlled, there was no significant relationship between effect size and clinical representativeness, either at the global level (all 11 criteria summed) or at the individual criterion level:

> [These results suggest that] psychological therapies are robustly effective across conditions that range from research-oriented to clinically representative.... Previous findings that clinical representativeness leads to lower effect size are probably an artifact of other confounding variables, especially biased self-selection into treatment in many quasi-experiments that happen to be clinically representative. (Shadish et al., 2000, p. 522)

The meta-analytic evidence suggests that the use of manuals does not increase the benefits of psychotherapy. In the area of depression, manual-guided treatments do not result in superior outcomes to nonmanualized treatments. Moreover, it appears that treatments administered in clinically representative contexts are not inferior to treatments delivered in strictly controlled clinical trials, where adherence to treatment protocols is expected. These findings suggest that adherence to a treatment protocol is not related to the outcomes produced by the treatment, a phenomenon that indicates that specific ingredients are not critical to the success of psychotherapy.

Relationship Between Adherence and Outcome

Evidence for the role of adherence can be obtained by examining the relationship between adherence and outcome. Unfortunately, there are no meta-analyses investigating this relationship, and consequently evidence is acquired at the individual study level. As is so often the case when primary studies are examined, the evidence is not straightforward. Essentially, there are studies that have found a relationship between adherence and outcome, and there are studies that have not. Moreover, investigation of this relationship is prone to several complex threats to validity, and thus conclusions must be made tentatively. In the next sections, these studies are reviewed—first those that found no relationship and then those that did find a relationship.

Studies Finding No Relationship Between Adherence and Outcome. There are several exemplary studies that have failed to find a relationship between adherence to a manual and outcome. In the NIMH TDCRP (Elkin, 1994), adherence as well as competence were measured. In this study, the CSPRS was used to discriminate among the treatments. One of the subscales, the CSPRS-CB is a measure of adherence to the cognitive–behavioral protocol in the following areas: cognitive rationale, cognitive processes, evaluating and changing behavioral focus, homework, and collaborative structure (28 items). The other subscale, the CSPRS-FC, focused on facilitative conditions such as involvement, warmth, and support (8 items). If adherence to the manual is related to outcome, then the

CSPRS-CB should correlate with the dependent measures used in the NIMH TDCRP. Shaw et al. (1999) reported these correlations. The correlation between the CSPRS-CB and three outcome measures examined (the BDI; the HRSD; and the Symptom Checklist–90, or SCL-90) were not significantly different from zero. More informative, however, were the partial correlations obtained by entering pretest scores on the respective outcome measures into a hierarchical regression analysis. In these regressions, which are presented in Table 7.2, the pretest score was entered first, followed by the CSPRS-FC, and then the CSPRS-CB (the Cognitive Therapy Scale, or CTS, is discussed later in this section), and thus adherence is tested holding the level of severity (i.e., pretest score) and support given by the therapist (i.e., CSPRS-FC) constant. In these regressions, adherence (i.e., CSPRS-CB) accounted for zero or a negligible percentage of the variance in the outcome measures.[4] In these analyses, adherence to the treatment protocol appears to be trivially related to outcome.

There is another interesting finding in Shaw et al.'s (1999) analyses. In the NIMH TDCRP, competence was measured with the CTS. Competence, as measured by this scale, was not correlated with outcome. However, when adherence and FC were partialled out, the CTS was correlated with outcome, as measured by the HRSD (see Table 7.2). This is the classic suppressor variable in that when the variance due to adherence and facilitative conditions scores was removed from the variance due to competence scores, the remainder of the variance in the competence scores was related to outcome:

> Thus, it seems that the aspects of the CTS that are related to outcome are *not* those that overlap with either facilitative conditions or simple adherence to the treatment approach. (Shaw et al., 1999, p. 842).

This finding hints at the fact that adherence may have detrimental effects because it suppresses the effect of competence. As measured, competence becomes a predictor of outcome only if the adherence is removed.

There are other studies of cognitive therapy for depression that have not shown a relationship between adherence and outcome. Castonguay, Goldfried, Wiser, Raue, and Hayes (1996) compared the relative predictive ability of two common factors, working alliance and emotional experiencing, with an adherence variable, therapist's focus on the impact of distorted cognitions on depression (labeled "intrapersonal consequences"). In this study, four therapists, who received from 6 to 14 months of training and

---

[4]The CSPRS-FC is a common-factor-like scale and accounted for between 0 and 5% of the variance in outcomes in these regression analyses. However, the power of this scale is limited by the fact that raters do not agree on its application (intraclass correlations for rater agreement varied from .47 to .58, which are very low; Hill, O'Grady, and Elkin, 1992)

TABLE 7.2

Regression Analysis of Adherence and Competence on Dependent Measures
in the NIMH-TDCRP (From Shaw et al., 1999)

Variable (In Order of Entry)	Multiple R	R^2	ΔR^2	dfs	F	p
Termination HRSD						
HRSD prescore	.28	.08	.08	1, 34	2.97	.09
CSPRS-FC	.35	.13	.05	1, 33	1.71	.20
CSPRS-CB	.35	.13	.00	1, 32	0.01	.93
CTS	.53	.28	.15	1, 31	6.46	.02
Termination BDI						
BDI prescore	.43	.19	.19	1, 34	7.90	.00
CSPRS-FC	.43	.43	.00	1, 33	0.00	.95
CSPRS-CB	.45	.20	.01	1, 32	0.50	.49
CTS	.48	.23	.03	1, 31	1.22	.28
Termination SCL-90						
SCL-90 prescore	.30	.09	.09	1, 34	3.31	.08
CSPRS-FC	.35	.12	.03	1, 33	1.26	.27
CSPRS-CB	.35	.12	.00	1, 32	0.08	.78
CTS	.40	.16	.04	1, 31	1.40	.24

Note.   NIMH-TDCRP = National Institutes of Mental Health Treatment of Depression Collaborative Research Program; HRSD = Hamilton Rating Scale for Depression; BDI = Beck Depression Inventory; SCL-90 = Symptom Checklist–90; CSPRS = Collaborative Study Psychotherapy Rating Scale; FC = Facilitative Conditions subscale; CB = Adherence Subscale; CTS = Cognitive Therapy Scale. From "Therapist Competence Ratings in Relation to Clinical Outcome in Cognitive Therapy of Depression," by B. F. Shaw, I. Elkin, J. Yamaguchi, M. Olmsted, T. M. Vallis, K. S. Dobson, A. Lowery, S. M. Sotsky, J. T. Watkins, and S. D. Imber, 1999, *Journal of Consulting and Clinical Psychology, 67*, p. 842. Copyright © 1999 by the American Psychological Association. Adapted with permission.

who were supervised throughout the study, delivered cognitive therapy to 30 clients. The three predictor variables (viz., working alliance, experiencing, and intrapersonal consequences) were measured in the first half of treatment and then correlated with midtreatment and posttreatment outcome scores, partialling out pretreatment scores for each of the variables. Generally, the two common factors were correlated with outcome, as expected. However, the focus on intrapersonal consequences (i.e., the specific ingredient) was positively correlated with depressive symptoms; that is, there were higher rates of therapist focus on distorted cognitions in cases in which depressive symptoms were highest. Moreover, this latter relationship seemed to be accounted for by the working alliance, as the relationship was absent when working alliance scores were entered into the model. Descriptive analyses of representative cases with low alliance and high intrapersonal consequences revealed the following:

> Although therapists dealt with these alliance problems directly, they did not do so by investigating their potential source. Instead, they attempted to resolve the alliance problems by increasing their adherence to the cognitive therapy model.... Some therapists dealt with strains in the alliance by increasing their attempts to persuade the client of the validity of the cognitive therapy rationale, as the client showed more and more disagreement with this rationale and its related tasks. (Castanguay et al., 1996, pp. 501, 502)

In this study it appears that adherence to the protocol could be detrimental, especially when the relationship between the therapist and the client was poor.

Detrimental consequences of adherence were also detected by Henry and Strupp in studies of the effects of training therapists to deliver time-limited dynamic therapy (TLDP; Henry, Schacht, et al., 1993; Henry, Strupp, et al., 1993). In these studies, therapists were trained to comply with the TLDP manual. The training, which was administered by authors of the manual, consisted of 50 weekly 2-hour seminar and supervisory sessions. Training involved didactic presentations, readings, and intensive supervision. Assessments were made of adherence to the TLDP manual with the Vanderbilt Therapeutic Strategies Scale (VTSS); therapeutic process was assessed with the Vanderbilt Psychotherapy Process Scale (VPSS) and the Structural Analysis of Social Behavior (SASB). Although training successfully increased adherence to the TLDP manual, concomitant deterioration in the therapeutic process was noted:

> There were ... indications of unexpected deterioration in certain interpersonal and interactional aspects of therapy as measured by the VPPS and SASB ratings. This finding is disturbing because previous work has repeatedly demonstrated the significance of these variables to positive therapeutic process and outcome (Henry et al., 1986, 1990; O'Malley et al., 1983). The apparently negative effect of training on aspects of the therapeutic relationship is particularly ironic in light of the fact that TLDP focuses on intensive scrutiny and management of interpersonal patterns in the therapeutic relationship as the medium of change. In fact, TLDP was designed in part to reduce expression of therapist hostility toward difficult and negative patients. In light of these complex findings, we are forced to hypothesize that although the "treatment was delivered," the *therapy* (at least as envisioned) did not always occur.... Attempts at changing or dictating specific therapist behaviors may alter other therapeutic variables in unexpected and even counterproductive ways. (Henry, Strupp, et al., 1993, p. 438)

The findings of this study suggest that training therapists to adhere to a manual can result in deteriorating interpersonal relations between the therapist and the client.

Barber et al. (1996) examined therapist adherence and competence vis-à-vis outcome in depressed clients treated with supportive–expressive (SE) dynamic therapy. Adherence to and competence in the supportive and expressive components of SE therapy were assessed at session 3 and were then used to predict subsequent change in depression. Adherence to the supportive and to the expressive components did not predict subsequent change, but competent administration of the expressive ingredients did predict subsequent change. On the other hand, prior change (change before Session 3) predicted adherence: "These results support the clinical impression that the more the patient benefits from treatments, the easier it is, relatively, for the therapist to adhere to the SE treatment manual, although not necessarily to conduct competent therapy" (p. 620). This study raises the possibility that therapeutic success causes adherence, rather than vice-versa. However, others have not found that client characteristics or change were related to adherence (DeRubeis & Feeley, 1990; Feeley et al., 1999; Henry, Schacht, et al., 1993).

Tracey, Sherry, and Albright (1999) investigated the pattern of complimentarity during the course of CBT. Complimentarity is a construct derived from interpersonal theory and is defined as transactional responses that are opposite on the power dimension and matched on the affiliative dimension. Tracey et al. (1999) hypothesized a process model in which successful therapy would be characterized by high levels of complimentarity during the beginning and ending stages of therapy and low levels during the middle stage. In all analyses, adherence, as measured by the standard instrument Cognitive–Behavioral Treatment subscale of the Cognitive Therapy Scale (Shaw, 1984), was entered into the analysis to control for the relationship between adherence and outcome. Although the expected pattern related to complimentarity was related to outcome, adherence had no influence on any of the models tested because the correlation between adherence and outcome was negligible ($r = .11$; T. J. G. Tracey, personal communication, October 15, 1998).

Although the studies reviewed in this section have shown that adherence to the protocol is not related to outcome, and in some cases may be detrimental, there are other studies that have found a relationship between adherence and outcome. These studies are reviewed now.

Studies Finding Relationship Between Adherence and Outcome.

There are several studies that have found a relationship between adherence and outcome or between treatment purity, a construct related to adherence, and outcome. One of the earliest studies that examined adherence to a protocol was Luborsky, McLellan, Woody, O'Brien, and Auerbach's (1985) investigation of the determinants of therapist success. In this study, therapists either conducted SE therapy or CBT for the treatment of substance abuse. Clients also received drug counseling. The SE therapists were selected and supervised by Lester Luborsky, one of the developers of the SE therapy; CBT therapists were selected and supervised by Aaron Beck, the developer of CBT. Determinants of therapist effectiveness fell into several categories: patient qualities, therapist personal qualities as judged by peers, patient–therapist relationship qualities, and therapy qualities. Neither patient qualities nor therapist personal qualities were significantly related to outcome. The correlations between the working alliance, rated after the third session by the client, and the outcome measures (drug use, employment, legal status, and psychological functioning) ranged from .58 to .72, values consistent with those found in chapter 6.

Adherence in Luborsky et al.'s (1985) study was measured on a questionnaire that assessed "the degree to which the session fit the specification" of the therapy. These assessments were made on 15-min segments of randomly selected sessions. Treatment purity was defined as the ratio of (a) adherence to the administered treatment to (b) the adherence to the other treatment and to drug counseling. Thus, higher purity scores reflected greater adherence to the intended treatment, lower adherence to the other treatments, or both. The correlations between treatment purity and outcomes ranged from .36 to .50, indicating that successful cases were characterized by treatments that adhered to the administered treatment and not to the other treatments. However, the direction of causality is not clear, and the authors recognized that the working alliance may play a role:

> The high correlation between purity of technique and patient outcome suggests that once a helping alliance is formed, the therapists do what they are supposed to do [to] achieve their effectiveness in this way. However, an equally tenable, reverse-direction interpretation is that when a patient experiences a helping alliance, he enables the therapist to adhere to his intended technique. (Luborsky et al., 1985, p. 610).

The reverse-direction interpretation is supported by the variation in treatment purity across the therapists. That is, the therapist provided a purer treatment with some clients than with others, suggesting that the client influenced the purity of the treatment. Nevertheless, this study found a relationship between an adherence-related measure (i.e., treatment purity) and outcome, which must be taken as tentative evidence for the specific ingredients in each of these treatments.

Another study that found a relationship between treatment purity and outcome involved professional and paraprofessional group treatments for depression (Bright, Baker, & Neimeyer, 1999). The two treatments compared in this study were CBT, which is an established and empirically supported treatment for depression, and mutual support groups (MSGs), which are "based on the assumption that relief from personal problems may be achieved through discussion with others suffering from similar stress" (p. 493). The MSG condition was less structured and more focused on group members sharing their experiences. In terms of improvement, the two conditions were equally beneficial to the participants.

Purity was measured by assessing the degree to which four characteristics of CBT were present and the degree to which four characteristics of MSG were present. Scores were summed so that positive scores indicated delivery of a purer form of the administered treatment, and negative scores indicated delivery of the nonadministered treatment. Regardless of the training of the therapist, treatment purity was correlated with changes in depression as measured by the Hamilton Rating Scale for depression ($rs = .38$ and .41 for professional and paraprofessional, respectively). No correlations were found for the three remaining dependent variables. Thus, there was weak evidence (correlations for only one of four variables) for a relationship between treatment purity and outcome, suggesting that specific ingredients were responsible for the benefits of the treatments. However, it should be recognized that the MSG condition has few ingredients that would be identified as specifically remedial for depression, and thus adherence to MSG should not be particularly important. That is, the expected interaction between a treatment specific to depression (i.e., CBT) and one that is not (i.e., MSG), which is illustrated in Figure 7.1, was not found, weakening the case for specificity.

One of the problems that plagues studies of adherence, as discussed earlier, is that therapists will have an easier time adhering to a protocol when the client is cooperative, motivated, and progressing. The two studies on purity have not been able to rule out the possibility that clients facilitate therapists adherence. Two studies conducted by DeRubeis and Feeley (1990; Feeley et al., 1999) addressed this issue by examining the temporal relationship between adherence and outcome.

In the first study, DeRubeis and Feeley (1990) studied the change process of cognitive therapy for depression. Adherence, therapist-offered facilitative conditions (e.g., warmth, empathy), and the working alliance were assessed at an early session (Session 2 or 3) and in three sessions from the 2nd, 3rd, and 4th quarters of the therapy (labeled Quadrants 2, 3, and 4, respectively). Adherence was empirically separated into two factors. The first factor was composed of methods of CT that focused on "concrete" symptoms, such as assigning homework, asking clients to report cognitions verbatim, and labeling cognitive errors. The second factor was composed of more "abstract" discussions, such as encouraging distancing of beliefs, providing cognitive therapy rationale, and exploring underlying assumptions. Focus in this study was on the early session and Quadrant 2 because 90% of the change in BDI scores had occurred by then. Given this design, adherence, facilitative conditions, and working alliance could be related to prior change as well as subsequent change. In Quadrant 1, concrete cognitive therapy was unrelated to prior change, but related to subsequent change. Thus it appears that adherence to the concrete aspects of cognitive therapy in the early sessions is not a result of initial progress of the client but is important for progress in the early stages of cognitive therapy. No such relationship was found for adherence to the abstract principles of cognitive therapy, implying that it is the active, structural ingredients of cognitive therapy that may be therapeutic. However, concrete cognitive therapy, by Quadrant 2, was related to prior change but not related to subsequent change, detracting from the causal direction found in Quadrant 1. Contrary to previous studies, the working alliance was not related to outcome (see chap. 6).

The temporal relationship between change and concrete cognitive therapy was replicated by Feeley et al. (1999). In this later study of 32 depressed clients, concrete cognitive therapy was predictive of change subsequent to Session 2, whereas abstract cognitive therapy, facilitative conditions, and working alliance were not related to subsequent change. Prior change did not predict any of the process variables later in therapy.

The two studies by DeRubeis and Feeley that examined the temporal relationship of change and various process measures provide evidence that the active, focused aspects of cognitive therapy are critical for their success and that the facilitative conditions, working alliance, and abstract aspects of cognitive therapy are unimportant. The results that the concrete aspects of cognitive therapy are important has been suggested in other findings as well (e.g., see Shaw et al. 1999), but may reflect a variable related to the structure of therapy rather than aspects of cognitive therapy per se. As noted by Shaw et al., "Of key importance [is] the therapist's ability to deal competently with setting an agenda and assigning relevant homework while pacing the session appropriately" (p. 844), rather than competently delivering the specific ingredients of cognitive therapy.

Conclusions Regarding Adherence and Outcome. Two sets of studies have been reviewed regarding the relationship of adherence and outcome. Some studies have not detected any significant relationship between adherence and outcome but did find evidence that common factors were important. Some of these studies found detrimental effects for therapists who technically adhered to treatment protocols. However, some other studies have found that adherence or purity was related to outcome. In Luborsky et al.'s (1985) study, it was found that working alliance was a stronger predictor of outcome than was adherence. Nevertheless, in two studies that were commendable for examining temporal relationships, technical adherence to active, focused aspects of cognitive therapy, but not variables related to common factors, were predictive of subsequent change. In studies that have examined more than one treatment, it appears that purity is related to outcome for all treatments. In no case was there a pattern of adherence and outcome for two therapies of the type illustrated in Figure 7.1, which would indicate that adherence to protocols of beneficial therapies is related to outcome, whereas adherence to protocols of treatments not designed for the particular disorder would not be related to outcome. All told, the evidence related to adherence provides at best weak evidence for the therapeutic importance of specific ingredients.

CONCLUSIONS

In a critical test of the contextual model versus the medical model, examination of allegiance and adherence provides strong support for the contextual model. Allegiance effects, were consistently present and notably large. The contextual model emphasizes the person of the therapist and the therapist's belief that the therapy is beneficial for the client. When the therapist believes that the treatment is efficacious, he or she will enthusiastically communicate that belief to the client.

Adherence to treatment protocols was generally not associated with outcomes, although a few notable exceptions were found. Adherence to treatment protocols is absolutely required in a medical model of psychotherapy and underlies the bases of empirically supported treatments. Nevertheless, there is no compelling evidence that adherence is important. Even when adherence has been found to be related to outcomes, it was the structuring part of the adherence, rather than the core theoretical ingredients, that predicted outcome.

8

Therapist Effects:
An Ignored but Critical Factor

The qualities of the therapist that lead to beneficial outcomes has been of interest to psychotherapy researchers and clinicians since the origins of the field. It seems intuitive that some characteristics of therapists would be more desirable than others and that consequently some therapists would be more effective with clients than others. In this regard, therapists are similar to other professionals, as some lawyers win more cases than others, some artists create more memorable and creative sculptures than others, and some teachers facilitate greater student achievement than others.

To understand the many ways that therapists influence the psychotherapy process and outcome, Beutler, Machado, and Neufeld (1994) created a taxonomy of therapist variables, which is presented in Figure 8.1. They classified aspects related to the therapists as either (a) objective or subjective, and (b) cross-situation traits or therapy-specific states, thereby yielding four types of therapist variables. Many of the therapy-specific states have been discussed in previous chapters. For example, *therapist interventions* relate to adherence (chap. 7) and specific effects (chap. 5); *therapeutic relationships* relate to the working alliance (chap. 6); *therapeutic philosophy orientation* relates to relative efficacy (chap. 4). The cross-situational traits for therapists are characteristics of the therapist that are relatively constant across the various clients treated by the therapist.

Beutler et al. (1994) reviewed the research to identify therapist variables in the four classes that were related to psychotherapy outcome; the preponderance of the evidence was related to therapy-specific states and was con-

184

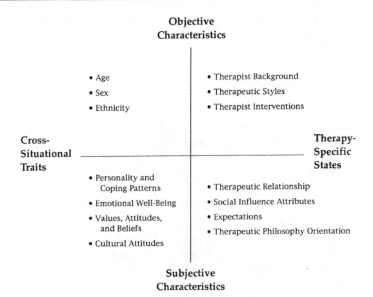

Objective
Characteristics

• Age   • Therapist Background

• Sex   • Therapeutic Styles

• Ethnicity   • Therapist Interventions

Cross-   **Therapy-**
Situational ────────────────────────────── **Specific**
Traits   **States**

• Personality and
  Coping Patterns   • Therapeutic Relationship

• Emotional Well-Being   • Social Influence Attributes

• Values, Attitudes,   • Expectations
  and Beliefs
                                   • Therapeutic Philosophy Orientation
• Cultural Attitudes

Subjective
Characteristics

FIG. 8.1.   Taxonomy of therapist variables. From "Therapist Variables," by L. E. Beutler, P. Machado, and S. Neufeld, in A. E. Bergin and S. L. Garfield (Eds.), *Handbook of Psychotherapy and Behavior Change* (4th ed., p. 231), 1994, New York: Wiley. Copyright © 1994 by John Wiley and Sons. Adapted with permission of John Wiley & Sons, Inc.

sistent with the evidence reviewed in earlier chapters. Although individual therapist variables (i.e., the cross-situational traits, such as personality of the therapist) are interesting and informative, this chapter considers the therapist as a holistic factor, spanning the array of possible variables.

The central issue for differentiating the medical model and the contextual model is to estimate the degree to which the therapist affects the outcome of therapy—stated as a question, "Is the particular therapist important?" The medical model posits that the specific ingredients are critical to the outcome of therapy, and therefore whether the ingredient is received by the client is more important than who delivers the ingredient. On the other hand, in the contextual model, the therapist is critical because it is recognized that there will be variability in the manner in which therapies are delivered—that is, the skill of therapists will vary greatly.

The portrayal of the contextual versus medical model differences relative to therapists is, however, more complex. Medical model proponents clearly recognize that some therapists will be more competent than others in delivering a specific treatment:

> *Competence* [refers] to the level of skill shown by the therapist in delivering the treatment. [Skill is] the extent to which the therapists conducting the intervention

took the relevant aspects of the therapeutic context into account and responded
to these contextual variables appropriately. Relevant aspects of the context include, but are by no means limited to, (a) client variables such as degree of impairment; (b) the particular problems manifested by a given client; (c) the client's
life situation and stress; (d) and factors such as stage in therapy, degree of improvement already achieved, and appropriate sensitivity to the timing of interventions within a therapy session. (Waltz et al., 1993, p. 620)

Competence, as defined in this way, typically is assessed by raters who are
expert therapists themselves. However, there is no guarantee that competence is related to outcome—that is, the characteristics of therapy measured
by expert raters may be irrelevant to outcome. Indeed, researchers are hard-
pressed to find correlations between measures of competence and outcome,
as exemplified by the NIMH TDCRP (Shaw et al., 1999; see chap.7).

The important issue for the medical versus contextual model debate,
however, is not how competence is measured, but whether there is much
variability among therapists with regard to outcomes. In clinical trials comparing treatments intended to be therapeutic, therapists are screened,
trained, supervised, and expected to reach an adequate level of competence.
Variability among therapists may be due to the characteristics of therapists
and therapy assessed by the scale or may be due to other less recognizable
characteristics. Nevertheless, the medical model supposition that some ingredients are better than others combined with minimization of therapists
differences in clinical trials suggests that the variability among treatments
should be greater than variability among therapists.

In this chapter, competence is defined by outcome. Simply put, more
competent therapists produce better outcomes than less competent therapists. Of course, it is productive to identify those characteristics that differentiate more competent from less competent therapists—yet surprisingly
little research has been directed toward this goal (see Blatt, Sanislow,
Zuroff, & Pilkonis, 1996, for an example of this type of research). When
competence is defined by outcomes, variability in outcomes due to therapists is equivalent to the variability due to competence. The contextual
model emphasizes variability in competence rather than variability in treatments, and thus variability among therapists should be greater than the variability among treatments. To summarize, the two models have divergent
hypotheses:

Medical model: variability of treatments > variability of therapists

Contextual model: variability of therapists > variability of treatments

The first section of this chapter discusses design issues relative to therapists effects. The second section examines studies that produce evidence
about the size of therapist effects.

DESIGN ISSUES

Consideration of therapists in any outcome study of psychotherapy is critical to proper conclusions about the efficacy of treatments. Unfortunately, there is no simple solution that can be applied universally to all outcome studies that will yield the proper conclusion without threats to validity. However, ignoring therapists in the design can lead to catastrophic errors, as is shown in this chapter; so understanding the nature of therapist effects in psychotherapy studies is vital. In this section, two alternatives for assigning therapists to treatments, nested and crossed designs, are presented.

Nested Design

In the nested experimental design, therapists are randomly assigned to treatments, as shown in Figure 8.2. That is, each therapist delivers one and only one treatment. Although nested designs are well-discussed in most experimental design texts (e.g., Kirk, 1995), the design is presented in some detail here because inappropriate analyses lead to incorrect conclusions.

Let n be the number of participants randomly assigned to each therapist, q be the number of therapists assigned to each treatment, and p be the number of treatments. Thus, there are nq participants in each treatment and npq participants total. When a nested design is used, typically the therapist factor is ignored (Crits-Christoph & Mintz, 1991; Wampold & Serlin, 2000); however, ignoring the therapist factor leads to gross Type I errors and overestimation of treatment effects (Wampold & Serlin, 2000).

Before examining the design further, it should be noted that therapists should be considered a random factor (Crits-Christoph & Mintz, 1991; Wampold & Serlin, 2000):

> In this model, the researchers are interested in making conclusions about the specific treatments chosen to be studied, and consequently treatment should be considered a fixed effect. On the other hand, rarely is the researcher interested in the particular [therapists] used in the study. The issue is whether [therapists] in general differ in the outcomes they produce. Therefore, [therapists] should be treated as a random factor so that conclusions can be made about [therapists] in

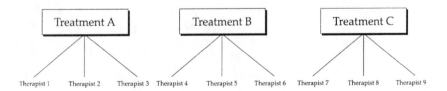

FIG. 8.2.   Therapists nested within treatments.

general. Ideally, [therapists] would be randomly selected from the population of [therapists] and then assigned to the treatments. In practice, [therapists] who have chosen a treatment or have an affinity to a treatment often are used to deliver that treatment, a condition that mirrors the real-world situation in which [therapists] are free to deliver their preferred treatment chosen from a set of professionally accepted treatments. In the latter case, the [therapists] are not randomly assigned to treatments, and the conclusions need to be restricted to "[therapists] who have an affinity to treatment X" rather than to [therapists] in general. (Wampold & Serlin, 2000, p. 427).

The nested model accommodates a factor related to therapists. If therapists vary in their effectiveness, the clients assigned to some therapists will have better outcomes than the clients assigned to other therapists, regardless of client variables (recall that participants are randomly assigned to therapists in the nested design) and treatment. The variance attributable to therapists must be taken into account in the nested design in order to estimate treatment differences. Differences among therapists can statistically be conceptualized as a correlation among the error terms of participants nested within therapists and is typically indexed by an intraclass correlation coefficient, which is defined as the ratio of variance due to therapists to total variance in the model (Kenny & Judd, 1986; Kirk, 1995; Wampold & Serlin, 2000). The greater the variance among therapists, the greater the correlation of error terms and the larger the intraclass correlation coefficient.

The correct analysis of the nested design in which therapist is considered a random factor is shown in Table 8.1. The details of the source table will not be examined in detail, but one feature of sampling theory for this design is absolutely critical to establish valid conclusions from outcome studies that use nested designs. Note that the expected value for the mean squares for treatments contains a term that includes the variance due to therapists (viz., $n\sigma^2_{\varepsilon_2}$), and thus the proper F is calculated as the ratio of the mean squares for treatment and the mean squares for therapists—that is, for treatments, mean square error is the incorrect denominator. The correct and incorrect (i.e., ignoring the therapist effect) is shown for a hypothetical example in Table 8.2. When the correct analysis is conducted using the correct denominator, the F value and degrees of freedom for the treatment effect are considerably less than the respective values for the incorrect analysis.

When the nested factor is ignored, it is assumed that the observations are independent, when indeed they are not because some therapists are more effective than others. The effect of ignoring the fact that observations are not independent has been derived, and the applied research community has been warned of the subsequent dire consequences (Barcikowski, 1981; Kenny & Judd, 1986; Kirk, 1995; Walsh, 1947; Wampold & Serlin, 2000). Unfortunately, the incorrect analysis yields an F that is unduly liberal, in that the probability of Type I error will be abnormally large, and the null hy-

TABLE 8.1

Source Table for Nested Design, Including Expectation of Mean Squares (Treatment Fixed, Therapist Random)

Source	SS	df	MS	E(MS)	F
Treatment	SSTx	$p - 1$	SSTx/$(p - 1)$	$\sigma^2_{\varepsilon_3} + n\sigma^2_{\varepsilon_2} + nq\Sigma\alpha^2_j/(p - 1)$	MSTx/MSTherapists
Therapist	SSTherapists	$p(q - 1)$	SSTherapists/$p(q - 1)$	$\sigma^2_{\varepsilon_3} + n\sigma^2_{\varepsilon_2}$	MSTherapists/MSWCell
WCell	SSWCell	$pq(n - 1)$	SSWCell/$pq(n - 1)$	$\sigma^2_{\varepsilon_3}$	
Total	SSTotal	$npq - 1$			

Note. $\sigma^2_{\varepsilon_3}$ = within-therapist variance; $\sigma^2_{\varepsilon_2}$ = Variance due to therapists; α_j = treatment effect for Treatment j. From "The Consequences of Ignoring a Nested Factor on Measures of Effect Size in Analysis of Variance Designs," by B. E. Wampold, and R. C. Serlin, 2000, *Psychological Methods, 4*, 425–433. Copyright © by the American Psychological Association. Reprinted with permission.

TABLE 8.2

Source Tables for Nested and Incorrect Designs
$(\omega^2 = .1, \rho_1 = .3, n = 4, p = 2, q = 5)$

Source	SS	df	MS	F	Effect Size
Nested design (correct analysis)					
Treatment	9.064	1	9.064	3.339	$\hat{\omega}^2 = .100$
Therapists	21.714	8	2.714	2.714	$\hat{\rho}_1 = .30$
WCell	30.000	30	1.000		
Total	60.778	39			
Design ignoring nested therapist factor (incorrect analysis)					
Treatment	9.064	1	9.064	6.660	$\hat{\omega}^{2\prime} = .124$
Error	51.714	38	1.361		
Total	60.778	39			

Note. From "The Consequences of Ignoring a Nested Factor on Measures of Effect Size in Analysis of Variance Designs," by B. E. Wampold and R. C. Serlin, 2000, 4, 425–433. *Psychological Methods*. Copyright © by the American Psychological Association. Reprinted by permission.

pothesis will be rejected frequently when there are no true treatment differences. On the basis of a Monte Carlo study, Wampold and Serlin derived the error rates for rejecting the null hypotheses when there are no true treatment differences, for different therapist effects, and client–therapist ratios; these error rates are found in Table 8.3. Consider a comparison between two treatments, with four therapists per treatment ($q = 4$), each seeing five clients ($n = 5$), where therapists account for 10% of the variance in outcomes; 15% of such comparisons will result in rejection of the null hypotheses when there is no true difference between the treatments. Given that few treatment comparisons yield statistically significant results (see chap.4), it is disturbing to find that 15% of such comparisons will yield spurious statistically significant findings when uniform efficacy is true.

The important determination in this chapter is the estimation of therapist effects. In the appropriate analysis of the nested design, the proportion of variance attributable to therapists (within treatments) can be estimated. Let ρ_1 be the population intraclass correlation coefficient for therapists with the interpretation that it represents the population proportion of variance accounted for by therapists within treatments. The estimator of this intraclass correlation coefficient, denoted by $\hat{\rho}_1$, can easily be calculated (see Wampold & Serlin, 2000). In the example shown in Table 8.2, $\hat{\rho}_1$ was equal to 0.30, indi-

TABLE 8.3

Error Rates When Nested Therapist Factor Is Ignored
(Nominal Error Rate Is .05, Two Treatments)

q, n	*Proportion of Variability Due to Therapist*					
	0.00	0.10	0.20	0.30	0.40	0.50
10, 2	0.053	0.065	0.079	0.092	0.105	0.119
5, 4	0.049	0.086	0.123	0.162	0.199	0.232
4, 5	0.051	0.100	0.150	0.199	0.243	0.283
2, 10	0.050	0.160	0.257	0.339	0.404	0.463

Note. From "The Consequences of Ignoring a Nested Factor on Measures of Effect Size in Analysis of Variance Designs," by B. E. Wampold and R. C. Serlin, 2000, 4, 425–433. *Psychological Methods.* Copyright © by the American Psychological Association. Reprinted with permission.

cating that the estimate of the proportion of the variance accounted for by therapists was 30%.

Discriminating between the medical and contextual models of psychotherapy has rested largely on the determination of effect size for various critical questions. In chapter 4, estimates of the effect size for the direct comparisons of two treatments were calculated. However, these estimates do not take into account therapist variance. It turns out that ignoring the nested factor results in an overestimation of effect sizes and makes the F test too liberal. Wampold and Serlin (2000) derived the degree to which failure to take into account dependence of observations affects the size of proportion of variance measures. Let ω^2 be the true proportion variance accounted for by treatments; further, denote $\hat{\omega}^2$ to be the correct estimator of ω^2 taking into account therapist effects, and denote $\hat{\omega}^{2'}$ to be the incorrect estimator (i.e., when therapists are ignored). As can be seen in Table 8.2, the correct estimate for the proportion of variability due to treatments was .100, whereas the incorrect estimate was .124, indicating that ignoring therapist inflates the size of the estimates of treatment effects. Thus, ignoring therapist effects results in an overestimation of the treatment effects. Table 8.4 shows the degree to which treatment effects are inflated in various instances. Take the case where there are absolutely no treatment effects (i.e., $\omega^2 = 0$), there are two therapists per treatment (i.e., $q = 2$), 10 participants per therapist (i.e., $n = 10$), and therapists account for 30% of the variance in outcomes (i.e., $\rho_I = .30$); the expected value of the incorrect estimate is 0.067. *That is, in this case, researchers would conclude that nearly 7% of the variability in outcomes was due to treatments, when in fact absolutely none of the variance was due to treatments (i.e., treatments are equally effi-cacious)!* Later in the chapter, the consequences for ignoring the therapist factor in psychotherapy are modeled.

The nested design has been presented in some detail in order to establish that ignoring the therapist factor results in grossly liberal tests of treatment differences and an overestimation of treatment effects. The bottom line is simple: Use the appropriate analysis when therapists are nested within treatments. Not only does it provide the correct conclusion, but it provides an estimate of therapist effects, which is extremely important information. When the incorrect analysis is conducted, the detrimental effects of ignoring therapist variance are increased when few therapists are used (see Tables 8.3 and 8.4).

The alternative to the nested design is the crossed design, which is discussed next.

Crossed Design

In the crossed design, therapists deliver each of the treatments being studied, as illustrated in Figure 8.3. As in the case of the nested design, therapists are considered a random factor because the researcher wishes to make conclusions about therapists in general rather than the specific therapists being studied.

Suppose that there are J therapists (randomly selected from a population of therapists) and K treatments; n participants are assigned to each of the JK combinations of therapists and treatments. The appropriate source table is given in Table 8.5. This factorial design is often called a mixed model, due to the inclusion of a fixed and a random factor. Details of this design are found in standard textbooks (see, e.g., Hays, 1988; Kirk, 1995; Wampold & Drew, 1990).

The analysis of the mixed model is similar to the nested design in that the expectation of the mean squares for treatments contains a term other than the error and treatment terms. In this context, the expected mean square contains a term involving the variance due to the interaction. If some therapists produce better outcomes with one therapy and other therapists produce better outcomes with another therapy, then the interaction effects will be large. The proper F ratio is determined with the mean squares interaction as the denominator rather than the mean squares error. Consequently, ignoring therapists in the design (and consequently ignoring the interaction) will result in a liberal test of treatment effects and an overestimation of the size of treatment effects, similar to the consequences of ignoring therapist effects in the nested design. Although the reader is spared a detailed discussion of the crossed design (see Hays, 1988; Kirk, 1995; Wampold & Drew, 1990), the bottom line is the same as in the nested design: Use the appropri-

TABLE 8.4

Incorrect Estimates of the Population Proportion of Variance Accounted for by Treatments

ρ_I	$q = 10$, $n = 2$	$q = 5$, $n = 4$	$q = 4$, $n = 5$	$q = 2$, $n = 10$
		$E(\hat{\omega}^2)$		
$\omega^2 = 0.00$ (no population treatment effect)				
0.0	.000	.000	.000	.000
0.1	.004	.008	.010	.022
0.2	.006	.015	.020	.044
0.3	.009	.023	.031	.067
0.4	.011	.031	.041	.090
0.5	.014	.039	.051	.115
$\omega^2 = 0.01$ (small population treatment effect)				
0.0	.010	.010	.010	.010
0.1	.013	.017	.019	.031
0.2	.016	.024	.029	.053
0.3	.018	.032	.039	.075
0.4	.021	.040	.049	.098
0.5	.024	.047	.060	.122
$\omega^2 = 0.059$ (medium population treatment effect)				
0.0	.059	.059	.059	.059
0.1	.059	.063	.065	.075
0.2	.060	.069	.073	.095
0.3	.062	.076	.082	.115
0.4	.064	.083	.091	.136
0.5	.066	.091	.101	.158
$\omega^2 = 0.138$ (large population treatment effect)				
0.0	.138	.138	.138	.138
0.1	.138	.138	.140	.148
0.2	.138	.143	.147	.163
0.3	.138	.149	.154	.181
0.4	.140	.154	.162	.198
0.5	.142	.161	.170	.219

Note. From "The Consequences of Ignoring a Nested Factor on Measures of Effect Size in Analysis of Variance Designs," by B. E. Wampold and R. C. Serlin, 2000, 4, 425–433. *Psychological Methods.* Copyright © by the American Psychological Association. Reprinted with permission.

	Tx A	Tx B	Tx C
Therapist 1	n subjects	n subjects	n subjects
Therapist 2	n subjects	n subjects	n subjects
Therapist 3	n subjects	n subjects	n subjects
Therapist 4	n subjects	n subjects	n subjects

FIG. 8.3.   Therapists and treatments crossed.

ate analysis when therapists are crossed with treatments. Not only does it provide the correct conclusion, but it provides an estimate of therapists effects, which is extremely important information.

Clearly, ignoring the variability of therapists, whether in a nested or a crossed design, produces a liberal F test and overestimates treatment effects. Nevertheless, in a review of 140 comparative studies, Crits-Christoph and Mintz (1991) found that none correctly analyzed the treatment effect by conducting the appropriate nested or crossed analysis. Thus, researchers are overestimating treatment effects in clinical trials.

Relative Advantages of the Nested and Crossed Design

One of the distinct advantages of the nested design is that one can compare treatments administered by therapists who are skilled in and have allegiance to each of the therapies being compared. Because allegiance is so important to successful outcome (see chap. 7), the nested design permits a comparison to treatments conducted by therapists who have allegiance to those treatments. A good example of a nested design is the NIMH TDCRP, which used 10 therapists in the IPT and pharmacotherapy conditions and 8 in the CBT condition. Skill and allegiance were controlled in the following way:

> All [therapists] had to meet specific background and experience criteria: at least two years of full-time clinical work following completion of professional training (ie, following the Ph.D. and clinical internship for clinical psychologists and following the MD and psychiatric residency for psychiatrists); treatment of at least ten depressed patients; and a special interest in and commitment to the thera-

TABLE 8.5

Source Table for Crossed Design, Including Expectation of Means Square (Treatment Fixed, Therapist Random)

Source	SS	df	MS	E(MS)	F
Treatment	SSTx	$K-1$	SSTx/$(K-1)$	$\sigma_\varepsilon^2 + Jn\Sigma\beta_k^2/(K-1) + n\sigma_{\text{Interaction}}^2$	MSTx/MSInteraction
Therapist	SSTherapists	$J-1$	SSTherapists/$(J-1)$	$\sigma_\varepsilon^2 + kn\sigma_A^2$	MSTherapist/MSWCell
Interaction	SSInter	$(J-1)(K-1)$	SSInter/$(J-1)(K-1)$	$\sigma_\varepsilon^2 + n\sigma_{\text{Interaction}}^2$	MSInteraction/MSE
WCell	SSWCell	$JK(n-1)$	SSWCell/$JK(n-1)$	σ_ε^2	
Total	SSTotal	$JKn-1$			

Note. σ_ε^2 = within-cell variance; β_k = treatment effect for Treatment k; σ_A^2 = variance due to therapists; $\sigma_{\text{Interaction}}^2$ = variance for the interaction of treatments and therapists.

peutic approach in which they were trained. In addition, IPT therapists had to have previous training in a psychodynamic oriented framework, CB therapists were to have had some cognitive and/or behavioral background, and the past training of pharmacotherapists had to include a considerable emphasis on psychotropic drug treatment.... Thus, the treatment conditions being compared in this study are, in actuality, "packages" of particular therapeutic approaches and the therapists who both choose to and are chosen to administer them. (Elkin, Parloff, Hadley, & Autry, 1985, p. 308)

The disadvantage of the nested design as used in psychotherapy research is that different therapists administer the treatments, so, technically, therapists and treatments are confounded. It may be that the therapists delivering one of the treatments are generally more skilled than the therapists delivering the other treatment.

In the crossed design, the general characteristics of the therapist are equivalent across treatments, but care must be taken to ensure that the training, skill, and allegiance are balanced. For example, in a study comparing behavior therapy and CBT, Butler, Fennell, Robson, and Gelder (1991) used clinical psychologists who had originally been trained in behavior therapy but who had received special training in CBT from the Center for Cognitive Therapy in Philadelphia. Although the psychologists initially may have had allegiance to behavior therapy, their special training would certainly increase their skill, if not their allegiance, to CBT. However, a comparison of cognitive therapy and applied relaxation conducted by Clark et al. (1994) demonstrated the problems with a crossed design. In this study, which was discussed in chapter 7, two of the authors, who clearly were proponents of cognitive therapy and skilled in its delivery, also administered both cognitive therapy and applied relaxation. Moreover, these two therapists were supervised by Clark, who was the first author and who had developed the cognitive therapy used in the study. In this study, treatment was confounded with allegiance, and therefore it is not possible to determine whether the observed superiority of cognitive therapy was due to the efficacy of cognitive therapy or to the allegiance and skill of the therapists.

Both of the methods for assigning therapists to treatments have confounds, and therefore the researcher must be cognizant of the threats and minimize the degree to which the conclusions will be invalidated. In either case, the appropriate analysis should be undertaken, as discussed earlier in this chapter.

SIZE OF THERAPIST EFFECTS

Although Crits-Christoph and Mintz (1991) could not find studies that correctly tested treatment differences by considering the variability in the therapists, there have been several attempts to estimate the size of therapist effects by reanalyzing data from the primary studies. In this section, these attempts are reviewed. These estimates are then used to understand the degree to which treatment effects have been overestimated.

Estimation of Therapist Effects

Luborsky et al.'s (1986) reanalysis of four studies initiated a series of attempts to determine the size of therapist effects. They obtained the raw data from four major psychotherapy studies: The Hopkins Psychotherapy Project (Hoehn-Saric, 1965), The VA-Penn Psychotherapy Project (Woody et al., 1983), The Pittsburgh Psychotherapy Project (Pilkonis et al., 1984), and the McGill Psychotherapy Project (Piper et al., 1984). In the reanalysis, Luborsky et al. correctly considered the therapist as a random factor and performed the appropriate analysis; consequently, the treatment effects found in the original studies were altered.

Although Luborsky et al. (1986) did not estimate the proportion of variance accounted for by therapists, the results clearly showed that there were large therapist effects, much in excess of the treatment effects. Luborsky et al. concluded:

> These results confirm our supposition about the generality of the effects in other studies [viz., that therapist effects were large]—in each reanalyzed study at least two statistically significant univariate therapist effects were revealed. This confirmation is consistent with the long-held view of Frank about the crucial importance of the therapist's contribution.... The frequency and size of the therapists' effects generally overshadowed any differences between different forms of treatment in these investigations. (pp. 508–509)

In 1991, Crits-Christoph et al., on the basis of the data from 15 previously published studies, estimated therapist effects. In the fifteen studies, they calculated the proportion of variance attributable to therapists within 27 different treatments. For all outcome measures and all treatments, the mean proportion was 0.086; that is, overall, nearly 9% of the variance was due to therapists. Translating this to an effect size measure *d* that is typically used to index psychotherapy treatment effects (see Table 2.4), the effect size for therapists is in excess of 0.60. Recalling that the effect sizes for the differences among treatments was at most 0.20, the magnitude of the therapists effect is impressively large. The range for the aggregate dependent variables in each treatment was 0.00–0.487—almost 50% of the variance in one of these treatments was accounted for by the therapists. When dependent variables were segregated, the mean proportion of variance accounted for by therapists for the dependent variable with the largest effect was 0.223, with a maximum of 0.729. The latter value indicates that for one dependent variable, over 70% of the variance was due to therapists!

Crits-Christoph and Mintz (1991) investigated the size of the treatment–therapist interaction effects in crossed designs in addition to the size of the therapist effect. This is important because, as discussed earlier, the interaction effect inflates the mean square for treatment. They found that 0–10% of the variance in outcomes, as determined by aggregating the dependent measures in a study, was due to the interaction. However, when individual variables were considered, the interaction accounted for up to 38 percent of the variance. These values indicate that failing to correctly analyze crossed designs will result in liberal F tests and overestimation of treatment effects, as the interaction term contained in the mean squares treatment is ignored.

There were other important findings in the reanalyses conducted by Crits-Christoph (Crits-Christoph et al., 1991; Crits-Christoph & Mintz, 1991). The better controlled studies that used treatment manuals and that were published more recently had smaller therapist effects than did the other studies. Crits-Christoph and Mintz concluded that "this implies that the quality control procedures commonly implemented in contemporary outcome trials (e.g., careful selection, training, and supervision of therapists and the use of treatment manuals) to control for differences among therapists may have been quite successful" (p. 24). Of course, the homogenization of therapists does not imply that their competence has been increased; recall that the use of manuals did not seem to benefit clients (see chap. 7). Moreover, reanalysis of well-conducted clinical trials that have been published since 1991 contradict the conclusion that therapists are homogenous when they are carefully selected, trained, and supervised, as shown in the final reanalyses considered next.

Blatt, Sanislow, Zuroff, and Pilkonis (1996) reanalyzed the data from the NIMH TDCRP to determine the characteristics of effective therapists. This is an important analysis, because the NIMH study was well-controlled, used manuals, and employed a nested design in which therapists were committed to and skilled in the delivery of each treatment (see earlier discussion). For the three active treatments (CBT, IPT, IMI-CM) and the pill placebo group (CM), Blatt et. al. divided therapists into three groups based on composite residualized gain scores: (a) more effective therapists, (b) moderately effective therapists, and (c) less effective therapists. Contrary to the Crits-Christoph conclusion (Crits-Christoph et al., 1991; Crits-Christoph & Mintz, 1991), there was significant variation among therapists in this well-controlled study. Blatt et al. came to the following conclusion:

> The present analyses of the data ... indicate that significant differences exist in therapeutic efficacy among therapists, even within the experienced and well-trained therapists in the [NIMH study]. Differences in therapeutic efficacy were independent of the type of treatment provided or the research site and not related to the therapists' level of general clinical experience or in treating de-

pressed patients. Differences in therapeutic efficacy, however, were associated with basic clinical orientation, especially about treatment. More effective therapists had a more psychological rather than biological orientation to the clinical process.... Additionally, more effective therapists, compared with less and moderately effective therapists, expect therapy to require more treatment sessions before patients begin to manifest therapeutic change.... Relatively few significant findings were obtained when comparing attitudes about the etiology of depression or about techniques considered essential to successful treatment. (Blatt et al., 1996, pp. 1281–1282)

Interestingly, two therapists who achieved therapeutic efficacy with medication in the IMI-CM group also achieved success in the clinical management condition, suggesting that the relationship between client and therapist is vitally important.

Luborsky, McLellan, Diguer, Woody, and Seligman (1997) conducted a reanalysis of seven samples of drug-addicted and depressed clients that is particularly informative because the same therapists were used in several of the samples. Although Luborsky et al. did not provide estimates of the therapist effects, their conclusions were clear cut:

Therapists in all seven samples differed widely in the mean level of improvement shown by the patients in their caseloads.... [The results] were somewhat surprising because (a) patients within each sample were similar in terms of diagnosis; (b) they were randomly assigned; (c) the therapists had been selected for their competence in their particular form of psychotherapy; and (d) the therapists were regularly supervised and were further guided by treatment manuals. Despite these steps that should have maximized skill and minimized differences, the range of percentages of improvement for the 22 therapists in the seven samples was from slightly negative change, to slightly more than 80% improvement. (Luborsky et al., 1997, p. 60).

An extremely important finding of this study is that therapists who were successful in one sample were also successful in other samples. Luborsky et al. attributed this finding, based on this and previous research, to the fact that "the most effective therapists are rated by their patients, even after a few sessions, as being helpful and part of an alliance with them" (p. 62).

The final reanalysis involves the treatment of alcohol problems in the multisite study conducted by Project MATCH (see chap. 5 for a description of this study; Project MATCH Research Group, 1997, 1998). This is a study in which therapists were selected for their competence and allegiance to the treatment and, as well, were well trained and supervised. Recall that there were few differences among the treatments (see chap. 5). However, in this reanalysis (Project MATCH Research Group, 1998), over 6% of the variance was due to therapists (range = 1–12%), a figure not too different from the 9% figure found by Crits-Christoph et al. (1991). Interestingly, the variance in each treatment was due primarily to one therapist, although the outlying therapist differed from one sample to another, a result that is contrary to that found by Luborsky et al. (1997).

The results of the several reanalyses reviewed here are clear. Although some studies can be found that demonstrate therapist homogeneity, a preponderance of the evidence indicates that there are large therapist effects (in the range of 6–9% of the variance in outcomes accounted for by therapists) and that these effects greatly exceed treatment effects, as predicted by the contextual model. These percentages are particularly impressive when compared with variability among treatments, which is at most 1% (see chap. 4). In addition, ignoring therapist effects inflates estimates of treatment effects, making the discrepancy between therapist and treatment effects all the more impressive. In the following sections, the degree to which treatment effects are overestimated is modeled.

Modeling Therapist and Treatment Effects

Wampold and Serlin (2000) modeled treatment and therapist effects for nested designs, and their results are summarized here, beginning with a general result followed by a reanalysis of a treatment comparison study.

Effects in General.   Recall from chapter 4 that the upper bound for treatment effects was $d = 0.20$, which translates into the fact that about 1% of the variance in outcomes is due to treatments. However, this estimate is the incorrect estimate because it is based on designs that did not appropriately model therapist variance and therefore is an overestimate; using the notation introduced in the beginning of this chapter, $\hat{\omega}^{2'} = .01$. Further, recall that Crits-Christoph et al. (1991) found that the mean proportion of variance attributable to therapists was 0.086; that is, $\hat{\rho}_1 = 0.086$. In the nested designs reviewed by Wampold, Mondin, Moody, Stich, et al. (1997), the median number of therapists was two per treatment (i.e., $q = 2$) with six participants per therapist (i.e., $n = 6$); because effect sizes were typically derived from comparisons of two treatments, $p = 2$. Using these values (viz., $n = 6$, $p = 2$, $q = 2$, $\hat{\omega}^{2'} = .01$, and $\rho_1 = .086$) and the formulas derived by Wampold and Serlin (in press), the estimate of the amount of variance attributable to treatments is zero (i.e, $\hat{\omega}^2$). *That is, if therapist effects had been properly modeled, the effect size of $d = .20$ for treatments is completely artifactual.* In reality, treatment effects appear to be zero.

Specific Example.   To understand how therapist effects change the conclusions that are made about treatments, Wampold and Serlin (2000) examined a study that compared two therapies for the treatment of anxiety disorders conducted by Durham et al. (1994). Although Durham et al. concluded that cognitive therapy was superior to analytic therapy, they failed to consider therapist effects. In this study, two therapists delivered each of the treatments to approximately 16 clients. In Table 8.6, the incorrect F values and effect sizes derived from Durham et al.'s study are given. In addition, Table 8.6 presents the correct values under two scenarios, $\rho_I = 0.10$ and $\rho_I = 0.30$, which are reasonable given the values obtained by Crits-Christoph et al. (1991) for individual variables. Wampold and Serlin came to the following conclusion:

> Ignoring provider effects, 8 of 12 dependent variables showed statistically significant treatment effects and the mean estimate of the proportion of variance due

TABLE 8.6

Reanalysis of Durham et al. (1994) Assuming Various Therapist Effects

Variable	Incorrect (published)		$\rho_I = .1$		$\rho_I = .3$	
	$F'(1, 60)$	$\hat{\omega}^{2'}$	$F(1, 2)$	$\hat{\omega}^2$	$F(1, 2)$	$\hat{\omega}^2$
Overall severity	2.9	.03	1.10	.01	0.45	.00
SAS	1.1	.00	0.42	.00	0.17	.00
HAS	9.7*	.12	3.69	.10	1.51	.06
BSI	11.8*	.14	4.49	.13	1.84	.09
STAI-T	16.2*	.19	6.17	.18	2.52	.15
BAI	17.9*	.21	6.81	.20	2.78	.17
BDI	13.2*	.16	5.02	.15	2.05	.12
Tension	3.8	.04	1.45	.02	0.59	.00
Panic	9.5*	.12	3.62	.10	1.48	.06
Irritability	0.2	.00	0.08	.00	0.03	.00
SES	5.9*	.07	2.25	.05	0.92	.00
DAS	9.6*	.12	3.65	.10	1.49	.06
M		.10		.09		.06

*$p < .05$; SAS = Social Adjustment Scale; HAS = Hamilton Anxiety Scale; BSI = Brief System Inventory; STAI-T + State-Trait Anxiety Inventory; BAI = Beck Anxiety Inventory; BDI = Beck Depression Inventory; SES = Self-Esteem Scale; DAS = Dysfunctional Attitude Scale.

Note. F′ from Durham et al. (1994), $\hat{\omega}^{2'}$ calculated à la Kirk (1995, p. 178), the remaining values calculated with the methods presented in Wampold and Serlin (2000). From "The Consequences of Ignoring a Nested Factor on Measures of Effect Size in Analysis of Variance Designs," by B. E. Wampold and R. C. Serlin, 2000, 4, 425–433. *Psychological Methods.* Copyright © 2000 by the American Psychological Association. Reprinted with permission.

to treatments was 10 percent. However, when $\hat{\rho}_I = .10$, none of the dependent measures were significant and the estimate of the proportion of variance due to treatments dropped to 9 percent. Even more dramatic was that when $\hat{\rho}_I = .30$, none of the dependent variables was statistically significant and treatment variance dropped to 6 percent.... The effects of provider variance on conclusions of this study are striking. That this study has been heralded as demonstrating the superiority of cognitive therapy (see e.g., DeRubeis & Crits-Christoph, 1998) demonstrates the need to consider provider variance before concluding that some treatments are more effective than others. (Wampold & Serlin, 2000, pp. 432–433)

CONCLUSIONS

The essence of therapy is embodied in the therapist. Earlier it was shown that the particular treatment that the therapist delivers does not affect outcomes. Moreover, adherence to the treatment protocol does not account for the variability in outcomes. Nevertheless, therapists within a given treatment account for a large proportion of the variance. Clearly, the person of the therapist is a critical factor in the success of therapy.

The medical model stipulates that it is the technical expertise of the therapist that should account for the variability in outcomes—How well does the therapist follow the treatment protocol, and Does the protocol reflect a valid and useful theoretical perspective? The evidence is clear that the type of treatment is irrelevant, and adherence to a protocol is misguided, but yet the therapist, within each of the treatments, makes a tremendous difference. It was shown previously that allegiance to the therapy was important. It is now clear that the particular therapist delivering the treatment is absolutely crucial, adding support for the contextual model of psychotherapy.

Implications of Rejecting
the Medical Model

In this book, evidence has been presented that demonstrates that the medical model does not adequately explain the benefits of psychotherapy. On the contrary, the evidence is largely consistent with a contextual model of psychotherapy. Corroborating the contextual model has enormous implications for research in psychotherapy and for the delivery of mental health services. It is scientifically interesting that the medical model is not explanatory. However, policy related to psychotherapy has increasingly assumed that psychotherapy can be conceptualized as a medical treatment, changing the nature of the endeavor and possibly destroying its usefulness. In this chapter, the urgency of dislodging psychotherapy from the chains of the medical establishment is discussed.

The first part of this chapter reviews the evidence and discusses the implications for the scientific understanding of psychotherapy. The second part discusses the implications of rejecting the medical model for the delivery of mental health services for the training and supervision of therapists.

IMPLICATIONS FOR THE SCIENCE
OF PSYCHOTHERAPY

Summary of the Evidence

In the various chapters of this book, the empirical evidence related to the benefits of psychotherapy was presented within a framework that contrasted the medical model to the contextual model. Recounting the conclu-

203

sions and comparing the various sources of the benefits of psychotherapy will serve to reinforce the conclusions that the specific ingredients of treatments are not responsible for the benefits of psychotherapy. The effect sizes derived from various sources are summarized in Table 9.1; these effects are discussed, summarized, and compared.

Since the late 1970s and early 1980s, the efficacy of psychotherapy has been well established. Estimates of the effect size for psychotherapeutic treatment, when compared with no treatment, converges to 0.80. Given that (a) outcome variables in psychotherapy are notoriously unreliable, (b) variance attributable to clients is great, (c) many disorders are resistant to interventions, and (d) research methods are fallible, the documented potency of psychotherapy in clinical trials is remarkably large and robust.

Having establishe[...]otherapy, the objective of this book has been to exa[...]tify the aspects of therapy that are responsible for t[...]enefits of psychotherapy. Two explanatory models [...]ical model and the contextual model. The medical [...]e client presents with a disorder, problem, or com[...]psychological explanation for the disorder, problem[...]hanism of change can be derived from the expla[...]peutic ingredients consistent with the explanation[...]n, or complaint and with the mechanism of change[...]lient; and (e) the specific ingredients are remedia[...]r, or complaint.

If the medical mo[...]nework for conceptualizing psychotherapy, then [...]that the specific ingredients are responsible for th[...]py. Precious little evidence exists for this proposi[...]model, it is expected that the efficacy of various tre[...]specific ingredients will be more remedial than ot[...]h designs that are able to isolate and establish the[...]pecific ingredients and outcomes should reveal [...]lead to change. Neither of these predictions has [...]there is strong evidence that treatments are unifor[...]component, mediating, and moderating studies h[...]find the theoretical connection between specific ingredients and outcomes. Table 9.1 summarizes the evidence from chapters 4, 5 and 8, from which it is concluded that little if any of the variability in outcomes in psychotherapy is due to specific ingredients. In fact, the evidence indicates that, at most, specific ingredients account for only 1% of the variance in outcomes. Decades of psychotherapy research have failed to find a scintilla of evidence that any specific ingredient is necessary for therapeutic change.

The contextual model explains the benefits of psychotherapy by postulating that the "aim of psychotherapy is to help people feel and function

TABLE 9.1

Effects for Various Psychotherapeutic Aspects

Source	Descriptor or Phenomenon	Design	Effect Size	Proportion of Variance	Chapter	Notes
Effects of psychotherapy	Absolute efficacy	Tx vs. Control	0.80	13%	3	Well-established point estimate of psychotherapeutic effects
Treatments	Relative efficacy	Tx A vs. Tx B	0.00 to 0.20	0% to 1%	4, 8	Best estimate for effect size is 0.00; 0.20 is upper bound under most liberal assumptions and inflated by not considering therapist effects
Specific ingredients	Specific effects	Component, mediating and moderating	0.00	0%	5	Little evidence found for specific effects from these designs
Common factor	Placebo effects	Placebo vs. control	0.40	4%	5	Lower bound for estimate of proportion of variance due to common factors in that placebo treatments contain some, but not all, common factors specified in contextual model
Common factor	Working alliance	Correlation of alliance and outcome	0.45	5%	6	A single common factor accounts for about 5% of the variance in outcomes
Common factor	Allegiance	Correlation of allegiance and outcome OR difference between treatments	Up to 0.65	Up to 10%	7	Allegiance of therapist has consistently been found to be related to outcome; estimates of effects from various meta-analyses range up to 0.65
Therapist effects	Competence	Nested or crossed	0.50 to 0.60	6% to 9%	8	Estimates for aggregate of outcome variables; proportion of variability due to therapists for individual variables ranges up to 70%

Note. Tx = treatment

205

better by encouraging appropriate modifications in their assumptive worlds, thereby transforming the meaning of their experiences to more favorable ones" (Frank & Frank, 1991, p. 30). The components common to all therapies include (a) an emotionally charged confiding relationship with a helping person; (b) a healing setting that involves the client's expectations that the professional helper will assist him or her; (c) a rationale, conceptual scheme, or myth that provides a plausible, although not necessarily true, explanation of the client's symptoms and how the client can overcome his or her demoralization; and (d) a ritual or procedure that requires the active participation of both client and therapist and is based on the rationale underlying the therapy.

If the contextual model explains the benefits of psychotherapy, then variability in outcomes should be attributable to one or more of the common factors. Table 9.1 summarizes evidence in several areas that demonstrates that indeed common factors are crucial to the psychotherapeutic endeavor. Placebo treatments, which contain some but not all common factors, account for 4% of the variability in outcomes. Thus, this subset of common factors explains a significant portion of the variance. However, the complete set of common factors (i.e., a treatment intended to be therapeutic) would account for a greater proportion of the variance; thus 4% is a lower bound for the effects of common factors. One prominent common factor studied is the working alliance; the proportion of variability in outcomes due to this one factor is substantial (about 5%). Moreover, allegiance, another common factor, accounts for up to 10% of the variability in outcomes. Finally, the variance due to therapists within treatments accounts for somewhere between 6 and 9% of the variance in outcomes.

The evidence compellingly supports the contextual model as the underlying conceptual basis for the benefits of psychotherapy. Scientifically, the medical model metaphor for psychotherapy is simply not congruent with the data produced by the corpus of studies in psychotherapy. In this book, two competing meta-models have been contrasted. One could quibble about the epistemological standing of these two models as the proper competing explanatory models for explaining the benefits of psychotherapy. Regardless of whether one could develop another explanatory model or whether the two models presented herein could be modified, the evidence, summarized in Table 9.1, has ponderous repercussions for the science and practice of psychotherapy.

Partitioning Variance to Specific Ingredients and Common Factors

From a scientific perspective, it is valuable to partition the variability in outcomes in psychotherapy to various sources. Although Table 9.1 summarizes the results of psychotherapy in terms of the proportion of variance attributable to various sources, comparisons across the sources are problematic. The fundamental issue is that the total variance in studies is a function of the design and the choice of comparisons (see Wampold & Serlin, 2000, for a discussion of this issue in terms of nested designs). For example, a comparison of two treatments intended to be therapeutic produces less variance than the comparison of a treatment and a poorly designed placebo. Although clearly unethical, one could manipulate the total variance by using a treatment that was intended to be harmful (e.g., the therapist badgered the client and was critical of any attempt to discuss the client's distress). The point here is that the estimates of the proportions of variance presented in Table 9.1 are not perfectly comparable across sources. Nevertheless, rough estimates of the variability in outcomes attributable to various sources provide direction for scientific inquiry.

An occasionally cited partition of the variability in improvement of psychotherapy clients was developed by Lambert (1992). Lambert's partition, which appears in Figure 9.1, attributes 30% of the variance to common factors and 15% to expectancy effects (which was equated with placebo effects) and 15% to techniques. Because both the expectancy effects and common factors are classified as incidental aspects of therapy in the medical model, the aggregation of these two sources accounts for three times the variance attributed to specific ingredients (i.e., techniques). However, these percentages are arbitrary as "no statistical procedures were used to derive the percentages that appear in [Figure 9.1], which appears [sic] somewhat more precise than is perhaps warranted" (Lambert, 1992, p. 98).

A more scientifically derived partition can be obtained by using the evidence found in Table 9.1. Consider that 13% of the variability in outcomes is due to psychotherapy. Then the proportion of the effects for psychotherapy due to factors incidental to the specific ingredients can be estimated by taking the proportion of variability due to therapists within treatments to the variability due to whether treatment is provided (viz., $0.09/0.13 = 0.70$). That is, at least 70% of the psychotherapeutic effects are general effects (i.e., effects due to common factors).[1] The variance due to specific ingredients (i.e., specific effects) can be estimated as the proportion of variability between treatments intended to be therapeutic to the variability due to whether treatment is provided. Consequently, specific effects account for at most 8% of the variance (viz., $0.01/0.13 = 0.08$). The remaining variability (viz., 22%), which is unexplained, is certainly due, in part, to client differences (see Garfield, 1994). Whatever the source of the unexplained variance, it is clearly not related to specific ingredients. These calculations are

---

[1]Certainly, all aspects of therapy incidental to a specific treatment are not embodied in the therapist, therefore 70% estimation of general effects is conservative.

- **Extratherapeutic Change:** Those factors that are a part of the client (such as ego strength and other homeostatic mechanisms) and part of the environment (such as fortuitous events, social support) that aid in recovery regardless of participation in therapy.

- **Expectancy** (placebo effects): That portion of improvements that results from the client's knowledge that he/she is being treated and from the differential credibility of specific treatment techniques and rationale.

- **Techniques:** Those factors unique to specific therapies (such as biofeedback, hypnosis, or systematic desensitization).

- **Common Factors:** include a host of variable that are found in a variety of therapies regardless of the therapists theoretical orientation: such as empathy, warmth, acceptance, encouragement of risk taking, et cetera.

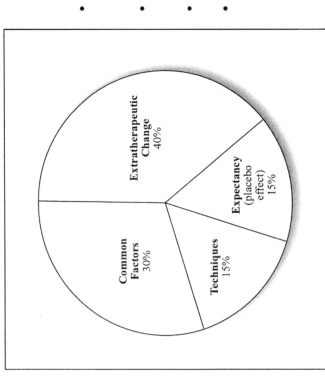

FIG. 9.1.   Percent of improvement in psychotherapy patients as a function of therapeutic factors. From "Psychotherapy Outcome Research: Implications for Integrative and Eclectic Therapists," by M. J. Lambert, in J. C. Norcross and M. R. Goldfried (Eds.), *Handbook of Psychotherapy Integration* (p. 97), 1992, New York: Basic Books. Copyright © 1992 by Basic Books. Adapted with permission.

graphically presented in Figure 9.2, which takes the form used to present the general and specific effects in chapter 1 (see Figure 1.1). Lest there be any ambiguity about the profound contrast between general and specific effects, it must be noted that the 1% of the variability in outcomes due to specific ingredients is likely a gross upper bound (see chaps. 4 and 8). Clearly, the preponderance of the benefits of psychotherapy are due to factors incidental to the particular theoretical approach administered and dwarf the effects due to theoretically derived techniques.

Rejecting the medical model and understanding the nature of the contextual model has implications for how psychotherapy is studied, practiced, funded, and valued by society. In this section, the focus is on the science of psychotherapy, and thus recommendations for research are discussed next.

Research Recommendations

Recommendation 1: Limit Clinical Trials.   The clinical trial is a methodology derived from the medical model (Henry, 1998; Wampold, 1997). If specific ingredients were indeed important aspects of psychotherapy, then various types of clinical trials, such as treatment–control

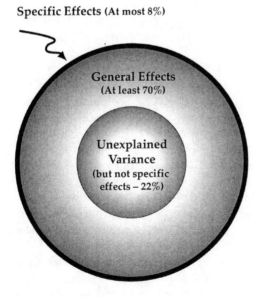

FIG. 9.2.   Effects of psychotherapy scientifically partitioned into specific and general effects (areas proportional to variability due to source).

group comparisons, component studies, and treatment comparisons, would yield results supportive of the medical model. Through the years, the results of various types of clinical trials have overwhelmingly produced evidence that the particular specific ingredients of various therapies are not the aspects of therapy producing benefits. If the contextual model is indeed explanatory, then continued use of clinical trials will continue to produce results that replicate the unwavering pattern of the previous decades. In 1975, Sloane et al. found that behavioral and analytically oriented psychotherapies were superior to the control group, but generally equivalent to each other (see chap. 4). Since that time, the preponderance of studies using a comparative outcome design have found the same result—the treatments compared are superior to no treatment (or to a treatment not intended to be therapeutic), but are approximately equally efficacious. Moreover, there is no trend toward finding treatment differences in more recent studies (Wampold, Mondin, Moody, Stich, et al., 1997).

How is it that comparative outcome studies continue to be funded and conducted? If one ascribes to the medical model, then there is always hope that evidence will turn up showing that a particular treatment is demonstrably better than another and that the specific ingredients of that treatment are particularly potent. However, as has been shown throughout this book, the evidence is overwhelmingly unsupportive of the medical model and the specificity of unique ingredients of any therapy. The saying "searching for a needle in a haystack" might be apropos, but the missing object (i.e., the efficacious specific ingredient) is more of a mirage than an object to be found.

Recommendation 2: Focus on Aspects of Treatment That Can Explain the General Effects or the Unexplained Variance.   Figure 9.2 demonstrates dramatically that unexplained variance and general effects account for almost all of the variance due to treatments. Consequently, it seems prudent to focus research on these sources. There are a great many unknowns in the 92% (or more) of variance that is either unexplained or is unambiguously due to factors incidental to the particular treatments.

Over the years, a number of speculations have been made about the nature of the general effects. Kirsch (1985) argued that behavior change is primarily an expectancy effect. Others see the process of psychotherapy as one of social influence and perception (Frank & Frank, 1991; Garfield, 1995; Heppner & Claiborn, 1989; Strong 1968). The therapeutic relationship is primary to many (Bachelor & Horvath, 1999; Gelso & Carter, 1985; Safran & Muran, 1995). Rogers focused on the person of the therapist as expressed as his or her congruence, unconditional positive regard, and empathy, which facilitates the clients' intrinsic desire for change (i.e., self-actualization). Many theoreticians have attempted to define uniquely the essence of the common factors that lead to change. For example, Hanna (Hanna & Puhakka, 1991; Hanna & Ritchie, 1995) developed the construct of *resolute perception*:

> *Resolute perception* is defined as the steady and deliberate observation of or attending to something that is intimidating, painful, or stultifying with therapeutic intent. Resolute perception ... can be directed toward anything, whether in one's inner experience or in the environment, that one would ordinarily avoid, shun, withdraw from, or react to. Implicit in this deliberateness and steadiness is an openness to experience what truly and actually is coupled with a readiness to honestly examine it, evaluate it, and, if need be, to change it with therapeutic intent. By *therapeutic intent* is meant that the resoluteness is toward a promotion of well-being variously described as personal growth, adaptive behavior, authenticity, release of stress or tension, and so on. (Hanna & Puhakka, 1991, p. 599)

Clearly, the constructs used to investigate the commonalities of therapies are not independent. Empathy and the formation of the working alliance, for example, are intricately and inextricably connected. Nevertheless, continued conceptualization of and research on the commonalities of therapy are critical to understanding the scientific bases of psychotherapy and to augmenting the benefits of these treatments.

It is indeed curious that one of the most apparent sources of variability, the therapist, is so little understood. In chapter 8, the evidence demonstrated that therapists accounted for around 6–9% of the variability in outcomes within treatment when variables were aggregated; when variables were segregated, individual variables accounted for up to 22% of the variability within treatments. Yet very little is known about the qualities and actions of therapists who are eminently successful. Recall from chapter 8 that Blatt et al. (1996) found that in the NIMH TDCRP, the more effective therapists were more psychologically minded, eschewed biological treatments, and expected treatments to take longer. These results clearly do not provide much direction for selecting therapist trainees or for training therapists.

To further understand how psychotherapy works and how psychotherapists should be trained, research on the common factors should be supported. Review panels that fund psychotherapy research at the NIMH are composed primarily of physicians and psychologists who conceptualize psychotherapy as an analogue of a medical treatment. However, the evidence in this book suggests strongly that research funds should be spent on psychotherapy process research that attends to the contribution of the common factors to outcomes.

Recommendation 3: Relax Emphasis on Treatment Manuals.
Since the late 1980s, treatment manuals have been universally required to obtain funding for psychotherapy outcome research. Many have em-

braced this dictate as an advance of science: "The treatment manual requirement, imposed as a routine design demand, chiseled permanently into the edifice of psychotherapy efficacy research the basic canon of standardization" (Kiesler, 1994). Although standardization is an important aspect of group designs, care must be taken around the aspects of therapy that are standardized. The focus of manuals, which emanate from a medical model conceptualization of psychotherapy (see chap. 1), is on the specific ingredients. There is evidence that adherence to a manual attenuates the quality of aspects of therapy incidental to the theoretically conceived notions of what should transpire in therapy (Henry, Schacht, et al., 1993; Henry, Strupp, et al., 1993) and that the use of manuals reduces variability among therapists (Crits-Christoph & Mintz, 1991). It may well be that standardization decreases the performance of the best therapists, thereby eliminating from study the most efficacious exemplars, which should be the focus of research endeavors that wish to examine excellence.

Manuals standardize treatments so that attention can be directed toward differences among treatments, but they place emphasis on a source that has historically been unproductive. Thus, manuals focus attention toward a wasteland and away from the fertile ground. Using a basketball analogy, Wampold (1997) described the misdirection of attention as follows:

> We suspect that a great deal of the variance in success of teams is due to players' ability, institutional support, and motivation and very little is due to whether the teams play man-to-man defense or zone defense. If the goal is to identify the most important factors related to winning records so that coaches could build the best teams possible, it would make little sense to arrange studies that examine the type of defense used by homogenizing players' abilities, institutional support, and so forth. Why then are we trying to homogenize therapy and therapists, when we know that these vary variables contribute to much variance in outcomes, so that we can examine differences between treatments, when treatment differences historically have accounted for so little variance? (pp. 34–35)

Manuals may reduce the variance within treatments, increasing the power to detect between group differences, but the price is very high. In the medical model, the holy grail involves the specific ingredients, and it is worth any sacrifice to find the tiniest fragment of this precious commodity. However, the important source of variance is within-treatments rather than between-treatments. The point is simple: If the goal is to detect differences among treatments, à la the medical model, then standardization of treatments with manuals is scientifically justified. However, from a contextual model perspective, standardization of treatment may eliminate from consideration the lovely aspects of therapy that, by their very essence, create change.

Recommendation 4: Focus on Effectiveness Rather Than Efficacy.
In chapter 7, the distinction between efficacy and effectiveness was discussed. Efficacy and effectiveness refer to the degree to which a treatment is beneficial within the clinical trial context and the clinical
setting, respectively (Seligman, 1995). From a practical standpoint, effectiveness is critical to the delivery of services to clients in the real
world, and thus establishment of effectiveness is obviously important.
Because treatments in clinical trials involve manuals, intensively
trained therapists, supervision, and monitoring, it has been thought that
the size of effects in clinical trials will be larger than those produced
when the same treatment is administered to more heterogeneous clients
by therapists who are typically not supervised or monitored. However,
this does not appear to be true, at least for adults (see chap. 7). However,
the evidence in this regard is indirect, and several important questions
are unanswered.

There has never been a direct comparison between a treatment practiced
in the clinical trial context (training, manual, supervision, and monitoring)
and the same treatment delivered in the clinical practice setting (no extra
training, no manual, and no monitoring). In addition, there has never been a
comparison of an empirically supported treatment (see chap. 1 and the discussion later in this chapter) and eclectically practiced treatment in the clinical practice context. Consider a study of treatment for depression
containing the following groups:

1. CBT as practiced in the clinical practice setting (no manual, no training, no supervision).
2. CBT as practiced in clinical trails (manual, training, and supervision)
3. Eclectic therapy as practiced in the clinical practice context
4. Eclectic therapy with supervision and training equal to that of Group 2

This design would address several important questions:

A. Is an empirically supported treatment superior to one that is not em-
   pirically supported (Group 1 + 2 vs. Group 3 + 4)?
B. Is an empirically supported treatment in a clinical trial context supe-
   rior to the same treatment practiced in the clinical practice setting
   (Group 1 vs. Group 2)?
C. Does supervision improve therapeutic outcomes, a question of great
   importance in the supervision area (Holloway & Neufeld, 1995;
   Group 3 vs. Group 4)?

Although this research would answer these important (and orthogonal) questions, it must be realized that it would not be funded under current policy because several of the treatments would be administered without manuals. Clearly, there are a great many designs that could be used to investigate assumptions made under the medical model about the benefits of psychotherapy, but any investigation of psychotherapy as it is practiced in the community would not be funded because of the medical model research design bias.

IMPLICATIONS FOR PRACTICE AND TRAINING

Accepting the contextual model as the scientific conceptual basis for the benefits of psychotherapy has enormous implications for the practice of psychotherapy, for the delivery of mental health services, and for training. Some of these recommendations have been made through the years, but it should be kept in mind that they are now supported by the best available science.

Empirically Supported Treatments

As discussed in chapter 1, identification of a set of ESTs was necessary "if clinical psychology is to survive in this heyday of biological psychiatry" (Task Force on Promotion and Dissemination of Psychological Procedures, 1995, p. 3). The criteria for determining whether a treatment is classified as an EST, the most recent of which are presented in Table 9.2, are patterned after the Food and Drug Administration's criteria for certifying drugs and consequently favor treatments that conform to the medical model and are analogues of medications. For example, the criteria require that a manual be used to guide the treatment, thus favoring behavioral and cognitive treatments, which have focused on the manualization of treatment. Moreover, the criteria were developed so as to favor treatments that contain relatively discrete components. Simply stated, the conceptual basis of the EST movement is embedded in the medical model of psychotherapy and thus favors treatments more closely aligned with the medical model, such as behavioral and cognitive treatments. Not surprisingly, the preponderance of ESTs are cognitive and behavioral treatments—15 of 16 Efficacious Treatments in 1998 were behavioral or cognitive–behavioral oriented (Chambless et al., 1998). As a result of this medical model bias, humanistic and dynamic treatments are at a distinct disadvantage, regardless of their effectiveness. The scientific and conceptual problems with ESTs have been discussed elsewhere (see e.g., Henry, 1998; Wampold, 1997).

The evidence presented in this book has undermined the scientific basis of the medical model of psychotherapy, thus destroying the foundation on which ESTs are built. Scientifically, it is informative to establish that a treat-

TABLE 9.2

Criteria for Empirically Validated Treatments

Well-established treatments

I. At least two good between-groups design experiments demonstrating efficacy in one or more of the following ways:

A. Superior (statistically significantly so) to pill or psychological placebo or to another treatment

B. Equivalent to an already established treatment in experiments with adequate sample sizes

OR

II. A large series of single case design experiments (n > 9) demonstrating efficacy. These experiments must:

A. Use good experimental designs, and

B. Compare the intervention to another treatment, as in IA.

Further criteria for both I and II:

III. Experiments must be conducted with treatment manuals.

IV. Characteristics of the client samples must be clearly specified.

V. Effects must have been demonstrated by at least two different investigators or investigating teams.

Probably efficacious treatments

I. Two experiments showing the treatment is superior (statistically significantly so) to a waiting-list control group

OR

II. One or more experiments meeting the Well-established criteria IA or IB, III, and IV, but not V.

OR

III. A small series of single-case-design experiments (n ≥ 3) otherwise meeting Well-established treatment criteria.

Note.   From "Update on Empirically Validated Therapies, II," by D. L. Chambless et al., 1998, *The Clinical Psychologist, 51,* p. 4. Copyright © 1998 by Division 12 of the American Psychological Association, Washington, DC. Adapted with permission.

ment, say CBT for depression, is empirically supported by demonstrating that it is more effective than no treatment or a placebo treatment, when administered with a manual. In the larger context, however, giving primacy to an EST ignores the scientific finding that all treatments studied appear to be uniformly beneficial as long as they are intended to be therapeutic (see chap.

4). Although apparently harmless, the EST movement has immense detrimental effects on the science and practice of psychotherapy, as it legitimizes the medical model of psychotherapy and suggests that some treatments are more effective than others when in fact treatments are equally effective.

It might seem that ESTs are a valid means to prevent acceptance of treatments that have weak, nonexistent, or contratheoretical psychological bases. Such is not the case. If treatment efficacy is established via factors incidental to the specific ingredients, then superfluous ingredients can be added, producing a treatment that can nevertheless be promoted for its "unique and efficacious ingredients." Much publicity has been directed toward eye movement desensitization and reprogramming (EMDR) for PTSD (F. Shapiro, 1989), a treatment that has been designated as "possibly efficacious" (DeRubeis & Crits-Christoph, 1998). EMDR contains an ingredient in which rapid saccadic eye movements are elicited as the client repeatedly imagines the traumatic event, and this ingredient is proposed by EMDR developers as unique and essential. However, there is evidence that the rapid eye movement is not necessary for improvement (e.g., Lohr, Kleinknecht, Tolin, & Barrett, 1995), and indeed there are many clinical researchers who consider the rapid eye movement component of EMDR ludicrous. However, if the medical model is accepted but is not explanatory, then any treatment that contains absolutely worthless or even ludicrous specific ingredients will meet the criteria of an EST provided it is conducted with a manual and is twice compared with placebo or other EST treatments by different teams of researchers (and who have specified the characteristics of the subjects). Recall that there is little evidence that the cognitive procedures of CBT for depression are needed to reduce depression (see chap. 5); consequently EMDR cannot be ruled out as an EST on the basis of lack of evidence for specificity. Similarly, many seemingly unscientific-appearing therapies can meet the efficacy criteria. For example, dance therapy has shown consistently large treatment effects (Ritter & Low, 1996). The point is that in the long run, adoption of EST criteria will lead to the identification of ESTs with dubious specific ingredients.

Clinical Implications of the Contextual Model:
If Not Empirically Supported Treatments, Then What?

If the medical model is not explanatory and identification of ESTs should be abolished, then what are the criteria for determining which treatments are appropriate for psychologists to use? Some interpret adoption of the contextual model as "anything goes" because the specific ingredients are irrelevant. Others go so far as to believe that if specific ingredients are irrelevant, there is no reason to include them in a treatment. The purpose of this section is to clarify the clinical implications of the contextual model.

Status of Techniques.   The first point to address is that the contextual model places great emphasis on procedures that are consistent with the rationale for treatment. When the contextual model was described in chapter 1, emphasis was placed on the "ritual or procedure" that requires the active participation of the client and the therapist and that each believes that the procedure (in the context of the healing setting) will be beneficial to the client. Jerome Frank, in the introduction to the latest edition of *Persuasion and Healing* (Frank & Frank, 1991), clearly indicated the importance of technique:

> My position is not that technique is irrelevant to outcome. Rather, I maintain that, as developed in the text, the success of all techniques depends on the patient's sense of alliance with an actual or symbolic healer. This position implies that ideally therapists should select for each patient the therapy that accords, or can be brought to accord, with the patient's personal characteristics and view of the problem. Also implied is that therapists should seek to learn as many approaches as they find congenial and convincing. Creating a good therapeutic match may involve both educating the patient about the therapist's conceptual scheme and, if necessary, modifying the scheme to take into account the concepts the patient brings to therapy." (p. xv).

Clearly, techniques consistent with a theoretical explanation of the disorder, problem, or complaint are needed in a contextual model conceptualization of psychotherapy. A therapist cannot form a therapeutic relationship without having a well-conceived mode of therapeutic action.

Relative Worth of Treatments and Epistemology of Specific Ingredients.   It should be emphasized that the contextual model is silent about the relative worth of treatments. Cognitive and behavioral treatments are more deeply imbedded in the medical model of psychotherapy in which specific ingredients are primary than are the humanistic or experiential therapies. Yet recognition that the therapies must contain procedures and that the nature of the procedures are by and large irrelevant to outcomes gives no edge to the humanistic or experiential treatments. Nothing in this book should be interpreted as partiality to humanistic or experiential therapies or as prejudice against cognitive or cognitive–behavioral treatments that predominate ESTs.

Even though specific effects are extremely small and probably nonexistent, the status of specific ingredients is critically important. The evidence in this book has shown that specific ingredients are not active in and of themselves. Therapists need to realize that the specific ingredients are necessary but active only in the sense that they are a component of the healing context. Slavish adherence to a theoretical protocol and maniacal promotion of a single theoretical approach are utterly in opposition to science.

Therapists need to have a healthy sense of humility with regard to the techniques they use.

Ironically, it is the clients who appear to have a healthy perspective in that they report that they value the relationship and other common factors, which is in contrast to therapists, who focus on skills. In the 1960s, when therapists and clients were asked about helpful areas of therapy, it was found that it was therapists vis-à-vis clients who indicated that therapeutic skills and techniques were helpful (Feifel & Eells, 1963). In 1984, Murphy, Cramer, and Lillie (1984) determined that clients reported that talking with someone who understands them and is interested in their problems and therapist advice were the most helpful aspects of treatment. Eugster and Wampold (1996) asked Diplomates of the American Board of Professional Psychology and their clients to rate a session on a number of constructs and, in addition, to evaluate the session overall. Therapist expertise was related to session evaluation for therapists but not for clients. On the other hand, the real relationship was positively related to clients' evaluation of sessions, but negatively related for therapists (when other constructs were considered simultaneously). Moreover, therapist interpersonal style was related to clients' but not therapists' session evaluation.

Therapist Perspective Toward Specific Ingredients.

What perspective should a therapist take relative to specific ingredients given the knowledge that they must necessarily be part of therapy but that they do not lead to the benefits of the treatment? The first part of the answer to this question is that the therapist needs to realize that the client's belief in the explanation for their disorder, problem, or complaint is paramount, as are the concomitant specific ingredients. Occasionally, even proponents of an approach have a glimmer of recognition of this fact. For example, Donald Meichenbaum (1986) clearly a zealous advocate and proponent of cognitive therapies, described the laudatory actions of a therapist:

> As part of the therapy rationale, the therapist conceptualized each client's anxiety in terms of Schacter's model of emotional arousal (Schachter, 1966). That is, the therapist stated that the client's fear reaction seemed to involve two major elements: (a) heightened physiological arousal, and (b) a set of anxiety-producing, avoidant thoughts and self-statements (e.g., disgust evoked by the phobic object, a sense of helplessness, panic thoughts of being overwhelmed by anxiety, a desire to flee). After laying this groundwork, the therapist noted that the client's fear seemed to fit Schachter's theory that an emotional state such as fear is in large part determined by the thoughts in which the client engages when physically aroused. It should be noted that the Schachter and Singer (1962) theory of emotion was used for purposes of conceptualization only. Although the theory and research upon which it is based have been criticized (Lazurus, Averill, & Opton, 1971; Plutchik & Ax, 1967), the theory has an aura of plausibility that the clients

tend to accept: The logic of the treatment plan is clear to clients in light of this conceptualization. (p. 370).

Part of the plausibility of an explanation and of techniques derives from the coherence of the treatment. An eclectic therapist who randomly selects techniques from a bag of techniques or a therapist who fails to act strategically at all will be as ineffective as a therapist who slavishly adheres to a protocol regardless of the clients' belief in the rationale for that treatment.

A component of the contextual model is the therapists' belief in the treatment. But how can a therapist, who has reviewed the empirical literature and adopted the contextual model, believe in any particular treatment, given the fact that the benefits of this treatment are not due to the specific ingredients? Does not the contextual model destroy belief in any and all treatments? On the contrary, the contextual model should promote belief in treatments, albeit at a different level. The contextual model therapist understands that it is the healing context and the meaning that the client gives to the experience that are important. A humanist therapist could administer systematic desensitization and believe in its efficacy because the therapist understands that it is the client's belief that is paramount—this therapist would administer the systematic desensitization with enthusiasm, faith, and allegiance. Under the contextual model, the following equation holds:

Client belief + healing context = therapist belief

Compatibility of Treatment With Client Attitudes, Values, and Culture. If the particular specific ingredient of any treatment is not responsible for the benefits of the treatment, how should therapists decide which approach to use? Frank, in the earlier quotation, provided an answer: "Ideally therapists should select for each patient the therapy that accords, or can be brought to accord, with the patient's personal characteristics and view of the problem" (p. xv). It would therefore seem that the compatibility of treatment with the client's worldview would be important.

In chapter 5, the results of studies that investigated the interaction of client characteristics and treatment were reviewed. The evidence for theoretical interactions between client deficits and the mechanism of change were conspicuously absent. However, there were a number of studies that demonstrated that there were person characteristics (other than those theoretically predicted) that moderated treatment efficacy. In Simons et al.'s (1985) study reviewed in chapter 5, the following observation was made with regard to cognitive therapy for depression and client's belief in the rationale for treatment:

Cognitive therapy relies on a specific explanation for the development and treatment of depressive symptoms. The model is based on the belief that the thoughts, attitudes, and interpretations mediate feelings and behavior. The cognitive therapist offers this set of assumptions to the patient and helps the behaviors. Examination of the [Self-Control Schedule] items reveals that in order to achieve a high score, a patient must already endorse this explanatory model.... The congruence between the patient's and the therapist's conceptualization of the problems and how they are best approached may be a powerful facilitator of treatment response (Frank, 1971; Garfield, 1973). In contrast, patients with low [Self-Control Schedule] scores may find it difficult to accept the self-help quality of cognitive therapy. Rather they may prefer a therapeutic situation in which they assume a more passive role and leave the therapy to the therapist. (Simons et al., 1985, p. 86)

Numerous other studies can be found to support the moderating effects of client characteristics unrelated to psychological deficits responsible for the client's disorder, problem, or complaint. Larry Beutler (e.g., Beutler & Clarkin, 1990; Beutler, Engle, et al., 1991; Beutler, Mohr, Grawe, Engle, & MacDonald, 1991) has systematically and successfully searched for many of these moderating characteristics.

William J. Lyddon tested the hypothesis that a client's personal epistemology would predict preferences for theoretical approaches to psychotherapy (Lyddon, 1989, 1991). On the basis of Royce's theory of knowledge (see Royce & Powell, 1983), Lyddon (1991) classified participants into one of three epistemic styles: rational style, metaphoric style, or empirical style. Similarly, using the scheme developed by Mahoney (see, e.g., Mahoney & Gabriel, 1987), Lyddon classified treatments into three corresponding types: rationalist (e.g., Ellis's rational–emotive therapy), constructivist cognitive therapies (e.g., the therapies of Guidano, Liotti, and Mahoney), and behavioral therapies. As shown in Table 9.3, participants overwhelmingly preferred therapies that matched their epistemic style. This result fits with the clinical intuition that different types of clients prefer different types of treatment.

Another model of matching a client's worldview and therapy has been presented by Rabinowitz, Zevon, and Karuza (1988) and is presented in Table 9.4. An important aspect of this model is that there are many people who, because of their attributions, are unlikely to present for psychological help. When they do, however, the treatment they receive should be consistent with the client's attributional style. For example, client-centered therapy would be contraindicated for those who have an enlightenment model of mental health, as shown in Table 9.4.

Although neither Lyddon's nor Rabinowitz et al.'s models may be the best way to conceptualize clients' worldviews and their match to therapy, it is clear that matching therapy to a client's attitudes and values is an area where greater inquiry is needed.

One of the most important considerations regarding attitudes and values is the racial, ethnic, and cultural characteristics of the client. Because the

TABLE 9.3

Percentage of First-Choice Counseling Preference as a Function
of Dominant Epistemology

Dominant epistemology	Therapy Approach		
	Constructivist	*Behaviorist*	*Rationalist*
Metaphorism	91.0	4.5	4.5
Empiricism	12.5	67.5	20.0
Rationalism	10.0	20.0	70.0

TABLE 9.4

Consequences of Attribution of Responsibility in Four Models of Helping
and Coping

Attribution to Self of Responsibility for Problems	Attribution to Self of Responsibility for Solution	
High	*High* (*Moral model*)	*Low* (*Enlightenment model*)
Perception of self	Lazy	Guilty
Actions expected of self	Striving	Submission
Others besides self who must act	Peers	Authorities
Actions expected of others	Exhortation	Discipline
Implicit view of human nature	Strong	Bad
Pathology	Loneliness	Fanaticism
Low	(*Compensatory Model*)	(*Medical model*)
Perception of self	Deprived	Ill
Actions expected of self	Assertion	Acceptance
Others besides self who must act	Subordinates	Experts
Actions expected of others	Mobilization	Treatment
Implicit view of human nature	Good	Weak
Pathology	Alienation	Dependency

Note. The term *medical model* as used by Brickman et al. is different from the use of the term in this book. From "Models of coping and helping," by Brickman, P., Rabinowitz, V. C., Karuza, J., Jr., Coates, D., Cohn, E., & Kidder, L., 1982, *American Psychologist, 37*, p. 370. Copyright © 1982 by the American Psychological Association. Adapted with permission.

specific ingredients of most treatments, particularly ESTs, are designed and implemented without consideration of race, ethnicity, or culture, these treatments are recommended for a disorder, problem, or complaint blind to the client's cultural values. In an entire special issue of the *Journal of Consulting and Clinical Psychology* on ESTs, not one mention was made of client race, ethnicity, or culture, as if these constructs were irrelevant to the delivery of services.

An example will serve to make the point. A young Asian woman who was earning her Ph.D. in the United States was depressed as a result of marital difficulties. Her marriage, which was arranged in the traditional manner of her country of origin, was a commuter marriage, as her husband was earning his Ph.D. at another university. One of his hobbies was tennis, so during their separation she took tennis lessons. On her arrival to visit him during a holiday, he was bemused by her carrying a tennis racket—bemused because she was to cook a traditional meal for him and his friends while they played tennis rather than join them for a tennis match. She recognized that her education and professional goals would never be realized in the way she imagined if she remained in a traditional marriage where her professional aspirations were subordinate to his.

This young woman, who spoke fluent English, having spent part of her childhood in the United States, presented to her therapist as a highly acculturated Asian. The therapist treated her depression with CBT, assessing her core schemas with regard to her depression around her decision to seek a divorce. The therapist investigated issues of individuality; her reluctance to think first of her education, professional goals, and personal happiness; and her right to have an egalitarian marriage if that were her wish. Her ambivalence to seek a divorce was rooted, however, in the fact that she was of two cultures. The part of her that was acculturated to American values resonated with the intervention. On the other hand, she was deeply connected to her family of origin, where divorce would bring shame to her family, causing her much unhappiness due to the collectivist nature of the society. Moreover, divorce in her Asian culture would ruin the chances that her sister would be able to have a husband of good standing. Reluctantly, she informed the therapist of these considerations but he persisted in altering her core schema with regard to her reluctance to commit to her education, professional goals, and personal happiness. It was impossible for him to consider that this was a dilemma created by living in two cultures and having to choose one (commitment to family, traditional values, and the collective happiness) over the other (self-actualization, personal happiness, and egalitarian marriage). She terminated therapy, struggled with her decision, but after making the difficult and courageous choice to pursue divorce, her depression lifted, although she continued to work through the psychological consequences of deviating from traditional cultural values.

Approaching therapy through a contextual model embraces a multicultural counseling perspective. As individuals in a multicultural society, many psychological issues are related to one's racial, ethnic, and cultural values, issues of oppression and privilege, and racism and discrimination. Many psychologists trained in predominantly majority contexts with ESTs and other traditional therapies abandon the orthodoxy of those treatments in lieu of culturally relevant treatments that are acceptable and appropriate for the populations with whom they are working.

Boundaries of Appropriate Psychological Treatments.   Acceptance of the contextual model does not imply that psychologists can use any treatment. Jerome Frank indicated that "therapists should seek to learn as many approaches as they find congenial and convincing" (Frank & Frank, 1991, p. xv). Psychologists should only find treatments that are well-grounded in psychological principles to be congenial and convincing. That is, theoretical approaches and the concomitant techniques must be consistent with knowledge in psychology. Recovered memory treatments died a horrible death not because they failed a clinical trial or because such treatments were shown, in controlled research, to be ineffective or harmful; rather they were discredited by basic psychological research and clinical analogues that showed that recovered memories can be induced (e.g., Loftus and Pickrell, 1995; Mazzoni, Loftus, Seitz, & Lynn, 1999; Mazzoni, Lombardo, Malvagia, & Loftus, 1999). As mentioned earlier, EMDR has met many of the criteria for an EST but nevertheless involves rapid eye movement, which has a dubious basis in neuropsychology. It may be easier to rule out EMDR as a psychological treatment within the contextual model context than it is in the medical model context.

Psychologists are bound by a profession imbedded in the science of psychology, and professional psychologists should act accordingly. Interventions administered by clergy, indigenous healers, occult practitioners, motivational speakers, or other nontraditional practitioners may be effective and even as effective as psychological treatments. Nevertheless, such treatments are not allowed within the set of psychological treatments, and therefore the contextual model should not be criticized on the basis that it would contain such treatments.

There are many examples of therapies that psychologists should find as an anathema. A brochure (and Web site) advertising a holistic therapy described the therapeutic ingredients for treating depression, PTSD, and various physical complaints (including infertility) as containing the following:

Soothing touch, in a safe and supportive atmosphere, invites you to let go into deep levels of relaxation, so essential to healing; bodywork loosens physical constriction around trauma; psychotherapeutic techniques dislodge unconscious attitudes and beliefs locking the trauma in place and distorting the viewpoint; and energy therapy help heal the body, mind and energy field from the original wound. Together, these approaches allow you to release and repattern unconscious negative dynamics and in that process, you become healthier, stronger and more authentic. Because this work addresses many levels, in addition to easing physical or emotional difficulties, it is also effective in furthering the spiritual journey.

Not all nonstandard therapies are found on the fringes, as some are discussed in professional journals. Consider an article titled "Including the Body in Couple Therapy: Bioenergetic Analysis" (Astor, 1996), describing bioenergetic treatment for a couple, the husband and wife of which were diagnosed, respectively, as "schizoid and masochistic" and "psychopathic narcissist." The treatment, consisted in part, of the following components:

Grounding exercises involved getting the [husband] to stand properly on his own two feet and to learn literally to resist being a pushover. These exercises also taught him to take energy up from the ground by pushing himself up straight from a squatting posture.... He was encouraged to express his rage and his frustration though kicking and hitting [fortunately, a punching bag].... The [wife] was asked to do difficult, painful exercises that would lead to both frustration and exhaustion.... Her exercises included standing on one leg, knee deeply bent, with the other leg held high in the air. She stood this way for an indefinite time, until she collapsed.... These difficult and painful exercises served to help break up her old rigidities" (Astor, 1996, p. 260).

Fortunately, no one subjected bioenergetic analysis to clinical tests that might have validated it through the criteria for an EST. Indeed, the case described by Astor was a success, although "bioenergetic analysis in couple therapy may not be a cure-all or be compared with a full blown psychoanalysis, it still serves as an extremely effective adjunct to the couple therapy process" (Astor, 1996, p. 261).

Although many interventions are ruled out by the fact that they have no psychological basis or contradict psychological knowledge, psychologists may use strategies that appear to contradict this rule. For example, cognitive therapists treating religious persons may need to structure their interventions to be consistent with biblical interpretations. Propst et al. (1992) developed and tested a religious version of cognitive therapy for depression that "gave Christian religious rationales for the procedures, used religious arguments to counter irrational thoughts, and used religious imagery procedures" (p. 96). Clearly, religious imagery does not have a basis in psychology in that no basic research exists on religious imagery and behavior change; nevertheless, at a higher level the therapist realizes that compatibility with the attitudes and values of the client is important, and thus imbedding cognitive techniques in a religious cloak may be therapeutic.

Therapists, whether administering an EST, a well-established therapy, an eclectic therapy, or a therapy outside of the psychological boundary, must exercise caution. Therapies that have been shown to be efficacious, therapies that appear to be at least benign, or therapies that seem "crazy" can be harmful if serious problems are ignored or adequately addressed . Often psychological complaints are signs of organic disorders or reactions to medications, and therapists using any therapeutic approach should be trained to detect such disorders and make the appropriate referrals.

Therapy practice is both a science and an art. The skilled musician has substantial training in music theory (i.e., science) and then uses artistry to create innovative and creative performances (i.e., art). The performer's grounding in music theory is invisible to the audience unless the canons of composition are violated in such a way as the performance is discordant. Similarly, the master therapist, informed by psychological knowledge and theory and guided by experience, produces an artistry that assists clients to move ahead in their lives with meaning and health. Treating clients as if they were medical patients receiving mandated treatments conducted with manuals will stifle the artistry.

Recommendations

Recommendation 5: Abolish the EST Movement as Presently Conceptualized. As originated by Division 12 of the American Psychological Association (Task Force on Promotion and Dissemination of Psychological Procedures, 1995) and as promulgated by proponents (Chambless et al., 1996, 1998; Chambless & Hollon, 1998), the EST criteria and the list of therapies so designated are saturated with the medical model conceptualization of psychotherapy. The bias is distinctly toward behavioral and cognitive–behavioral treatments, reducing the likelihood of acceptance of humanistic, experiential, or psychodynamic therapies. Because clinical trials are shaped by the medical model as well as the EST criteria, there exists further prejudice against therapies other than behavioral and cognitive therapies. Clinical scientists, in the hopes of promoting what are the 'scientific therapies' (i.e., behavioral and cognitive–behavioral therapies), have developed criteria that, from a medical model perspective, would be valid and informative, but, when taken in light of the evidence presented in this book, are ill-conceived and misleading. Designated empirically supported treatments should not be used to mandate services, reimburse service providers, or restrict or guide the training of therapists.

It should be noted that Division 17 (Counseling Psychology) of the American Psychological Association has taken a different approach to empirically supported treatments. In lieu of criteria for designating treatments as ESTs, Division 17 has developed principles for presenting empirical evidence relative to particular interventions (Wampold, Lichtenberg, &

Waehler, in press). Reviews of empirical studies that follow these principles provide practitioners with needed knowledge to inform their practice. To date, reviews following the principles have been developed in the areas of family-based treatments (Sexton & Alexander, in press), career counseling (Whiston, in press), and anger management (Deffenbacher, Oetting, & DiGiuseppe, in press). It is interesting to note that none of these interventions would be considered for EST status as they are not interventions for specific disorders; that is, they don't fit the medical model paradigm.

Recommendation 6: Choose the Best Therapist.   The evidence is clear: Dramatically more variance is due to therapists within treatments than to treatments. Consequently, a person with a disorder, problem, or complaint should seek the most competent therapist possible without regard to the relative effectiveness of the various therapies. Recommendations by friends with similar attitudes, values, and culture, or referrals by those knowledgeable of the competence of therapists are superb sources. If after concerted and honest effort, progress is not obtained, change therapists before changing the approach to therapy.

Recommendation 7: Choose the Therapy That Accords With Client's Worldview.   Help seekers should select a therapy that accords with their worldview. Two (of many) systems for understanding this fit were presented earlier in this chapter (viz., Lyddon, 1989, 1991; Rabinowitz et al., 1988). Given the influence of race, ethnicity, and culture on behavior and mental health, and the pervasiveness of issues of race, ethnicity, and culture in American society, selecting a therapeutic approach that considers multiculturalism is important for all clients. Clients from populations of historically oppressed persons will benefit particularly from therapists who understand this dynamic, who are credible to the client, who can build an alliance with a client who may mistrust therapists representing institutional authority, who are multiculturally competent, and who use an approach that incorporates the tenets of multicultural counseling (Atkinson, Thompson, & Grant, 1993). Moreover, therapists must understand that beliefs about the causes of and solutions for mental health problems are a function of culture (Kleinman & Sung, 1979; Torrey, 1972).

Recommendation 8: Freedom of Choice.   Clients should have the freedom to select the theoretical approach of their choice, and this freedom should not be abrogated by health maintenance organizations, third party payers, or employers. If institutions are interested in restricting treatments in some ways, they should focus on the sources that account for differences, which are the therapists. That is, institutions should ensure that mental health agencies offer a range of treatments by competent providers. For example, college and university counseling centers should not hire psychologists who fit a "center" theoretical approach, but should have psychologists of many orientations.

Recommendation 9: Local Evaluation of Services.   Because therapists account for much of the variability of outcomes, some therapists are consistently facilitating better outcomes than others. It is incumbent on agencies, institutions, and individual therapists to objectively monitor therapy outcomes at the local level. Therapists consistently producing poor outcomes should receive additional training and supervision.

Recommendation 10: Reconceptualize the Relationship of Psychotherapy to the Established Health Care Delivery System.   Psychotherapy, as a field, has had a tenuous relationship with medicine and the established health care delivery system. Although the origins of psychotherapy are found in medicine, the culture of psychotherapy has been distinct from medicine. There was a time when the "talking cure" was practiced predominantly by psychiatrists, but psychotherapy is now primarily in the domain of psychologists, social workers, and counselors. Nevertheless, psychotherapy is pressured to exist in close proximity to medicine, if for no other reason than the fact that reimbursement for services is a component of the health care delivery system in the United States. In a way, psychotherapy is a minority culture forced into co-existence with a dominant culture with different values. There are a number of strategies that any minority culture can use to adapt to such a situation (e.g., see LaFromboise, Coleman, & Gerton, 1993); examination of the strategies will help to understand the dilemmas facing psychotherapy.

One strategy that a minority culture can use in response to a dominant culture is to assimilate into the dominant culture: "One model for explaining the psychological state of a person living within two cultures assumes an ongoing process of absorption into the culture that is perceived as dominant or more desirable" (LaFromboise et al., 1993, p. 396). Those who espouse a medical model of psychotherapy are attempting to assimilate into the dominant health care system and take on the trappings of that culture. For example, in the area of reimbursement for services, psychologists are attempting to compete on the same playing field by suggesting that psychotherapies and psychological services are analogues of medicine. The quotation cited earlier embodies this competition for resources: "If clinical psychology is to survive in this heyday of biological psychiatry, [the American Psychological Association] must act to emphasize the strength of what we have to offer—a variety of psychotherapies of proven efficacy" (Task Force on Promotion and Dissemination of Psychological Procedures, 1995, p. 3). The attempt to obtain prescription privileges is the quintessential statement about acquiring the attitudes and values of the dominant culture. Of course, there are disadvantages to an assimilation strategy.

From a pragmatic view, this is a competition that psychology will never win. Medicine, which includes the pharmaceutical companies, is a bold gorilla that will crush the warm, fuzzy psychotherapy Teddy Bear. Presently, psychological services compete against medical services for precious dollars generated primarily by the health insurance and provider organizations. Allocations to mental health services reduce the monies available for physical health services. Health maintenance organizations, preferred provider organizations, and Federal Programs will yield to the logic of the pharmaceutical companies that desire to treat all mental disorders pharmacologically, even in the face of scientific efficacy that supports the superiority (or at least the equality) and cost effectiveness of psychological services (e.g., Antonuccio, Thomas, & Danton, 1997). One is infinitely more likely to see television advertisements for SSRIs (e.g., Prozac, Zoloft, etc.) for depression than for psychotherapy for depression. Scientifically, the medical model of psychotherapy is wanting; pragmatically, the medical model adherents are stepping onto a playing field (to mix the metaphor) for a game they are sure to loose.

From a philosophical standpoint, assimilation into the medical culture will change the nature of psychotherapy. Short-term treatments, restricted to medically necessary conditions (i.e., select mental disorders), selected from a list of empirically supported treatments, and conducted by therapists approved by HMOs and other medical institutions will predominate. Psychotherapy, as a means to give meaning to one's life, to face and conquer psychological issues, to make fundamental changes in one's life, will become remnants of memories from a dying culture. Although there may be little scientific evidence to place psychotherapy in a medical context, the desire to be accepted by the dominant culture may be too strong to resist assimilation.

A second strategy that minority cultures can use involves separation. The minority culture, according to this strategy, attempts to stand apart, fiercely holding on to their attitudes and values in the face of pressure to conform. Acceptance of the contextual model assumes a view of psychotherapy that is distinct from medicine and the established health care delivery system. Such a position implies that psychotherapy should exist under a separate system, with reimbursement through means separate from the medical system. That is, there would be a system for physical health care and another for mental health care. Interestingly, many Asian countries have dual health care systems, involving seemingly incompatible systems of Western and Eastern medicine. For some disorders, patients will present to a Western medicine practitioner and for other disorders to an Eastern medicine practitioner. Both systems are recognized as effective, and both are supported by the governments of those countries.

In the United States, psychotherapy could be supported through a system separate from traditional medicine to acknowledge that it is not a medical analogue. Some clients may prefer to have their depression treated pharmacologically, in which case they could use the medical system and its structure for paying for those services. Other clients may wish to acheive benefits through confronting their core issues, changing their sense of the world, grieving for the dissolution of their marriages, facing the changes in their lives that accompany aging, or learning how to interact honestly and intimately with others. Psychotherapy, remember, is remarkably efficacious (see chap. 3), so this alternative would not be an indulgence of peoples' interest in "pop psychology"—rather it would involve real work with documented benefits.

A separation strategy involves significant risks. First, it separates physical and mental health, when it is known that there is a significant connection between mind and body. Second, psychotherapy, as the minority culture, could become "oppressed" and have little power to secure the resources needed to exist independently and would then be relegated to an inferior status.

A third strategy involves having two cultures stand side by side, as equals:

> The multicultural model promotes a pluralistic approach to understanding the relationship between two or more cultures. The model addresses the feasibility of cultures maintaining distinct identities while individuals from one culture work with those of other cultures to serve common national or economic needs.... Berry (1986) claimed that a multicultural society encourages all groups to (a) maintain and develop group identities, (b) develop other-group acceptance and tolerance, (c) engage in intergroup contact and sharing, and (d) learn each other's language. (LaFromboise et al., 1993, p. 401).

Clearly, the multicultural strategy has many advantages for psychotherapy. According to this strategy, medicine and psychotherapy would come to value what each has to offer, to understand the similarities, and respect the differences. To put this strategy into practice, the medical institution would need to come to understand how psychotherapy works and that its benefits cannot be forced to conform to the medical model. Multiculturalism takes time, patience, understanding, and an honest examination of one's attitudes and values. At the present time, the dominant forces in psychotherapy and medicine do not seem eager to pursue a multicultural strategy.

Recommendation 11: Train Psychotherapists to Appreciate and Be Skilled in the Common Core Aspects of Psychotherapy.   The
Guidelines and Principles of Accreditation of the American Psychological Association for doctoral and internship training (APA, 2000) makes the following statement about how science and practice should be integrated:

Science and practice are not opposing poles; rather, together they equally contribute to excellence in training in professional psychology. Therefore, education and training in preparation for entry practice, and in preparation for advanced level practice in a substantive traditional or practice area as a psychologist should be based on the existing and evolving body of general knowledge and methods in the science and practice of psychology. This more general knowledge should be well integrated with the specific knowledge, skills, and attitudes that define an area of interest in professional psychology. The relative emphasis a particular program places on science and practice should be consistent with its training objectives. However, all programs should enable their students to understand the value of science for the practice of psychology and the value of practice for the science of psychology, recognizing that the value of science for the practice of psychology requires attention to the empirical basis for all methods involved in psychological practice.

The implication of this statement, taken in the context of the evidence presented in this book, is that the emphasis in training should be placed on core therapeutic skills, including empathic listening and responding, developing a working alliance, working through one's own issues, understanding and conceptualizing interpersonal and intrapsychic dynamics, and learning to be self-reflective about one's work. As students acquire these skills, they should add expertise in particular approaches—this expertise includes mastery of the theory as well as the techniques of various approaches.

Although there is no scientific evidence that training should place emphasis on ESTs, the Guidelines and Principles of Accreditation prescribe competencies in ESTs. For example, the Guidelines and Principles for internship sites states that "all interns [should] demonstrate an intermediate to advanced knowledge of professional skills, abilities, proficiencies, competencies, and knowledge in the area of theories and methods of ... effective intervention (*including empirically supported treatments*)." Although learning an EST is not contraindicated, there is no evidence that trainees should learn an EST over another legitimate treatment. Some students are more attracted to some approaches to therapy and will be better therapists practicing those approaches than they would be practicing an approach dictated by a training program. Detrimental is the practice of training therapists by having them learn a series of ESTs, totally ignoring the acquisition of the core therapeutic skills that form the basis of therapy and therapeutic effect. Many psychotherapy trainees prefer to learn a series of ESTs because they wish to avoid the frightening prospect of being present with a client and examining themselves and their interpersonal qualities.

CONCLUSION

Critics of psychotherapy as a treatment modality have cited the lack of specificity as undermining the scientific basis of the endeavor. Donald F.

Klein, a proponent of psychopharmacological treatments, summarized the evidence against specificity for treatments of depression:

> [The results of the NIMH study and other studies] are inexplicable on the basis of the therapeutic action theories propounded by the creators of IPT and CBT. However, they are entirely compatible with the hypothesis (championed by Jerome Frank; see Frank & Frank, 1991) that psychotherapies are not doing anything specific: rather, they are nonspecifically beneficial to the final common pathway of demoralization, to the degree they are effective at all. (Klein, 1996, p. 82)

To Klein, the lack of specificity of psychotherapy was sufficiently damning to advocate the use of pharmacological agents: "The bottom line is that if the Food and Drug Administration (FDA) was responsible for the evaluation of psychotherapy, then no current psychotherapy would be approvable, whereas particular medications are clearly approvable" (p. 211). Robyn M. Dawes, an eminent psychologist and statistician, took a similar tack in his book *House of Cards: Psychology and Psychotherapy Built on Myth*. The thesis of his book is that psychotherapy does not work as proposed and therefore is a myth:

> The most defensible answer to the question of why therapy works is, We don't know. We should do research to find out, and indeed many people are devoting careers to just such research. (p. 62)

To Dawes, the type of research necessary is the medical model clinical trials that can confirm the specificity of treatments. That treatments work through common pathways is anathema to clinical scientists inculcated in the medical model.

Psychotherapy is indeed effective, but not in the manner one would expect from a medical model conceptualization. Contrary to Dawes' conclusion, *We do know why psychotherapy works*. The evidence presented in this book demonstrates that the contextual model of psychotherapy explains the benefits of psychotherapy.

As clients involved in psychotherapy make meaning of their lives, one should be reminded that the history of psychotherapy has indeed been brief. In many Western cultures, psychotherapy is valued as a helping modality, one that can reduce symptoms, improve the quality of life, and give meaning to one's actions. Perhaps, as Jerome Frank has intimated, psychotherapy is indeed a myth, created by Freud and maintained by peoples' belief in the endeavor. In any event, it is a valuable myth and one that should be revered, cherished, and nourished—and not folded into the field of medicine, where it will be suffocated.

References

Abelson, R. P. (1995). *Statistics as principled argument*. Hillsdale, NJ: Lawrence Erlbaum Associates.

Abramowitz, J. S. (1996). Variants of exposure and response prevention in the treatment of obsessive–compulsive disorder: A meta-analysis. *Behavior Therapy, 27,* 583–600.

Abramowitz, J. S. (1997). Effectiveness of psychological and pharmacological treatments for obsessive–compulsive disorder: A quantitative review. *Journal of Consulting and Clinical Psychology, 65,* 44–52.

Adams, V. (1979, July 10). Consensus is reached: Psychotherapy works. *New York Times,* p. C1.

Ahn, H., & Wampold, B. E. (in press). Where oh where are the specific ingredients?: A meta-analysis of component studies in counseling and psychotherapy. *Journal of Counseling Psychology.*

American Psychiatric Association. (1994). *Diagnostic and statistical manual of mental disorders* (4th ed.). Washington, D.C.: American Psychiatric Association.

American Psychological Association. (2000). *Guidelines and principles for accreditation of programs in professional psychology* [On-line]. Available: http://www.apa.org/ed/gp2000.html

Andrews, G., & Harvey, R. (1981). Does psychotherapy benefit neurotic patients? A reanalysis of the Smith, Glass, & Miller data. *Archives of General Psychiatry, 38,* 1203–1208.

Antonuccio, D. O., Thomas, M., & Danton, W. G. (1997). A cost-effectiveness analysis of cognitive behavior therapy and fluoxetine (Prozac) in the treatment of depression. *Behavior Therapy, 28,* 187–210.

Appelbaum, K. A., Blanchard, E. B., Nicholson, N. L., Radnitz, C., Kirsch, C., Michultka, D., Attanasio, V., Andrasik, F., & Dentinger, M. P. (1990). *Behavior Therapy, 21,* 293–303.

Arkowitz, H. (1992). Integrative theories of therapy. In H. J. Freudenberger, J. W. Kessler, S. B. Messer, D. R. Petersen, H. H. Strupp, & P. L. Wachtel (Eds.), *A history of psychotherapy: A century of change* (pp. 261–303). Washington, DC: American Psychological Association.

Astor, M. (1996). Including the body in couple therapy: Bioenergetic analysis. *The Family Journal: Counseling and Therapy for Couples and Families, 4,* 257–261.

Atkinson, D. R., Thompson, C. E., & Grant, S. K. (1993). A three-dimensional model for counseling racial/ethnic minorities. *The Counseling Psychologist, 21,* 257–277.

Auerbach, A. (1963). An application of Strupp's method of content analysis of psychotherapy. *Psychiatry, 26,* 137–146.

Bachelor, A., & Horvath, A. (1999). The therapeutic relationship In M. A. Hubble, B. L. Duncan, & S. D. Miller, (Eds.), *The heart and soul of change: What works in therapy* (pp. 133-178).Washington, DC: American Psychological Association.

Barber, J. P., Crits-Christoph, P., & Luborsky, L. (1996). Effects of therapist adherence and competence on patient outcome in brief dynamic therapy. *Journal of Consulting and Clinical Psychology, 64,* 619–622.

Barber, J. P., & Muenz, L. R. (1996). The role of avoidance and obsessiveness in matching patients to cognitive and interpersonal psychotherapy: Empirical findings from the treatment for depression collaborative research program. *Journal of Consulting and Clinical Psychology, 5,* 951–958.

Barcikowski, R. S. (1981). Statistical power with group means as the unit of analysis. *Journal of Educational Statistics, 6,* 267–285.

Barker, S. L., Funk, S. C., & Houston, B. K. (1988). Psychological treatment versus nonspecific factors: A meta-analysis of conditions that engender comparable expectations for improvement. *Clinical Psychology Review, 8,* 579–594.

Barlow, D. H., Rapee, R. M., & Brown, T. A. (1992). Behavioral treatment of generalized anxiety disorder. *Behavior Therapy, 23,* 551–570.

Baron, R. M., & Kenny, D. A. (1986). The moderator–mediator distinction in social psychological research: Conceptual, strategic, and statistical considerations. *Journal of Personality and Social Psychology, 51,* 1173–1182.

Baucom, D. H., Sayers, S. L., & Sher, T. G. (1990). Supplementing behavioral marital therapy with cognitive restructuring and emotional expressiveness training: An outcome investigation. *Journal of Consulting and Clinical Psychology, 58,* 636–645.

Baucom, D. H., Shoham, V., Mueser, K. T., Daiuto, A. D., & Stickle, T. R. (1998). Empirically supported couple and family interventions for marital distress and adult mental health problems. *Journal of Consulting and Clinical Psychology, 66,* 53–88.

Baxter, L. R., Schwartz, J. M., Bergman, K. S., Szuba, M. P., Guze, B. H., Mazziotta, J. C., Alazraki, A., Selin, C. E., Ferng, H., Munford, P., & Phelps, M. E. (1992). Caudate glucose metabolic rate changes with both drug and behavior therapy for obsessive–compulsive disorder. *Archives of General Psychiatry, 49,* 681–689.

Beck, A. T., Rush, A. J., Shaw, B. F., & Emery, G. (1979). *Cognitive therapy of depression.* New York: Guilford.

Beck, A. T., Ward, C., Mendelson, M., & Erbaugh, J. (1961). An inventory for measuring depression. *Archives of General Psychiatry, 6,* 561–571.

Bergin, A. E. (1971). The evaluation of therapeutic outcomes. In A. E. Bergin & S. L. Garfield (Eds.), *Handbook of psychotherapy and behavior change* (pp. 217–270). New York: Wiley.

Bergin, A. E., & Lambert, M. J. (1978). The evaluation of therapeutic outcomes. In S. L. Garfield & A. E. Bergin (Eds.), *Handbook of psychotherapy and behavior change: An empirical analysis* (2nd ed., pp. 139–190). New York: Wiley.

Berman, J. S., Miller, C., & Massman, P. J. (1985). Cognitive therapy versus systematic desensitization: Is one treatment superior? *Psychological Bulletin, 97,* 451–461.

Beutler, L. E., & Baker, M. (1998). The movement toward empirical validation. In K. S. Dobson & K. D. Craig (Eds.), *Empirically supported therapies: Best practice in professional psychology* (pp. 43–65). Thousand Oaks, CA: Sage.

Beutler, L. E., & Clarkin, J. (1990). *Differential treatment selection: Toward targeted therapeutic interventions.* New York: Brunner/Mazel.

Beutler, L. E., Engle, D., Mohr, D., Daldrup, R. J., Bergan, J., Meredith, K., & Merry, W. (1991). Predictors of differential response to cognitive, experiential, and self-directed psychotherapeutic procedures. *Journal of Consulting and Clinical Psychology, 39,* 333–340.

Beutler, L. E., Machado, P., & Neufeld, S. (1994). Therapist variables. In A. E. Bergin & S. L. Garfield (Eds.), *Handbook of psychotherapy and behavior change* (4th ed., pp. 229–269). New York: Wiley.

Beutler, L. E., Mohr, D. C., Grawe, K., Engle, D., & MacDonald, R. (1991). Looking for differential treatment effects: Cross-cultural predictors of differential psychotherapy efficacy. *Journal of Psychotherapy Integration, 1,* 121–141.

Binder, J. L. (1993). Observations on the training of therapists in time-limited dynamic psychotherapy. *Psychotherapy, 30,* 592–598.

Blanchard, E. B., Appelbaum, K. A., Radnitz, C. L., Michultka, D., Morrill, B., Kirsch, C., Hillhouse, J., Evans, D. D., Guarnieri, P., Attanasio, V., Andrasik, F., Jaccard, J., & Dentinger, M. P. (1990). Placebo-controlled evaluation of abbreviated progressive muscle relaxation and of relaxation combined with cognitive therapy in the treatment of tension headache. *Journal of Consulting and Clinical Psychology, 58,* 210–215.

Blatt, S. J., Sanislow, C. A., Zuroff, D. C., & Pilkonis, P. A. (1996). Characteristics of effective therapists: Further analyses of data from the National Institute of Mental Health treatment of depression collaborative research program. *Journal of Consulting and Clinical Psychology, 64,* 1276–1284.

Blatt, S. J., Zuroff, D. C., Quinlan, D. M., & Pilkonis, P. A. (1996). Interpersonal factors in brief treatment of depression: Further analysis of the National Institute of Mental Health treatment of depression collaborative research program. *Journal of Consulting and Clinical Psychology, 64,* 162–171.

Borkovec, T. D. (1990). Control groups and comparison groups in psychotherapy outcome research. *National Institute on Drug Abuse Research Monograph, 104,* 50–65.

Borkovec, T. D., & Castonguay, L. G. (1998). What is the scientific meaning of empirically supported therapy? *Journal of Consulting and Clinical Psychology, 66,* 136–142.

Borkovec, T. D., & Costello, E. (1993). Efficacy of applied relaxation and cognitive-behavioral therapy in the treatment of generalized anxiety disorder. *Journal of Consulting and Clinical Psychology, 61,* 611–619.

Bowers, T. G., & Clum, G. A. (1988). Relative contributions of specific and nonspecific treatment effects: Meta-analysis of placebo-controlled behavior therapy research. *Psychological Bulletin, 103,* 315–323.

Brickman, P., Rabinowitz, V. C., Karuza, J., Jr., Coates, D., Cohn, E., & Kidder, L. (1982). Models of helping and coping. *American Psychologist, 37,* 368–384.

Bright, J. I., Baker, K. D., & Neimeyer, R. A. (1999). Professional and paraprofessional treatments for depression: A comparison of cognitive–behavioral and mutual support for interventions. *Journal of Consulting and Clinical Psychology, 67,* 491–501.

Brock, T. C., Green, M. C., Reich, D. A., & Evans, L. M. (1996). The Consumer Reports study of psychotherapy: Invalid is invalid. *American Psychologist, 51,* 1083.

Brody, N. (1980). *Placebos and the philosophy of medicine: Clinical, conceptual, and ethical issues.* Chicago: The University of Chicago Press.

Brunink, S., & Schroeder, H. (1979). Verbal therapeutic behavior of expert psychoanalytic oriented, Gestalt, and behavior therapists. *Journal of Consulting and Clinical Psychology, 47,* 567–574.

Burns, D. D., & Nolen-Hoeksema, S. (1992). Therapeutic empathy and recovery from depression in cognitive–behavioral therapy: A structural equation model. *Journal of Consulting and Clinical Psychology, 60,* 441–449.

Butler, G., Fennell, M., Robson, P., & Gelder, M. (1991). Comparison of behavior therapy and cognitive behavior therapy in the treatment of generalized anxiety disorder. *Journal of Consulting and Clinical Psychology, 59,* 137–175.

Calhoun, K. S., Moras, K., Pilkonis, P. A., & Rehm, L. (1998). Empirically supported treatments: Implications for training. *Journal of Consulting and Clinical Psychology, 66,* 151–161.

Campbell, D. T., & Kenny, D. A. (1999). *A primer on regression artifacts.* New York: Guilford.

Carroll, K. M., Rounsaville, B. J., & Nich, C. (1994). Blind man's bluff: Effectiveness and significance of psychotherapy and pharmacotherapy blinding procedures in a clinical trial. *Journal of Consulting and Clinical Psychology, 62,* 276–280.

Castonguay, L. G. (1993). "Common factors" and "nonspecific variables": Clarification of the two concepts and recommendations for research. *Journal of Psychotherapy Integration, 3,* 267–286.

Castonguay, L. G., Goldfried, M. R., Wiser, S., Raue, P. J., & Hayes, A. M. (1996). Predicting the effect of cognitive therapy for depression: A study of unique and common factors. *Journal of Consulting and Clinical Psychology, 64,* 497–504.

Chambless, D. L., Baker, M. J., Baucom, D. H., Beutler, L. E., Calhoun, K. S., Daiuto, A., DeRubeis, R., Detweiler, J., Haaga, D. A. F., Johnson, S. B., McCurry, S., Mueser, K. T., Pope, K. S., Sanderson, W. C., Shoham, V., Stickle, T., Williams, D. A., & Woody, S. R. (1998). Update on empirically validated therapies, II. *The Clinical Psychologist, 51,* 3–16.

Chambless, D. L., & Gillis, M. M. (1993). Cognitive therapy of anxiety disorders. *Journal of Consulting and Clinical Psychology, 61,* 248–260.

Chambless, D. L., & Hollon, S. D. (1998). Defining empirically supported therapies. *Journal of Consulting and Clinical Psychology, 66,* 7–18.

Chambless, D. L., Sanderson, W. C., Shoham, V., Johnson, S. B., Pope, K. S., Crits-Christoph, P., Baker, M., Johnson, B., Woody, S. R., Sue, S., Beutler, L., Williams, D. A., & McCurry, S. (1996). An update on empirically validated therapies. *The Clinical Psychologist, 49*(2), 5–18.

Clark, D. M., Salkovskis, P. M., Hackmann, A., Middleton, H., Anastasiades, P., & Gelder, M. (1994). A comparison of cognitive therapy, applied relaxation, and imipramine in the treatment of panic disorder. *British Journal of Psychiatry, 164,* 759–769.

Clum, G. A., Clum, G. A., & Surls, R. (1993). A meta-analysis of treatments for panic disorder. *Journal of Consulting and Clinical Psychology, 61,* 317–326.

Cohen, J. (1988). *Statistical power analysis for the behavioral sciences* (2nd ed.). Hillsdale, NJ: Lawrence Erlbaum Associates.

Compas, B. E., Haaga, D. A. F., Keefe, F. J., Leitenberg, H., & Williams, D. A. (1998). Sampling of empirically supported psychological treatments from health psychology: Smoking, chronic pain, cancer, and bulimia nervosa. *Journal of Consulting and Clinical Psychology, 66,* 89–112.

Cook, T. D., & Campbell, D. T. (1979). *Quasi-experimentation: Design and analysis for field settings.* Chicago: Rand McNally.

Cooper, H., & Hedges, L. V. (Eds.). (1994). *The handbook of research synthesis.* New York: Russell Sage Foundation.

Critelli, J. W., & Neumann, K. F. (1984). The placebo: Conceptual analysis of a construct in transition. *American Psychologist, 39,* 32–39.

Crits-Christoph, P. (1997). Limitations of the dodo bird verdict and the role of clinical trials in psychotherapy research: Comment on Wampold et al. (1997). *Psychological Bulletin, 122.* 216–220.

Crits-Christoph, P., Baranackie, K., Kurcias, J. S., Carroll, K., Luborsky, L., McLellan, T., Woody, G., Thompson, L., Gallagier, D., & Zitrin, C. (1991). Meta-analysis of therapist effects in psychotherapy outcome studies. *Psychotherapy Research, 1,* 81–91.

Crits-Christoph, P., & Mintz, J. (1991). Implications of therapist effects for the design and analysis of comparative studies of psychotherapies. *Journal of Consulting and Clinical Psychology, 59,* 20–26.

Cushman, P. (1992). Psychotherapy to 1992: A history situated interpretation. In D. K. Freedman (Ed.), *History of psychotherapy: A century of change* (pp. 21–64). Washington, DC: American Psychological Association.

Dadds, M. R., & McHugh, T. A. (1992). Social support and treatment outcome in behavioral family therapy for child conduct problems. *Journal of Consulting and Clinical Psychology, 60,* 252–259.

Dance, K. A., & Neufeld, R. W. J. (1988). Aptitude–treatment interaction research in the clinic setting: A review of attempts to dispel the "patient uniformity" myth. *Psychological Bulletin, 104,* 192–213.

Davison, G. C. (1998). Being bolder with the Boulder Model: The challenge of education and training in empirically supported treatments. *Journal of Consulting and Clinical Psychology, 66,* 163–167.

Dawes, R. M. (1994). *House of cards: Psychology and psychotherapy built on myth.* New York: Free Press.

Deffenbacher, J. L., Oetting, E. R., & DiGiuseppe, R. (in press). Principles of empirically supported interventions applied to anger management. *The Counseling Psychologist.*

Deffenbacher, J. L., & Stark, R. S. (1992). Relaxation and cognitive-relaxation treatments of general anger. *Journal of Counseling Psychology, 39,* 158–167.

DeRubeis, R. J., & Crits-Christoph, P. (1998). Empirically supported individual and group psychological treatments for mental disorders. *Journal of Consulting and Clinical Psychology, 66,* 37–52.

DeRubeis, R. J., & Feeley, M. (1990). Determinants of change in cognitive therapy for depression. *Cognitive Therapy and Research, 14,* 469–482.

Dobson, K. S. (1989). A meta-analysis of the efficacy of cognitive therapy for depression. *Journal of Consulting and Clinical Psychology, 57,* 414–419.

Dollard, J., & Miller, N. E. (1950). *Personality and psychotherapy: An analysis in terms of learning, thinking, and culture.* New York: McGraw-Hill.

Durham, R. C., Murphy, T., Allan, T., Richard, K., Treliving, L. R., & Fenton, G. W. (1994). Cognitive therapy, analytic therapy and anxiety management training for generalised anxiety disorder. *British Journal of Psychiatry, 165,* 315–323.

Dush, D. M., Hirt, M. L., & Schroeder, H. (1983). Self-statement modification with adults: A meta-analysis. *Psychological Bulletin, 94,* 408–422.

Elkin, I. (1994). The NIMH Treatment of Depression Collaborative Research Program: Where we began and where we are. In A. E. Bergin & S. L. Garfield (Eds.), *Handbook of psychotherapy and behavior change* (4th ed., pp. 114–139). New York: Wiley.

Elkin, I., Gibbons, R. D., Shea, M. T., & Shaw, B. F. (1996). Science is not a trial (but it can sometimes be a tribulation). *Journal of Consulting and Clinical Psychology, 64,* 92–103.

Elkin, I., Parloff, M. B., Hadley, S. W., & Autry, J. H. (1985). NIMH Treatment of Depression Collaborative Research Program: Background and research plan. *Archives of General Psychiatry, 42,* 305–316.

Elkin, I., Shea, T., Watkins, J. T., Imber, S. D., Sotsky, S. M., Collins, J. F., Glass, D. R., Pilkonis, P. A., Leber, W. R., Docherty, J. P., Fiester, S. J., & Parloff, M. B. (1989). National Institute of Mental Health treatment of depression collaborative research program: General effectiveness of treatments. *Archives of General Psychiatry, 46,* 971–982.

Ellis, A. (1957). Outcome of employing three techniques of psychotherapy. *Journal of Clinical Psychology, 13,* 344–350.

Ellis, A. (1993). Reflections on rational-emotive therapy. *Journal of Consulting and Clinical Psychology, 61,* 199–201.

Emmelkamp, P. M. G. (1994). Behavior therapy with adults. In A. E. Bergin & S. L. Garfield (Eds.), *Handbook of psychotherapy and behavior change* (4th ed., pp. 379–427). New York: Wiley.

Eugster, S. L., & Wampold, B. E. (1996). Systematic effects of participant role on the evaluation of the psychotherapy session. *Journal of Consulting and Clinical Psychology, 64,* 1020–1028.

Eysenck, H. J. (1952). The effects of psychotherapy: An evaluation. *Journal of Consulting Psychology, 16,* 319–324.

Eysenck, H. J. (1954). A reply to Luborsky's note. *British Journal of Psychology, 45,* 132–133.

Eysenck, H. J. (1961). The effects of psychotherapy. In H. J. Eysenck (Ed.), *Handbook of abnormal psychology* (pp. 697–725). New York: Basic Books.

Eysenck, H. J. (1966). *The effects of psychotherapy.* New York: International science press.

Eysenck, H. J. (1978). An exercise in meta-silliness. *American Psychologist, 33,* 517.

Eysenck, H. J. (1984). Meta-analysis: An abuse of research integration. *The Journal of Special Education, 18,* 41–59.

Feeley, M., DeRubeis, R. J., & Gelfand, L. A. (1999). The temporal relation of adherence and alliance to symptom change in cognitive therapy for depression. *Journal of Consulting and Clinical Psychology, 67,* 578–582.

Feifel, H., & Eells, J. (1963). Patient and therapists assess the same psychotherapy. *Journal of Consulting Psychology, 27,* 310–318.

Feske, U., & Goldstein, A. J. (1997). Eye movement desensitization and reprocessing treatment for panic disorder: A controlled outcome and partial dismantling study. *Journal Consulting and Clinical Psychology, 65,* 1026–1035.

Fisher, S., & Greenberg, R. P. (1997). The curse of the placebo: Fanciful pursuit of a pure biological therapy. In S. Fisher & R. P. Greenberg (Eds.), *From placebo to panacea: Putting psychiatric drugs to the test* (pp. 3–56). New York: Wiley.

Foa, E. B., Rothbaum, B. O., Riggs, D. S., & Murdock, T. B. (1991). Treatment of post-traumatic stress disorder in rape victims: A comparison between cognitive–behavioral procedures and counseling. *Journal of Consulting and Clinical Psychology, 59,* 715–723.

Follette, W. C., & Houts, A. C. (1996). Models of scientific progress and the role of theory in taxonomy development: A case study of the DSM. *Journal of Consulting and Clinical Psychology, 64,* 1120–1132.

Frank, J. D., & Frank, J. B. (1991). *Persuasion and healing: A comparative study of psychotherapy* (3rd ed.). Baltimore: Johns Hopkins University Press.

Free, M. L., & Oei, T. P. (1989). Biological and psychological processes in the treatment and maintenance of depression. *Clinical Psychology Review, 9,* 653–688.

Gaffan, E. A., Tsaousis, I., & Kemp-Wheeler, S. M. (1995). Researcher allegiance and meta-analysis: The case of cognitive therapy for depression. *Journal of Consulting and Clinical Psychology, 63,* 966–980.

Garfield, S. L. (1992). Eclectic psychotherapy: A common factors approach. In J. C. Norcross & M. R. Goldfried (Eds.), *Handbook of psychotherapy integration* (pp. 169–201). New York: Basic Books.

Garfield, S. L. (1994). Research on client variables in psychotherapy. In A. E. Bergin & S. L. Garfield (Eds.), *Handbook of psychotherapy and behavior change* (4th ed., pp. 191–228). New York: Wiley.

Garfield, S. L. (1995). *Psychotherapy: An eclectic–integrative approach.* New York: Wiley & Sons.

Garfield, S. L. (1998). Some comments on empirically supported treatments. *Journal of Consulting and Clinical Psychology, 66,* 121–125.

Garfield, S. L., & Bergin, A. E. (1994). Introduction and historical overview. In A. E. Bergin & S. L. Garfield (Eds.), *Handbook of psychotherapy and behavior change* (4th ed., pp. 3–18). New York: Wiley.

Gaston, L. (1990). The concept of the alliance and its role in psychotherapy: Theoretical and empirical considerations. *Psychotherapy, 27,* 143–153.

Gelso, C. J. & Carter, J. A. (1985). The relationship in counseling and psychotherapy: Components, consequences, and theoretical antecedents. *The Counseling Psychologist, 13,* 155–243.

Glass, G. V (1976). Primary, secondary, and meta-analysis of research. *Educational Researcher, 5,* 3–8.

Gloaguen, V., Cottraux, J., Cucherat, M., & Blackburn, I. (1998). A meta-analysis of the effects of cognitive therapy in depressed patients. *Journal of Affective Disorders, 49,* 59–72.

Goldfried, M. R. (1980). Toward the delineation of therapeutic change principles. *American Psychologist, 35,* 9911–999.

Goldfried, M. R., Castonguay, L. G., Hayes, A. M., Drozd, J. F., & Shapiro, D. A. (1997). A comparative analysis of the therapeutic focus in cognitive–behavioral and psychodynamic–interpersonal sessions. *Journal of Consulting and Clinical Psychology, 65,* 740–748.

Goldfried, M. R., & Wolfe, B. E. (1996). Psychotherapy practice and research: Repairing a strained alliance. *Journal of Consulting and Clinical Psychology, 51,* 1007–1016.

Goldman, A., & Greenberg, L. (1992). Comparison of integrated systemic and emotionally focused approaches to couples therapy. *Journal of Consulting and Clinical Psychology, 60,* 962–969.

Greenberg, L. S., Elliott, R. K., & Lietaer, G. (1994). Research on experiential psychotherapies. In A. E. Bergin & S. L. Garfield (Eds.), *Handbook of psychotherapy and behavior change* (4th ed., pp. 509–531). New York: Wiley.

Grencavage, L. M., & Norcross, J. C. (1990). Where are the commonalities among the therapeutic common factors? *Professional Psychology: Research and Practice, 21,* 372–378.

Grissom, R. J. (1996). The magical number .7 +- .2: Meta-meta-analysis of the probability of superior outcome in comparisons involving therapy, placebo, and control. *Journal of Consulting and Clinical Psychology, 64,* 973–982.

Grünbaum, A. (1981). The placebo concept. *Behaviour Research and Therapy, 19,* 157–167.

Halford, W. K., Sanders, M. R., & Behrens, B. C. (1993). A comparison of the generalization of behavioral martial therapy and enhanced behavioral marital therapy. *Journal of Consulting and Clinical Psychology, 61,* 51–60.

Hanna, F. J., & Puhakka, K. (1991). When psychotherapy works: Pinpointing an element of change. *Psychotherapy, 28,* 598–607.

Hanna, F. J., & Ritchie, M. H. (1995). Seeking the active ingredients of psychotherapeutic change: Within and outside the context of therapy. *Professional Psychology: Research and Practice, 26,* 176–183.

Hays, W. L. (1988). *Statistics.* New York: Holt, Rinehart & Winston.

Hedges, L. V., & Olkin, I. (1985). *Statistical methods for meta-analysis.* San Diego, CA: Academic Press.

Henry, W. P. (1998). Science, politics, and the politics of science: The use and misuse of empirically validated treatments. *Psychotherapy Research, 8,* 126–140.

Henry, W. P., Schacht, T. E., Strupp, H. H., Butler, S. F., & Binder, J. (1993). Effects of training in time-limited dynamic psychotherapy: Mediators of therapists' responses to training. *Journal of Consulting and Clinical Psychology, 61,* 441–447.

Henry, W. P., Strupp, H. H., Butler, S. F., Schacht, T. E., & Binder, J. (1993). Effects of training in time-limited psychotherapy: Changes in therapist behavior. *Journal of Consulting and Clinical Psychology, 61,* 434–440.

Henry, W. P., Strupp, H. H., Schacht, T. E., & Gaston, L. (1994). Psychodynamic approahces. In A. E. Bergin & S. L. Garfield (Eds.), *Handbook of psychotherapy and behavior change* (4th ed., pp. 467–508). New York: Wiley.

Heppner, P. P., & Claiborn, C. D. (1989). Social influence research in counseling: A review and critique. *Journal of Counseling Psychology, 36,* 365–387.

Heppner, P. P., Kivlighan, D. M., Jr., & Wampold, B. E. (1999). *Research design in counseling* (2nd ed.). Belmont, CA: Brooks/Cole.

Hill, C. E., O'Grady, K. E., & Elkin, I. (1992). Applying the Collaborative Study Psychotherapy Rating Scale to rate therapist adherence in cognitive–behavior therapy, interpersonal therapy, and clinical management. *Journal of Consulting and Clinical Psychology, 60,* 73–79.

Hoehn-Saric, R., Frank, J. D., Imber, S. D., Nash, E. H., Stone, A. R., & Battle, C. C. (1964). Systematic prepreparation of patients for short-term psychotherapy–II: Relation to characteristics of patient, therapist and the psychotherapeutic process. *Journal of Nervous and Mental Disorders, 140,* 374–383.

Hollon, S. D., & Beck, A. T. (1994). Cognitive and cognitive–behavioral therapies. In A. E. Bergin & S. L. Garfield (Eds.), *Handbook of psychotherapy and behavior change* (pp. 428–466). New York: Wiley.

Hollon, S. D., DeRubeis, R. J., & Evans, M. D. (1987). Causal mediation of change in treatment for depression: Discriminating between nonspecificity and noncausality. *Psychological Bulletin, 102,* 139–149.

Holloway, E. L., & Neufeld, S. A. (1995). Supervision: Its contributions to treatment efficacy. *Journal of Consulting and Clinical Psychology, 63,* 207–213.

Hope, D. A., Heimberg, R. G., & Bruch, M. A. (1995). Dismantling cognitive–behavioural group therapy for social phobia. *Behavioral Research and Therapy, 33,* 637–650.

Horvath, A. O., & Luborsky, L. (1993). The role of the therapeutic alliance in psychotherapy. *Journal of Consulting and Clinical Psychology, 61,* 561–573.

Horvath, A. O., & Symonds, B. D. (1991). Relation between working alliance and outcome in psychotherapy: A meta-analysis. *Journal of Counseling Psychology, 38,* 139–149.

Horvath, P. (1988). Placebos and common factors in two decades of psychotherapy research. *Psychological Bulletin, 104,* 214–225.

Howard, K. I., Krause, M. S., & Orlinsky, D. E. (1986). The attrition dilemma: Toward a new strategy for psychotherapy research. *Journal of Consulting and Clinical Psychology, 54,* 106–110.

Howard, K. I., Krause, M. S., Saunders, S. M., & Kopta, S. M. (1997). Trials and tribulations in the meta-analysis of treatment differences: Comment on Wampold et al. (1997). *Psychological Bulletin, 122,* 221–225.

Hoyt, W. T. (2000). Rater bias in psychological research: When is it a problem and what can we do about it? *Psychological Methods, 5,* 64–86.

Hoyt, W. T., & Kerns, M. D. (1999). Magnitude and moderators of bias in observer ratings: A meta-analysis. *Psychological Methods, 4,* 403–424.

Hubble, M. A., Duncan, B. L., & Miller, S. D. (Eds.). (1999). *The heart & soul of change: What works in therapy.* Washington, DC: American Psychological Association.

Hunt, E. (1996). Errors in Seligman's "The effectiveness of psychotherapy: The Consumer Reports study." *American Psychologist, 51,* 1082.

Hunt, M. (1997). *How science takes stock: The story of meta-analysis.* New York: Russell Sage Foundation.

Hunter, J. E., & Schmidt, F. L. (1990). *Methods of meta-analysis: Correcting error bias in research findings.* Newbury Park, CA: Sage.

Ilardi, S. S., & Craighead, W. E. (1994). The role of nonspecific factors in cognitive–behavior therapy for depression. *Clinical Psychology, 1,* 138–156.

Imber, S. D., Pilkonis, P. A., Sotsky, S. M., Elkin, I., Watkins, J. T., Collins, J. F., Shea, M. T., Leber, W. R., & Glass, D. R. (1990). Mode-specific effects among three treatments for depression. *Journal of Consulting and Clinical Psychology, 58,* 352–359.

Jacobson, N. S. (1991). Behavioral versus insight-oriented martial therapy: Labels can be misleading. *Journal of Consulting and Clinical Psychology, 59,* 142–145.

Jacobson, N. S., Dobson, K. S., Truax, P. A., Addis, M. E., Koerner, K., Gollan, J. K., Gortner, E., & Price, S. E. (1996). A component analysis of cognitive–behavioral treatment for depression. *Journal of Consulting and Clinical Psychology, 64,* 295–304.

Jacobson, N. S., & Hollon, S. D. (1996a). Cognitive–behavior therapy versus pharmacotherapy: Now that the jury's returned its verdict, it's time to present the rest of evidence. *Journal of Consulting and Clinical Psychology, 64,* 74–80.

Jacobson, N. S., & Hollon, S. D. (1996b). Prospects for future comparisons between drugs and psychotherapy: Lessons from the CBT-versus-pharmacotherapy exchange. *Journal of Consulting and Clinical Psychology, 64,* 104–108.

Jensen, J. P., & Bergin, A. E. (1990). The meaning of eclecticism: New survey and analysis of components. *Professional Psychology: Research and Practice, 21,* 124–130.

Jones, E. E., & Pulos, S. M. (1993). Comparing the process in psychodynamic and cognitive–behavioral therapies. *Journal of Consulting and Clinical Psychology, 61,* 306–316.

Kazdin, A. E. (1994). Methodology, design, and evaluation in psychotherapy research. In A. E. Bergin & S. L. Garfield (Eds.), *Handbook of psychotherapy and behavior change* (4th ed., pp. 19–71). New York: Wiley.

Kazdin, A. E. (1998). *Research design in clinical psychology* (3rd ed.). Boston: Allyn & Bacon.

Kazdin, A. E., & Bass, D. (1989). Power to detect differences between alternative treatments in comparative psychotherapy outcome research. *Journal of Consulting and Clinical Psychology, 57,* 138–147.

Kendall, P. C. (1998). Empirically supported psychological therapies. *Journal of Consulting and Clinical Psychology, 66,* 3–6.

Kenny, D. A., & Judd, C. M. (1986). Consequence of violating the independence assumption in analysis of variance. *Psychological Bulletin, 99,* 422–431.

Kiesler, D. J. (1994). Standardization of intervention: The tie that binds psychotherapy research and practice. In P. F. Talley, H. H. Strupp, & S. F. Butler (Eds.), *Psychotherapy research and practice: Bridging the gap* (pp. 143–153): Basic Books.

Kirk, R. E. (1995). *Experimental design: Procedures for the behavioral sciences* (3rd ed.). Pacific Grove, CA: Brooks/Cole.

Kirsch, I. (1985). Response expectancy as a determinant of experience and behavior. *American Psychologist, 40,* 1189–1202.

Klein, D. F. (1996). Preventing hung juries about therapy studies. *Journal of Consulting and Clinical Psychology, 64,* 81–87.

Kleinman, A., & Sung, L. H. (1979). Why do indigenous practitioners successfully heal? *Social Sciencs & Medicine, 13B,* 7–26.

Klerman, G. L., Weissman, M. M., Rounsaville, B. J., & Chevron, E. S. (1984). *Interpersonal psychotherapy of depression.* New York: Basic Books.

Kotkin, M., Daviet, C., & Gurin, J. (1996). The Consumer Reports mental health survey. *American Psychologist, 51,* 1080–1088.

Krupnick, J. L., Simmens, S., Moyer, J., Elkin, I., Watkins, J. T., & Pilkonis, P. A. (1996). The role of the therapeutic alliance in psychotherapy and pharmacotherapy outcome: Findings in the National Institute of Mental Health treatment of depression collaborative research program. *Journal of Consulting and Clinical Psychology, 64,* 532–539.

LaFromboise, T., Coleman, H. K. L., & Gerton, J. (1993). Psychological impact of biculturalsim: Evidence and theory. *Psychological Bulletin, 114,* 395–412.

Lambert, M. J. (1992). Psychotherapy outcome research: Implications for integrative and eclectic therapists. In J. C. Norcross & M. R. Goldfried (Eds.), *Handbook of psychotherapy integration* (pp. 94–129). New York: Basic Books.

Lambert, M. J., & Bergin, A. E. (1994). The effectiveness of psychotherapy. In A. E. Bergin & S. L. Garfield (Eds.), *Handbook of psychotherapy and behavior change* (4th ed., pp. 143–189). New York: Wiley.

Landman, J. T., & Dawes, R. M. (1982). Psychotherapy outcome: Smith and Glass' conclusions stand up under scrutiny. *American Psychologist, 37,* 504–516.

Lazarus, A. A. (1981). *The practice of multimodal therapy.* New York: McGraw-Hill.

Lipsey, M. W., & Wilson, D. B. (1993). The efficacy of psychological, educational, and behavioral treatment: Confirmation from meta-analysis. *American Psychologist, 48,* 1181–1209.

Loftus, E. F., & Pickrell, J. E. (1995). The formation of false memories. *Psychiatric Annals, 25,* 720–725.

Lohr, J. M., Kleinknecht, R. A., Tolin, D. F., & Barrett, R. H. (1995). The empirical status of the clinical application of eye movement desensitization and reprocessing. *Journal of Behavioral Therapy and Experimental Psychology, 26,* 285–302.

Luborsky, L. (1954). A note on Eysenck's article "The effect of psychotherapy: An evaluation." *British Journal of Psychology, 45,* 129–131.

Luborsky, L., Crits-Christoph, P., McLellan, A. T., Woody, G., Piper, W., Liberman, B., Imber, S., & Pilkonis, P. (1986). Do therapists vary much in their success? Findings from four outcome studies. *American Journal of Orthopsychiatry, 56,* 501–512.

Luborsky, L., & DeRubeis, R. J. (1984). The use of psychotherapy treatment manuals: A small revolution in psychotherapy research style. *Clinical Psychology Review, 4,* 5–14.

Luborsky, L., McLellan, A. T., Diguer, L., Woody, G., & Seligman, D. A. (1997). The psychotherapist matters: Comparison of outcomes across twenty-two therapists and seven patient samples. *Clinical Psychology: Science and Practice, 4,* 53–65.

Luborsky, L., McLellan, A. T., Woody, G., O'Brien, C. P., & Auerbach, A. (1985). Therapist success and is determinants. *Archives of General Psychiatry, 42,* 602–611.

Luborsky, L., Singer, B., & Luborsky, L. (1975). Comparative studies of psychotherapies: Is it true that "Everyone has won and all must have prizes?". *Archives of General Psychiatry, 32,* 995–1008.

Luborsky, L., Woody, G. E., McLellan, A. T., O'Brien, C. P., & Rosenzweig, J. (1982). Can independent judges recognize different psychotherapies? An experience with manual guided therapies. *Journal of Consulting and Clinical Psychology, 50,* 49–62.

Lyddon, W. J. (1989). Personal epistemology and preference for counseling. *Journal of Counseling Psychology, 36,* 423–429.

Lyddon, W. J. (1991). Epistemic style: Implications for cognitive psychotherapy. *Psychotherapy, 28,* 588–597.

Mahoney, M. J., & Gabriel, T. J. (1987). Psychotherapy and the cognitive sciences: An evolving alliance. *Journal of cognitive psychotherapy: An international quarterly, 1,* 39–59.

Mann, C. C. (1994). Can meta-analysis make policy? *Science, 266,* 960–962.

Markowitz, J. C., Klerman, G. L., Clougherty, K. F., Spielman, L. A., Jacobsberg, L. B., Fishman, B., Frances, A. J., Kocsis, J. H., & Perry, S. W. (1995). Individual psychotherapies for depressed HIV-positive patients. *American Journal of Psychiatry, 152,* 1504–1509.

Martin, D. J., Garske, J. P., & Davis, M. K. (2000). Relation of the therapeutic alliance with outcome and other variables: A meta-analytic review. *Journal of Consulting and Clinical Psychology, 68,* 438–450.

Mattick, R. P., Andrews, G., Hadsi-Pavlovick, D., & Christensen, H. (1990). Treatment of panic and agoraphobia: An integrative review. *The Journal of Nervous and Mental Disease, 9,* 567–576.

Maude-Griffin, P. M., Hohenstein, J. M., Humfleet, G. L., Reilly, P. M., Tusel, D. J., & Hall, S. M. (1998). Superior efficacy of cognitive behavioral therapy of urban crack cocaine abusers: Main and matching effects. *Journal of Consulting and Clinical Psychology, 66,* 832–837.

Maxwell, S. E., & Delaney, H. D. (1993). Bivariate median split and spurious statistical significance. *Psychological Bulletin, 113,* 181–190.

Mazzoni, G. A. L., Loftus, E. F., Seitz, A., & Lynn, S. J. (1999). Changing beliefs and memories through dream interpretation. *Applied cognitive psychology, 13,* 125–144.

Mazzoni, G. A. L., Lombardo, P., Malvagia, S., & Loftus, E. F. (1999). Dream interpretation and false beliefs. *Professional Psychology: Research and Practice, 30,* 45–50.

McKnight, D. L., Nelson-Gray, R. O., & Barnhill, J. (1992). Dexamethasone suppression test and response to cognitive therapy and antidepressant medication. *Behavior Therapy, 23,* 99–111.

Meichenbaum, D. (1986). Cognitive–behavior modification. In F. H. Kanfer & A. P. Goldstein (Eds.), *Helping people change: A textbook of methods* (3rd ed., pp. 346–380). New York: Pergamon Press.

Meltzoff, J., & Kornreich, M. (1970). *Research in psychotherapy.* Chicago: Adline.

Miller, R. C., & Berman, J. S. (1983). The efficacy of cognitive behavior therapies: A quantitative review of the research evidence. *Psychological Bulletin, 94,* 39–53.

Mintz, J., Drake, R., & Crits-Christoph, P. (1996). Efficacy and effectiveness of psychotherapy: Two paradigms, one science. *American Psychologist, 51,* 1084–1085.

Murphy, P. M., Cramer, D., & Lillie, F. J. (1984). The relationship between curative factors perceived by patients and their psychotherapy and treatment outcome: An exploratory study. *British Journal of Medical Psychology, 57,* 187–192.

Nicholas, M. K., Wilson, P. H.., & Goyen, J. (1991). Operant–behavioural and cognitive–behavioural treatment for chronic low back pain. *Behavioural Research and Therapy, 29,* 225–238.

Norcross, J. C., & Newman, C. F. (1992). Psychotherapy integration: Setting the context. In J. C. Norcross & M. R. Goldfried (Eds.), *Handbook of psychotherapy integration* (pp. 3–45). New York: Basic Books.

Norcross, J. C., Prochaska, J. O., & Farber, J. A. (1993). Psychologists conducting psychotherapy: New findings and historical comparisons on the psychotherapy division membership. *Psychotherapy, 30,* 692–697.

Oei, T. P. S., & Free, M. L. (1995). Do cognitive behaviour therapies validate cognitive models of mood disorders? A review of the empirical evidence. *International Journal of Psychology, 30,* 145–179.

Öst, L-G., Fellenius, J., & Sterner, U. (1991). Applied tension, exposure in vivo, and tension-only in the treatment of blood phobia. *Behavioural Research and Therapy, 29,* 561–574.

Parloff, M. B. (1986). Frank's "common elements" in psychotherapy: Nonspecific factors and placebos. *American Journal of Orthopsychiatry, 56,* 521–529.

Paul, G. L. (1969). Behavior modification research: Design and tactics. In C. M. Franks (Ed.), *Behavior therapy: Appraisal and status* (pp. 29–62). New York: McGraw-Hill.

Persons, J. B., Burns, D. D., & Perloff, J. M. (1988). Predictors of dropout and outcome in cognitive therapy for depression in a private practice setting. *Cognitive Therapy and Research, 12,* 557–575.

Persons, J. B., & Silberschatz, G. (1998). Are results of randomized controlled trials useful to psychotherapists? *Journal of Consulting and Clinical Psychology, 66,* 126–135.

Phillips, E. L. (1957). *Psychotherapy: A modern theory and practice.* London: Staples.

Pilkonis, P. A., Imber, S. D., Lewis, P., & Rubinsky, P. (1984). A comparative outcome study of individual, group, and conjoint psychotherapy. *Archives of General Psychiatry, 41,* 431–437.

Piper, W. E., Debbane, E. G., Bienvenu, J. P., & Garant, J. (1984). A comparative study of four forms of psychotherapy. *Journal of Consulting and Clinical Psychology, 52,* 268–279.

Porter, A. C., & Raudenbush, S. W. (1987). Analysis of covariance: Its model and use in psychological research. *Journal of Counseling Psychology, 34,* 383–392.

Porzelius, L. K., Houston, C., Smith, M., Arfken, C., & Fisher, E. Jr. (1995). Comparison of a standard behavioral weight loss treatment and a binge eating loss treatment. *Behavior Therapy, 26,*119–134.

Project MATCH Research Group. (1997). Matching alcoholism treatments to client heterogeneity: Project MATCH Posttreatment drinking outcomes. *Journal of Studies on Alcohol, 58*(1), 7–29.

Project MATCH Research Group. (1998). Therapist effects in three treatments for alcohol problems. *Psychotherapy Research, 8,* 455–474.

Propst, L. R., Ostrom, R., Watkins, P., Dean, T., & Mashburn, D. (1992). Comparative efficacy of religious and nonreligious cognitive–behavioral therapy for the treatment of clinical depression in religious individuals. *Journal of Consulting and Clinical Psychology, 60,* 94–103.

Rabinowitz, R. C., Zevon, M. A., & Karuza, J., Jr. (1988). Psychotherapy as helping: An attributional analysis. In L. Y. Abramson (Ed.), *Social cognition and clinical psychology: A synthesis* (pp. 177–203). New York: Guilford.

Rachman, S. (1971). *The effects of psychotherapy.* Oxford, England: Pergammon Press.

Rachman, S. (1977). Double standards and single standards. *Bulletin of the British Psychological Society, 30,* 295.

Rachman, S. J., & Wilson, G. T. (1980). *The effects of psychological therapy* (2nd ed.). New York: Pergamon.

Radojevic, V., Nicassion, P. M., & Weisman, M. H. (1992). Behavioral intervention with and without family support for rheumatoid arthritis. *Behavior Therapy, 23,*13–30.

Ritter, M., & Low, K. G. (1996). Effects of dance/movement therapy: A meta-analysis. *The arts in psychotherapy, 23,* 249–260.

Robinson, L. A., Berman, J. S., & Neimeyer, R. A. (1990). Psychotherapy for the treatment of depression: A comprehensive review of controlled outcome research. *Psychological Bulletin, 108,* 30–49.

Rogers, C. R. (1951). *Client-centered therapy.* Boston: Houghton Mifflin.

Rogers, C. R., Gendlin, E. T., Kiesler, D. V., & Truax, C. (Eds.). (1967). *The therapeutic relationship and its impact: A study of psychotherapy with schizophrenics.* Madison, WI: University of Wisconsin Press.

Rosen, J. C., Cado, S., Silberg, N. T., Srebnik, D., & Wendt, S. (1990). Cognitive behavior therapy with and without size perception training for women with body image disturbance. *Behavior Therapy, 21,* 481–498.

Rosenthal, R. (1994). Parametric measures of effect size. In H. Cooper & L. V. Hedges (Eds.), *The handbook of research synthesis* (pp. 231–260). New York: Russell Sage Foundations.

Rosenthal, R., & Rubin, D. B. (1982). A simple, general purpose display of magnitude of experimental effect. *Journal of Educational Psychology, 74,* 166–169.

Rosenthal, R., & Rubin, D. B. (1984). *Meta-analytic procedures for the social sciences.* Beverly Hills, CA: Sage.

Rosenzweig, S. (1936). Some implicit common factors in diverse methods of psychotherapy: "At last the Dodo said, 'Everybody has won and all must have prizes.'" *American Journal of Orthopsychiatry, 6,* 412–415.

Rosenzweig, S. (1954). A transvaluation of psychotherapy: A reply to Hans Eysenck. *Journal of Abnormal and Social Psychology, 49,* 298–304.

Royce, J. R., & Powell, A. (1983). *Theory of personality and individual differences: Factors, systems, and processes.* Englewood Cliffs, NJ: Prentice-Hall.

Safran, J. D., & Muran, J. C. (Eds.). (1995) The therapeutic alliance [Special Issue]. *In Session: Psychotherapy in Practice, 1*(1).

Seligman, M. E. P. (1995). The effectiveness of psychotherapy: The Consumer Reports study. *American Psychologist, 50,* 965–974.

Sexton, T. L., & Alexander, J. F. (in press). Family-based empirically supported intervention programs. *The Counseling Psychologist.*

Shadish, W. R., Matt, G. E., Navarro, A. M., & Phillips, G. (2000). The effects of psychological therapies in clinically representative conditions: A meta-analysis. *Psychological Bulletin, 126,* 512–529.

Shadish, W. R., Matt, G. E., Navarro, A. M., Siegle, G., Crits-Christoph, P., Hazelrigg, M. D., Jorm, A. F., Lyons, L. C., Nietzel, M. T., Prout, H. T., Robinson, L., Smith, M. L., Svartberg, M., & Weiss, B. (1997). Evidence that therapy works in clinically representative conditions. *Journal of Consulting and Clinical Psychology, 65,* 355–365.

Shadish, W. R., Montgomery, L. M., Wilson, P., Wilson, M. R., Bright, I., & Okwumabua, M. R. (1993). Effects of family and marital psychotherapies: A meta-analysis. *Journal of Consulting and Clinical Psychology, 61,* 992–1002.

Shadish, W. R., & Sweeney, R. B. (1991). Mediators and moderators in meta-analysis: There's a reason we don't let dodo birds tell us which psychotherapies should have prizes. *Journal of Consulting and Clinical Psychology, 59,* 883–893.

Shapiro, A. K., & Morris, L. A. (1978). The placebo effect in medical and psychological therapies. In S. L. Garfield & A. E. Bergin (Eds.), *Handbook of psychotherapy and behavior change* (2nd ed., pp. 369–410). New York: Wiley.

Shapiro, D. A., & Shapiro, D. (1982). Meta-analysis of comparative therapy outcome studies: A replication and refinement. *Psychological Bulletin, 92,* 581–604.

Shapiro, F. (1989). Efficacy of eye movement desensitization procedure in the treatment of traumatic memories. *Journal of Traumatic Stress, 2,* 199–203.

Shaw, B. F. (1984). Specification of the training and evaluation of cognitive therapists for outcome studies. In J. B. W. Williams & R. L. Spitzer (Eds.), *Psychotherapy research: Where are we and where should we go?: Proceedings of the 73rd Annual Meeting of the American Psychopathological Association, New York City, March 3–5, 1983* (pp. 173–188). New York: Guilford Press.

Shaw, B. F., Elkin, I., Yamaguchi, J., Olmsted, M., Vallis, T. M., Dobson, K. S., Lowery, A., Sotsky, S. M., Watkins, J. T., & Imber, S. D. (1999). Therapist competence ratings in relation to clinical outcome in cognitive therapy of depression. *Journal of Consulting and Clinical Psychology, 67,* 837–846.

Shepherd, M. (1993). The placebo: From specificity to the non-specific and back. *Psychological Medicine, 23,* 569–578.

Sherman, J. J. (1998). Effects of psychotherapeutic treatments for PTSD: A meta-analysis of controlled clinical trials. *Journal of Traumatic Stress, 11,* 413–435.

Simons, A. D., Garfield, S. L., & Murphy, G. E. (1984). The process of change in cognitive therapy and pharmacotherapy for depression. *Archives of General Psychiatry, 41,* 45–51.

Simons, A. D., Lustman, P. J., Wetzel, R. D., & Murphy, G. E. (1985). Predicting response to cognitive therapy of depression: The role of learned resourcefulness. *Cognitive Therapy and Research, 9,* 79–89.

Sloane, R. B., Staples, F. R., Cristol, A. H., Yorkston, N. J., & Whipple, K. (1975). *Psychotherapy versus behavior therapy.* Cambridge, MA: Harvard University Press.

Smith, B., & Sechrest, L. (1991). Treatment of Aptitude × Treatment interactions. *Journal of Consulting and Clinical Psychology, 59,* 233–244.

Smith, M. L., & Glass, G. V. (1977). Meta-analysis of psychotherapy outcome studies. *American Psychologist, 32,* 752–760.

Smith, M. L., Glass, G. V, & Miller, T. I. (1980). *The benefits of psychotherapy.* Baltimore: The Johns Hopkins University Press.

Snyder, D. K., & Wills, R. M. (1989). Behavioral versus insight-oriented marital therapy: Effects on individual and interpersonal functioning. *Journal of Consulting and Clinical Psychology, 57,* 39–46.

Snyder, D. K., Wills, R. M., & Grady-Fletcher, A. (1991). Long-term effectiveness of behavioral versus insight oriented martial therapy: A 4-year follow-up study. *Journal of Consulting and Clinical Psychology, 59,* 138–141.

Stiles, W. B., Shapiro, D. A., & Elliott, R. (1986). "Are all psychotherapies equivalent?" *American Psychologist, 41,* 165–180.

Stiles, W. B., Shapiro, D. A., & Firth-Cozens, J. A. (1989). Therapist differences in the use of verbal response mode forms and intents. *Psychotherapy, 26,* 314–322.

Strong, S. R. (1968). Counseling: An interpersonal influence process. *Journal of Counseling Psychology, 15,* 215–224.

Strupp, H. (1958). The performance of psychoanalytic and client-centered therapists in an initial interview. *Journal of Consulting Psychology, 22,* 265–274.

Tarrier, N., Pilgrim, H., Sommerfield, C., Faragher, B., Reynolds, M., Graham, E., & Barrowclough, C. (1999). A randomized trial of cognitive therapy and imaginal exposure in the treatment of chronic posttraumatic stress disorder. *Journal of Consulting and Clinical Psychology, 67,* 13–18.

Task Force on Promotion and Dissemination of Psychological Procedures. (1995). Training in and dissemination of empirically-validated psychological treatment: Report and recommendations. *The Clinical Psychologist, 48,* 2–23.

Taylor, S. (1996). Meta-analysis of cognitive–behavioral treatments for social phobia. *Journal of Behaviour Therapy and Experimental Psychiatry, 27,* 1–9.

Thackwray, D. E., Smith, M. C., Bodfish, J. W., & Meyers, A. W.(1993). A comparison of behavioral and cognitive–behavioral interventions for bulimia nervosa. *Journal of Consulting and Clinical Psychology, 61,* 639–645.

Tichenor, V., & Hill, C. E. (1989). A comparison of six measures of the working alliance. *Psychotherapy: Theory, Research and Practice, 36,* 195–199.

Torrey, E. F. (1972). What Western psychotherapists can learn from witchdoctors. *American Journal of Orthopsychiatry, 42,* 69–76.

Tracey, T. J. G., Sherry, P., & Albright, J. M. (1999). The interpersonal process of cognitive–behavioral therapy: An examination of complementarity over the course of treatment. *Journal of Counseling Psychology, 46,* 80–91.

van Balkom, A. J. L. M., van Oppen, P., Vermeulen, A. W. A., van Dyck, R., Nauta, M. C. E., & Vorst, H. C. M. (1994). A meta-analysis on the treatment of obsessive compulsive disorder: A comparison of antidepressants, behavior, and cognitive therapy. *Clinical Psychology Review, 14,* 359–381.

Wachtel, P. L. (1977). *Psychoanalysis and behavior therapy: Toward an integration.* New York: Basic Books.

Walsh, J. E. (1947). Concerning the effect of intraclass correlation on certain significance tests. *Annals of Mathematical Statistics, 18,* 88–96.

Waltz, J., Addis, M. E., Koerner, K., & Jacobson, N. S. (1993). Testing the integrity of a psychotherapy protocol: Assessment of adherence and competence. *Journal of Consulting and Clinical Psychology, 61,* 620–630.

Wampold, B. E. (1997). Methodological problems in identifying efficacious psychotherapies. *Psychotherapy Research, 7,* 21–43.

Wampold, B. E., & Drew, C. J. (1990). *Theory and application of statistics.* New York: McGraw-Hill.

Wampold, B. E., Lichtenberg, J. W., & Waehler, C. A. (in press). Principles of empirically supported interventions in counseling psychology. *The Counseling Psychologist.*

Wampold, B. E., Minami, T., Baskin, T. W., & Tierney, S. C. (in press). A meta-(re)analysis of the effects of cognitive therapy versus other therapies for depression. *Journal of Affective Disorders, 61.*

Wampold, B. E., Mondin, G. W., Moody, M., & Ahn, H. (1997). The flat earth as a metaphor for the evidence for uniform efficacy of bona fide psychotherapies: Reply to Crits-Christoph (1997) and Howard et al. (1997). *Psychological Bulletin, 122,* 226–230. ·

Wampold, B. E., Mondin, G. W., Moody, M., Stich, F., Benson, K., & Ahn, H. (1997). A meta-analysis of outcome studies comparing bona fide psychotherapies: Empirically, "All must have prizes." *Psychological Bulletin, 122*, 203–215.

Wampold, B. E., & Serlin, R. C. (2000). The consequences of ignoring a nested factor on measures of effect size in analysis of variance designs. *Psychological Methods, 4*, 425–433.

Watson, J. B., & Rayner, R. (1920). Conditioned emotional reactions. *Experimental psychology, 3*, 1–14.

Webster-Stratton, C. (1994). Advancing videotape parent training: A comparison study. *Journal of Consulting and Clinical Psychology, 62*, 583–593.

Weisz, J. R., Weiss, B., & Donenberg, G. R. (1992). The lab versus the clinic: Effects of child and adolescent psychotherapy. *American Psychologist, 47*, 1578–1585.

Weisz, J. R., Weiss, B., Han, S. S., Granger, D. A., & Morton, T. (1995). Effects of psychotherapy with children and adolescents revisited: A meta-analysis of treatment outcome studies. *Psychological Bulletin, 117*, 450–468.

Whiston, S. C. (in press). Application of the principles: Career counseling and interventions. *The Counseling Psychologist.*

Wilkins, W. (1983). Failure of placebo groups to control for nonspecific events in therapy outcome research. *Psychotherapy: Theory, Research and Practice, 20*, 31–37.

Wilkins, W. (1984). Psychotherapy: The powerful placebo. *Journal of Consulting and Clinical Psychology, 52*, 570–573.

Williams, S. L., & Falbo, J. (1996). Cognitive and performance-based treatments for panic attacks in people with varying degrees of agoraphobic disability. *Behavioural Research and Therapy, 34*, 253–264.

Wilson, G. T. (1982). How useful is meta-analysis in evaluating the effects of different psychological therapies? *Behavioural Psychotherapy, 10*, 221–231.

Wilson, G. T. (1996). Manual-based treatments: The clinical application of research findings. *Behaviour Research and Therapy, 34*, 295–314.

Wilson, G. T., & Rachman, S. J. (1983). Meta-analysis and the evaluation of psychotherapy outcome: Limitations and liabilities. *Journal of Consulting and Clinical Psychology, 51*, 54–64.

Wiser, S., & Goldfried, M. R. (1993). Comparative study of emotional experiencing in psychodynamic–interpersonal and cognitive–behavioral therapies. *Journal of Consulting and Clinical Psychology, 61*, 892–895.

Wolfe, B. E., & Goldfried, M. R. (1988). Research on psychotherapy integration: Recommendations and conclusions from an NIMH workshop. *Journal of Consulting and Clinical Psychology, 56*, 448–451.

Wolpe, J. (1952a). Experimental neuroses as learned behavior. *British Journal of Psychology, 43*, 243–268.

Wolpe, J. (1952b). Objective psychotherapy of the neuroses. *South African Medical Journal, 26*, 825–829.

Wolpe, J. (1954). Reciprocal inhibition as the main basis of psychotherapeutic effects. *American Medical Association Archives of Neurological Psychiatry, 72*, 205–226.

Wolpe, J. (1958). *Psychotherapy by reciprocal inhibition.* Palo Alto, CA: Stanford University.

Woody, G. E., Luborsky, L., McLellan, A. T., O'Brien, C. P., Beck, A. T., Blaine, J., Herman, I., & Hole, A. (1983). Psychotherapy for opiate addicts: Does it help? *Archives of General Psychiatry, 40*, 639–645.

Author Index

A

Abelson, R. P., 42
Abramowitz, J. S., 109, 110–114
Adams, V., 70
Addis, M. E., 4–6, 40, 122, 124, 137, 139, 159, 169, 186
Ahn, H., 77, 83, 84, 92–99, 107, 108, 115, 118, 123, 124, 133, 200, 210
Alazraki, A., 16
Albright, J. M., 179
Alexander, J. F., 226
Allan, T., 200
American Psychiatric Association, 13
American Psychological Association, 229
Anastasiades, P., 164, 196
Andrasik, F., 124
Andrews, G., 68, 69, 70, 109, 110, 112
Antonuccio, C. O., 228
Appelbaum, K. A., 124
Arfken, C., 125
Arkowitz, H., 10, 20, 21, 23
Astor, M., 224
Atkinson, D. R., 226
Attanasio, V., 124
Auerbach, A., 170, 180, 182
Autry, J. H., 141, 196

B

Bachelor, A., 210
Baker, K. D., 180
Baker, M., 22, 225
Baker, M. J., 18, 214, 215
Baranackie, K., 197–201
Barber, J. P., 145, 146, 169, 179
Barcikowski, R. S., 188
Barker, S. L., 134
Barlow, D. H., 124
Barnhill, J., 145, 151, 170
Baron, R. M., 135
Barrett, R. H., 216
Barrowclough, C., 114
Baskin, T. W., 105
Bass, D., 74
Battle, C. C., 197
Baucom, D. H., 18, 124, 125, 214
Baxter, L. R., 16
Beck, A. T., 8, 17, 44, 101, 106, 123, 135, 155, 172, 197
Behrens, B. C., 124
Benson, K., 83, 84, 92–99, 107, 108, 115, 117, 123, 200, 210
Bergan, J., 220
Bergin, A. E., 29, 58, 62, 63, 64, 70, 109, 134, 185

Subject Index